Imaging of Bone and Soft Tissue Tumors and Their Mimickers

Editor

HILLARY W. GARNER

RADIOLOGIC CLINICS OF NORTH AMERICA

www.radiologic.theclinics.com

Consulting Editor
FRANK H. MILLER

March 2022 • Volume 60 • Number 2

ELSEVIER

1600 John F. Kennedy Boulevard • Suite 1800 • Philadelphia, Pennsylvania, 19103-2899

http://www.theclinics.com

RADIOLOGIC CLINICS OF NORTH AMERICA Volume 60, Number 2
March 2022 ISSN 0033-8389, ISBN 13: 978-0-323-89748-8

Editor: John Vassallo (j.vassallo@elsevier.com)
Developmental Editor: Karen Solomon

Radiologic Clinics of North America (ISSN 0033-8389) is published bimonthly by Elsevier Inc., 360 Park Avenue South, New York, NY 10010-1710. Months of issue are January, March, May, July, September, and November. Periodicals postage paid at New York, NY and additional mailing offices. Subscription prices are USD 529 per year for US individuals, USD 1335 per year for US institutions, USD 100 per year for US students and residents, USD 624 per year for Canadian individuals, USD 1362 per year for Canadian institutions, USD 717 per year for international individuals, USD 1362 per year for international institutions, USD 100 per year for Canadian students/residents, and USD 315 per year for international students/residents. To receive student and resident rate, orders must be accompanied by name of affiliated institution, date of term and the signature of program/residency coordinatior on institution letterhead. Orders will be billed at individual rate until proof of status is received. Foreign air speed delivery is included in all *Clinics* subscription prices. All prices are subject to change without notice. **POSTMASTER:** Send address changes to *Radiologic Clinics of North America*, Elsevier Health Sciences Division, Subscription Customer Service, 3251 Riverport Lane, Maryland Heights, MO63043. **Customer Service: Telephone: 1-800-654-2452** (U.S. and Canada); **1-314-447-8871** (outside U.S. and Canada). **Fax: 1-314-447-8029. E-mail: journalscustomerservice-usa@elsevier.com (for print support); journalsonlinesupport-usa@elsevier.com (for online support)**.

Reprints. For copies of 100 or more of articles in this publication, please contact the Commercial Reprints Department, Elsevier Inc., 360 Park Avenue South, New York, New York 10010-1710. Tel.: +1-212-633-3874; Fax: +1-212-633-3820; E-mail: reprints@elsevier.com.

Radiologic Clinics of North America also published in Greek Paschalidis Medical Publications, Athens, Greece.

Radiologic Clinics of North America is covered in *MEDLINE/PubMed (Index Medicus), EMBASE/Excerpta Medica, Current Contents/Life Sciences, Current Contents/Clinical Medicine, RSNA Index to Imaging Literature, BIOSIS, Science Citation Index,* and *ISI/BIOMED.*

Contributors

CONSULTING EDITOR

FRANK H. MILLER, MD, FACR
Lee F. Rogers MD Professor of Medical
Education, Chief, Body Imaging Section and
Fellowship Program, Medical Director, MRI,
Department of Radiology, Northwestern
Memorial Hospital, Northwestern University,
Feinberg School of Medicine, Chicago, Illinois,
USA

EDITOR

HILLARY W. GARNER, MD
Assistant Professor, Department of Radiology,
Mayo Clinic, Jacksonville, Florida, USA

AUTHORS

SHIVANI AHLAWAT, MD
Associate Professor of Radiology and
Radiological Science, The Russell H. Morgan
Department of Radiology and Radiological
Science, Johns Hopkins University, Baltimore,
Maryland, USA

ZOHAIB Y. AHMAD, MD
Assistant Professor, Department of Radiology,
Columbia University Irving Medical Center,
New York, New York, USA

BEHRANG AMINI, MD, PhD
Associate Professor, Department of Radiology,
The University of Texas MD Anderson Cancer
Center, Houston, Texas, USA

ROBERT D. BOUTIN, MD
Department of Radiology, Stanford University
School of Medicine, Palo Alto, California,
USA

STEPHEN M. BROSKI, MD
Department of Radiology, Mayo Clinic,
Rochester, Minnesota, USA

FABIANO NASSAR CARDOSO, MD
Department of Radiology, Sylvester
Comprehensive Cancer Center, University of
Miami Miller School of Medicine/Jackson
Memorial Hospital, Miami, Florida, USA

CONNIE Y. CHANG, MD
Division of Musculoskeletal Imaging and
Intervention, Department of Radiology,
Massachusetts General Hospital, Boston,
Massachusetts, USA; Harvard Medical School,
Cambridge, Massachusetts, USA

CHASE CORTES
Department of Radiology, Sylvester
Comprehensive Cancer Center, University of
Miami Miller School of Medicine/Jackson
Memorial Hospital, Miami, Florida, USA

LAURA M. FAYAD, MD
Professor of Radiology, Orthopaedic Surgery
and Oncology, Chief of Musculoskeletal
Imaging, The Russell H. Morgan Department of
Radiology and Radiological Science, Johns
Hopkins University, Baltimore, Maryland, USA

HILLARY W. GARNER, MD
Assistant Professor, Department of Radiology, Mayo Clinic, Jacksonville, Florida, USA

KRISTA A. GOULDING, MD, MPH
Assistant Professor, Department of Orthopedic Surgery, Mayo Clinic, Phoenix, Arizona, USA

SINA HABIBOLLAHI, MD
Division of Musculoskeletal Imaging and Intervention, Department of Radiology, Massachusetts General Hospital, Boston, Massachusetts, USA

MATTHEW T. HOUDEK, MD
Associate Professor, Department of Orthopedic Surgery, Mayo Clinic, Rochester, Minnesota, USA

BENJAMIN M. HOWE, MD
Department of Radiology, Mayo Clinic, Rochester, Minnesota, USA

HAYLEY CORNWALL KIERNAN, BS
University of Arizona College of Medicine, Phoenix, Arizona, USA

PAUL E. KINAHAN, PhD
Professor, Department of Radiology and Bioengineering, Adjunct Professor of Physics and Radiation Oncology, University of Washington, Seattle, Washington, USA

STEVEN KWONG, MD
Department of Radiology, Stanford University School of Medicine, Palo Alto, California, USA

ADAM S. LEVIN, MD
Vice Chair of Faculty Development, Department of Orthopaedic Surgery, Associate Professor of Orthopaedic Surgery, Johns Hopkins University, Baltimore, Maryland, USA

DOROTA LINDA, MD, FRCPC
Toronto Joint Department of Medical Imaging, University of Toronto, Department of Medical Imaging, Mount Sinai Hospital, Toronto, Ontario, Canada

LAUREL A. LITTRELL, MD
Department of Radiology, Mayo Clinic, Rochester, Minnesota, USA

JEREMIAH R. LONG, MD
Assistant Professor, Department of Radiology, Mayo Clinic, Phoenix, Arizona, USA

SANTIAGO LOZANO-CALDERON, MD, PhD
Division of Orthopedics, Massachusetts General Hospital, Boston, Massachusetts, USA; Harvard Medical School, Cambridge, Massachusetts, USA

RAKESH MOHANKUMAR, FRCPC
Toronto Joint Department of Medical Imaging, University of Toronto, Department of Medical Imaging, Toronto Western Hospital, Toronto, Ontario, Canada

ALI M. NARAGHI, FRCR
Toronto Joint Department of Medical Imaging, University of Toronto, Department of Medical Imaging, Toronto Western Hospital, Toronto, Ontario, Canada

MICHAEL L. RICHARDSON, MD
Professor, Department of Radiology, Adjunct Professor of Orthopedics, University of Washington, Seattle, Washington, USA

GEOFFREY M. RILEY, MD
Department of Radiology, Stanford University School of Medicine, Palo Alto, California, USA

ANDREW ROSENBERG, MD
Department of Pathology, Sylvester Comprehensive Cancer Center, University of Miami Miller School of Medicine, Miami, Florida, USA

MOHAMMAD SAMIM, MD
NYU Langone Medical Center, New York University, NYU Orthopedic Hospital, New York, New York, USA

ALINE SERFATY, MD, PhD
Department of Radiology, Faculty of Medicine, Universidade Federal do Rio de Janeiro, Rio de Janeiro, Rio de Janeiro, Brazil; Medscanlagos Radiology, Cabo Frio, Rio de Janeiro, Brazil

COURTNEY E. SHERMAN, MD
Assistant Professor, Department of Orthopedic Surgery, Mayo Clinic, Jacksonville, Florida, USA

FELIPE SOUZA, MD
Department of Radiology, Sylvester Comprehensive Cancer Center, University of Miami Miller School of Medicine/Jackson Memorial Hospital, Miami, Florida, USA

RUPERT O. STANBOROUGH, MD
Assistant Professor, Department of Radiology,
Mayo Clinic, Jacksonville, Florida, USA

ROBERT STEFFNER, MD
Department of Orthopedic Musculoskeletal
Tumor Surgery, Stanford University School of
Medicine, Palo Alto, California, USA

TY K. SUBHAWONG, MD
Department of Radiology, Sylvester
Comprehensive Cancer Center, University of
Miami Miller School of Medicine/Jackson
Memorial Hospital, Miami, Florida, USA

DORIS E. WENGER, MD
Department of Radiology, Mayo Clinic,
Rochester, Minnesota, USA

LAWRENCE M. WHITE, MD, FRCPC
Toronto Joint Department of Medical Imaging,
University of Toronto, Department of Medical
Imaging, Mount Sinai Hospital, Toronto,
Ontario, Canada

BENJAMIN K. WILKE, MD
Assistant Professor, Department of Orthopedic
Surgery, Mayo Clinic, Jacksonville, Florida,
USA

Contents

This article focuses on soft tissue sarcomas, including the workup, management, and potential complications in dealing with these rare mesenchymal tumors. We present the information that is critical in the decision-making process for orthopedic oncologists to help facilitate a multidisciplinary approach to these complex cases.

The overwhelming majority of soft tissue masses encountered on routine imaging are incidental and benign. When incidental, the radiologist is usually limited to routine MR imaging sequences, often without contrast. In these situations, there are typical imaging features pointing to a single diagnosis or limited differential diagnosis. Although these imaging features can be helpful, many lesions are nonspecific and may require contrast administration, evaluation with other imaging modalities, follow-up imaging, or biopsy for diagnosis. This article will provide an overview of the most commonly encountered benign soft tissue masses along with some of their characteristic MR imaging features.

Imaging in soft tissue sarcomas (STS) plays a key role in diagnosis, surgical planning, and assessment of treatment response, and surveillance. In this review, we discuss the imaging features—with an emphasis on MR imaging—of nonvisceral STS, highlighting representative tumors from the various WHO subtypes. We focus on imaging findings that may aid the radiologist in categorizing tumor subtype and grade, and that affect disease staging.

Benign and malignant soft tissue tumors have many overlapping and potentially confusing imaging features. Here we discuss imaging and clinical features of 6 soft tissue tumor mimics: myositis ossificans, acute traumatic hematoma, geyser lesion, tumoral calcinosis, gout, and myonecrosis. These 6 lesions are some of the most common benign soft tissue mass-like lesions erroneously labeled as "malignancy." Familiarity with these lesions can potentially spare the patient biopsy, other invasive and noninvasive work-up, and anxiety.

Radiologists have an integral role in the diagnosis of bone and soft-tissue tumors beyond image interpretation. Image-guided biopsies are used to diagnose and stage musculoskeletal tumors. This article reviews the steps of minimally invasive image-guided biopsies, from prebiopsy planning through postbiopsy pathology follow-up. Helpful techniques to perform and troubleshoot these procedures adequately and safely are detailed. Radiologists are also expanding the treatment options available for many benign and malignant bone and soft-tissue tumors. Some of these more frequently performed procedures include percutaneous thermal ablation and cementoplasty. The evidence, indications, and basic principles of these interventional procedures are also discussed.

This article discusses how the radiologist should handle the imaging for the post-treatment sarcoma patient. This includes reviewing the timing of surveillance after therapy and the type of therapy used for sarcoma in order to better understand the typical post-treatment changes on imaging versus sarcoma recurrence. The type of imaging is reviewed, especially, magnetic resonance imaging and the relevant sequences, as well as the appearance of post-treatment changes, sarcoma recurrence, and post-treatment complications.

AI can improve the quality of CT, MR and PET/CT images, while simultaneously reducing imaging time, and doses of radiation and contrast. AI can improve radiologist workflow and decrease interpretation times. AI may someday be capable of accurately locating, classifying and segmenting bone and soft tissue tumors. The goal of radiomics is to use radiomic and other biomarkers to achieve "precision medicine", ie, to predict the right diagnosis and the right treatment of the right patient at the right time. Radiomic information may be helpful in guiding biopsies, classifying and grading tumors and predicting prognosis and treatment response.

PROGRAM OBJECTIVE

The objective of the Radiologic Clinics of North America is to keep practicing radiologists and radiology residents up to date with current clinical practice in radiology by providing timely articles reviewing the state of the art in patient care.

TARGET AUDIENCE

Practicing radiologists, radiology residents, and other healthcare professionals who provide patient care utilizing radiologic findings.

LEARNING OBJECTIVES

Upon completion of this activity, participants will be able to:

1. Describe the characteristics of benign ad malignant bone and soft tissue tumors and their mimickers and the various imaging diagnostics available.
2. Discuss the use of appropriate imaging diagnostics, both traditional and novel, pre- and post-operatively, to assist in identifying, diagnosing, and staging to develop treatment plans for benign and malignant bone and soft tissue tumors.
3. Recognize the importance of appropriate timing for evaluation of imaging diagnostics for staging, treatment planning, potential complications, and possible recurrence of benign and malignant bone and soft tissue tumors

ACCREDITATION

The Elsevier Office of Continuing Medical Education (EOCME) is accredited by the Accreditation Council for Continuing Medical Education (ACCME) to provide continuing medical education for physicians.

The EOCME designates this journal-based CME activity for a maximum of 11 *AMA PRA Category 1 Credit*(s)™. Physicians should claim only the credit commensurate with the extent of their participation in the activity.

All other healthcare professionals requesting continuing education credit for this enduring material will be issued a certificate of participation.

DISCLOSURE OF CONFLICTS OF INTEREST

The EOCME assesses conflict of interest with its instructors, faculty, planners, and other individuals who are in a position to control the content of CME activities. All relevant conflicts of interest that are identified are thoroughly vetted by EOCME for fair balance, scientific objectivity, and patient care recommendations. EOCME is committed to providing its learners with CME activities that promote improvements or quality in healthcare and not a specific proprietary business or a commercial interest.

The planning committee, staff, authors, and editors listed below have identified no financial relationships or relationships to products or devices they or their spouse/life partner have with commercial interest related to the content of this CME activity:

Shivani Ahlawat, MD; Zohaib Y. Ahmad, MD; Behrang Amini, MD, PhD; Robert D. Boutin, MD; Stephen M. Broski, MD; Fabiano Nassar Cardoso, MD; Connie Y. Chang, MD; Chase Cortes; Laura M. Fayad, MD; Hillary W. Garner, MD; Sina Habibollahi, MD; Benjamin M. Howe, MD; Pradeep Kuttysankaran; Steven Kwong, MD; Adam S. Levin, MD; Dorota Linda, MD, FRCPC; Laurel A. Littrell, MD; Jeremiah R. Long, MD; Santiago Lozano-Calderon, MD, PhD; Rakesh Mohankumar, FRCPC; Ali M. Naraghi, FRCR; Michael L. Richardson, MD; Geoffrey M. Riley, MD; Andrew Rosenberg, MD; Mohammad Samim, MD; Aline Serfaty, MD, PhD; Felipe Souza, MD; Rupert O. Stanborough, MD; Robert Steffner, MD; Doreen Thomas-Payne, MSN, BSN, RN, PMHNP-BC; Doris E. Wenger, MD; Lawrence M. White, MD, FRCPC

The planning committee, staff, authors, and editors listed below have identified financial relationships or relationships to products or devices they or their spouse/life partner have with commercial interest related to the content of this CME activity:

Krista A. Goulding, MD, MPH: *Research*: Summit Medical LLC

Matthew T. Houdek, MD: *Research*: Summit Medical LLC

Hayley Cornwall Kiernan, BS: *Research*: Summit Medical LLC

Paul E. Kinahan, PhD: *Research*: GE Healthcare

Courtney E. Sherman, MD: *Research*: Summit Medical LLC

Ty K. Subhawong, MD: *Consultant*: Agios Pharmaceuticals, Arog Pharmaceuticals

Benjamin K. Wilke, MD: *Research*: Summit Medical LLC

UNAPPROVED/OFF-LABEL USE DISCLOSURE

The EOCME requires CME faculty to disclose to the participants:

1. When products or procedures being discussed are off-label, unlabelled, experimental, and/or investigational (not US Food and Drug Administration [FDA] approved); and
2. Any limitations on the information presented, such as data that are preliminary or that represent ongoing research, interim analyses, and/or unsupported opinions. Faculty may discuss information about pharmaceutical agents that is outside of

FDA-approved labelling. This information is intended solely for CME and is not intended to promote off-label use of these medications. If you have any questions, contact the medical affairs department of the manufacturer for the most recent prescribing information.

TO ENROLL

To enroll in the Radiologic Clinics of North America Continuing Medical Education program, call customer service at 1-800-654-2452 or sign up online at http://www.theclinics.com/home/cme. The CME program is available to subscribers for an additional annual fee of USD 356.00.

METHOD OF PARTICIPATION

In order to claim credit, participants must complete the following:

1. Complete enrolment as indicated above.
2. Read the activity.
3. Complete the CME Test and Evaluation. Participants must achieve a score of 70% on the test. All CME Tests and Evaluations must be completed online.

CME INQUIRIES/SPECIAL NEEDS

For all CME inquiries or special needs, please contact elsevierCME@elsevier.com.

RADIOLOGIC CLINICS OF NORTH AMERICA

FORTHCOMING ISSUES

RECENT ISSUES

RELATED SERIES

Advances in Clinical Radiology
Available at: https://www.advancesinclinicalradiology.com/
Magnetic Resonance Imaging Clinics
Available at: https://www.mri.theclinics.com/
Neuroimaging Clinics
Available at: www.neuroimaging.theclinics.com
PET Clinics
Available at: www.pet.theclinics.com

THE CLINICS ARE AVAILABLE ONLINE!
Access your subscription at:
www.theclinics.com

Preface

Imaging of Bone and Soft Tissue Tumors and Their Mimickers

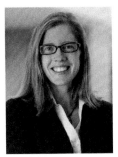

Hillary W. Garner, MD
Editor

The topic of musculoskeletal tumors encompasses a large heterogeneous group of both benign and malignant masses. These lesions are frequently encountered in clinical radiology practice, either as the primary reason for imaging presentation or as an incidental finding. As imaging experts, radiologists are counted on to characterize the mass, provide a differential diagnosis, provide recommendations for further evaluation, and in some cases perform image-guided tissue sampling and radiology-pathology correlation. Given the volume of imaging studies a radiologist encounters in daily practice, a fundamental working knowledge of the imaging features of the most common musculoskeletal masses is important to maintain diagnostic accuracy and efficiency.

In this issue of *Radiologic Clinics of North America*, the imaging findings and other relevant clinical information of frequently encountered benign and malignant tumors arising in both bone and soft tissue are reviewed. Separate reviews on common and potentially confusing tumor mimics of bone and soft tissue tumors are also provided. To best contextualize these reviews, orthopedic oncologists have contributed their valuable perspectives on how they incorporate the imaging information into their patient care plans. Comprehensive translation and communication of what we see into

what they need to know are essential to our role on the health care team. In addition, the clinical considerations and advanced techniques for interventional diagnostic and therapeutic management of musculoskeletal tumors as well as posttherapy imaging follow-up are discussed. Given the recent rapid growth in clinical interest and research on the roles of radiomics and artificial intelligence in musculoskeletal tumor imaging, the final article provides both an in-depth and an entertaining discussion on where we stand currently and what the future might bring in these realms.

I am deeply grateful for the time, effort, and expertise of the contributors to this issue. Herein, they have provided contemporary, digestible, relevant information that can be helpful for any radiologist working to refresh and update their knowledge and understanding on the broad topic of musculoskeletal tumors.

Hillary W. Garner, MD
Department of Radiology
Mayo Clinic Florida
4500 San Pablo Road
Jacksonville, FL 32224, USA

E-mail address:
garner.hillary@mayo.edu

0033-8389/22/© 2021 Published by Elsevier Inc.

Skeletal Sarcomas: Diagnosis, Treatment, and Follow-up from the Orthopedic Oncologist Perspective

Krista A. Goulding, MD, MPH[a],*, Benjamin K. Wilke, MD[b],
Hayley Cornwall Kiernan, BS[c], Matthew T. Houdek, MD[d],
Courtney E. Sherman, MD[b]

KEYWORDS

- Musculoskeletal • Sarcoma • Endoprosthesis • Custom implant • 3D-printed

KEY POINTS

- Local staging of a bone sarcoma should include whole-bone radiographs and cross-sectional imaging to evaluate tissue planes, identify skip metastases, joint involvement, and encasement of neurovascular structures to assist in surgical planning.
- Image-guided biopsies should be carried out with the guidance of an orthopedic oncologist to avoid tissue contamination and prevent unnecessarily invasive procedures or amputation.
- Advanced imaging diagnostics, computer-assisted navigation, and 3-D printed models, cutting guides and implants improve the planning and execution of resection and reconstruction in complex sarcoma surgery.
- Routine surveillance is key to timely diagnosis and treatment of local and distant relapse of sarcoma.

BACKGROUND

Primary bone sarcomas are a group of malignant tumors of mesenchymal origin, comprising less than 1% of all cancers.[1] Global incidence ranges from 3 to 7 per 100,000 individuals affected yearly.[2] The American Cancer Society estimates that 3610 new bone sarcomas were diagnosed in the United States in 2020.[3] More than 150 different subtypes of bone and soft tissue sarcoma have been reported. Osteosarcoma and Ewing sarcoma are the most prevalent subtypes in children and young adults, while chondrosarcoma is most common in older adults.

These malignant neoplasms display significant heterogeneity and variability in biological behavior, affecting connective tissue anywhere in the body.

As such, a team approach is required to maximize survival and function after treatment. This article provides an overview of the multi-disciplinary approach to the imaging, diagnosis, treatment, and surveillance of bone sarcomas from the perspective of the orthopedic oncologist.

CLINICAL PRESENTATION

Pain is the most common presenting symptom of primary bone cancers and is often described as deep, dull pain which progresses over time, and is often not responsive to simple analgesia.[4] Nighttime pain is occasionally present and is usually indicative of a more advanced tumor. A painful soft tissue mass may also be palpable on examination. Systemic symptoms are rare but are more common in

[a] Department of Orthopedic Surgery, Mayo Clinic Arizona, 5777 East Mayo Boulevard, Phoenix, AZ 85054, USA; [b] Department of Orthopedic Surgery, Mayo Clinic Florida, 4500 San Pablo Road. Jacksonville, FL 32224, USA; [c] University of Arizona College of Medicine, 475 North 5th, Street, Phoenix, AZ 85004, USA; [d] Department of Orthopedic Surgery, Mayo Clinic, 200 1st, Street Southwest, Rochester, MN 55905, USA
* Corresponding author.
E-mail address: goulding.krista@mayo.edu

Radiol Clin N Am 60 (2022) 193–203
https://doi.org/10.1016/j.rcl.2021.11.001
0033-8389/22/© 2021 Elsevier Inc. All rights reserved.

Ewing sarcoma and can include fever, fatigue, malaise, and weight loss. A history of trauma is important to consider. While acute trauma may lead to the development of a mass by the way of a hematoma, often patients will recount a remote history of trauma to the affected area. Usually, this has no relevance to the development of the mass. Pathologic fracture may be the first presentation of a primary bone sarcoma; these tumors have different molecular profiles and are associated with worse clinical outcomes than nonpathologic fracture-associated osteosarcoma.[5]

Physical examination should focus on the area of pain, tenderness, or mass. The area should be inspected and palpated, with size, consistency, mobility, depth, location of the mass, overlying skin changes, and presence of regional lymph nodes noted.[4] Previous incisions and biopsy sites are important to note as these will need to be incorporated in the final resection. Patients presenting with pathologic fractures should be immobilized and admitted to hospital, if necessary, during the workup of a skeletal mass.

PREOPERATIVE IMAGING MODALITIES

Preoperative imaging of bone tumors is a critical component of the evaluation. Radiographs of the whole bone in 2 planes are standard of care as they are inexpensive, readily available, and provide important diagnostic information that can be correlated with advanced cross-sectional imaging. Following radiographs, further evaluation is obtained with an MR imaging of the entire compartment and adjacent joints. It is critical to identify any skip metastases as this may preclude limb salvage or impact on the length of the bone resection. Likewise, identifying intraarticular tumor extension is crucial; tumors involving the joint require extraarticular resection or may necessitate limb ablative procedures. Joint contamination rarely occurs but may be due to tumor extension along intraarticular ligaments or tendons, pathologic fracture, direct joint extension, inappropriately placed biopsy, or unplanned intralesional resection.[6] Proximity of the mass to neurovascular structures is an important consideration in surgical planning, as vascular invasion or encasement of vascular structures may preclude limb salvage surgery and portends a worse prognosis (**Fig. 1**).

CT imaging can be performed to provide additional information, such as better visualization of calcifications, periosteal bone formation, and cortical destruction.[7]

Additionally, CT scans can facilitate the design and customization of joint sparing geometric resections and reconstructions with 3-dimensional

(3D) cutting guides. Three-dimensionally printed models are a valuable tool that we commonly use to assist in preoperative planning, particularly in multi-disciplinary cases involving difficult anatomic locations such as the pelvis, spine, and chest wall[8] (**Fig. 2**).

Advanced imaging should always be completed before biopsy to allow for the evaluation of the tumor in its most natural state without being confounded by postbiopsy inflammation or alteration of tissue planes.

DIFFERENTIAL DIAGNOSIS

Common bone sarcomas are listed in **Table 1**. The differential diagnoses for bone sarcoma are broad and based on patient age, location, and imaging characteristics. Common differentials can include[9]

- Bony metastatic disease
- Lymphoma
- Multiple myeloma
- Giant cell tumor
- Aneurysmal bone cyst
- Chondroblastoma
- Osteoblastoma
- Fibrous dysplasia
- Eosinophilic granuloma
- Enchondroma/atypical cartilage tumor
- Nonossifying fibroma
- Hyperparathyroidism (Brown tumor)
- Infection
- Solitary bone cyst
- Pseudocyst

BIOPSY BEWARE

Image-guided needle biopsy has been shown to be highly accurate for the diagnosis and staging of musculoskeletal sarcomas, with fewer complications and lower costs than open biopsy.[10] Biopsy planning is a crucial step in the diagnosis and treatment of bone sarcoma. When determining the best biopsy tract, the radiologist should consult with the orthopedic oncologist to select a biopsy entry site that will not interfere with the plan of incision for potential limb salvage surgery.[11] Anatomically-based guidelines for extremity sarcoma should be reviewed in conjunction with case-by-case surgeon consultation[12] to avoid the known hazards of biopsy, as poorly planned biopsies can potentially lead to unnecessary amputation or additional soft tissue reconstructive procedures.[10,13]

Rarely, a core biopsy is nondiagnostic, and a repeat needle biopsy or an open biopsy may be recommended. Respecting biopsy principles is crucial to minimizing contamination.[14] A small

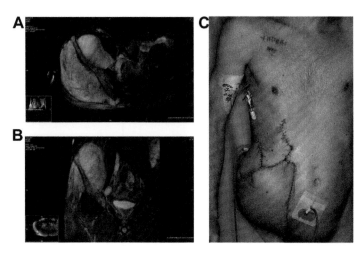

Fig. 1. Selected axial (*A*) and coronal (*B*) MR imaging sequences demonstrating a large, high-grade chondrosarcoma of the hemipelvis with vascular invasion. Red arrow depicts a large tumor thrombus within the right common iliac vein. This patient was treated with an extended external hemipelvectomy with en bloc hemisacrectomy, instrumented posterior spinal fusion, and a free fillet flap (*C*) taken from the ipsilateral lower limb.

incision should be created by the orthopedic oncologist performing the definitive resection in line with an extensile approach to the bone in question. Biopsies should be placed through one compartment only, avoiding critical neurovascular structures, and with meticulous hemostasis so that the biopsy tract can be excised en bloc with tumor. Any hematoma occurring after biopsy should be photographed and this should be communicated expediently to the orthopedic oncologist.

DIAGNOSTICS AND NOVEL APPROACHES

Accurate pretreatment diagnosis is essential to ensure appropriate oncological and surgical decision-making. The histopathological diagnosis of sarcoma is challenging due to the low incidence of disease and significant tumor heterogeneity. More than 150 different sarcoma subtypes have

been reported including both bone and soft tissue sarcomas.[15] Discordance between initial pathology diagnosis and expert second review occurs in more than 45% of cases,[2] and can result in modifications of tumor subtype and grade or major discrepancies in histologic type and invalidation of sarcoma diagnosis. Misdiagnosis can lead to inappropriate surgical and medical management at odds with published clinical practice guidelines.[7,16] Multidisciplinary case-by-case collaborative review is key to minimizing diagnostic error and optimizing oncological and functional outcomes for patients with bone sarcoma.

Novel diagnostic techniques have improved the reliability of sarcoma diagnosis with advances in immunohistochemical markers, fluorescence in situ hybridization (FISH), reverse transcription-polymerase chain reaction, and targeted next-generation sequencing (NGS).[17]

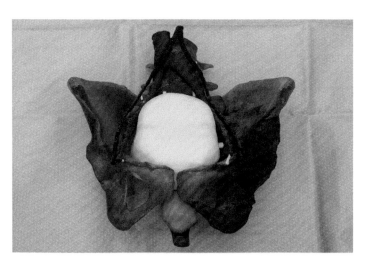

Fig. 2. Anatomic 3D-printed model of a left hemipelvis sarcoma (shown in *pink*) used in complex multidisciplinary surgical planning.

Table 1
Common bone sarcoma subtypes

Osteogenic	Chondrogenic	Undifferentiaed Small Round Cell Sarcomas (SRCS)	Fibrogenic	Vascular	Osteoclast/Giant Cell Rich	Notochordal	Other
Conventional osteosarcoma	Central ACT/chondrosarcoma grade 1	Ewing sarcoma	Desmoplastic fibroma of bone	Epithelioid haemangio-endothelioma	Malignant Giant Cell Tumor of bone	Conventional chordoma	Adamantinoma
Low grade central osteosarcoma	Central chondrosarcoma grade 2, 3	SRCS with EWSR-1-non-ETS fusions	Fibrosarcoma of bone	Angiosarcoma of bone		Dedifferentiated chordoma	Langerhans cell histiocytosis
Dedifferentiated osteosarcoma	Chondrosarcoma NOS	CIC-rearranged sarcoma					
Osteoblastoma-like osteosarcoma	Peripheral chondrosarcoma	BCOR-rearranged sarcoma					
Telangiectatic osteosarcoma	Periosteal chondrosarcoma						
Small cell osteosarcoma	Clear cell chondrosarcoma						
Osteosarcoma NOS	Mesenchymal chondrosarcoma						
Parosteal osteosarcoma	Dedifferentiated chondrosarcoma						
Periosteal osteosarcoma							
High-grade surface osteosarcoma							

Abbreviations: USRCS, undifferentiated small round cell sarcomas of bone and soft tissue; ACT, atypical cartilaginous tumor.

NGS has become an especially important diagnostic modality. In Ewing sarcoma, NGS has identified new gene segments previously undetected by FISH or PCR and has reduced the number of tumors previously categorized as undifferentiated.[18]

New DNA microarray technology and genomic hybridization techniques are able to screen several thousand DNA and mRNA sequences and identify genes relevant to the diagnosis and clinical features of certain tumors.[19] These studies have been able to identify several genes that may be involved in the development of osteosarcomas, and are therefore potential candidates for biomarkers.[19]

Recent advancements in proteomics and mass spectrometry allow for the rapid and accurate identification of thousands of proteins within a tumor. This technology can be used to identify potential protein markers related to the tumor profile and biologic behavior.[20] Many studies have also investigated liquid biopsies as a noninvasive approach to identifying biomarkers and advancing personalized treatments in common bone sarcomas.[21] Identifying treatment predictive and prognostic biomarkers are crucial in selecting targeted chemotherapeutics in the primary and relapsed setting.[18]

TUMOR STAGING

Staging studies are obtained when a tumor is determined to be malignant, before proceeding with surgical resection. Staging involves determining both local tumor extension as well as the extent of tumoral spread into regional lymph nodes or distant organs.

A PET-CT scan is commonly used to evaluate for regional and metastatic spread of disease. PET and CT images can be acquired simultaneously and combined spatially which allows for better localization of metabolic abnormalities, reduced scanning time, and improved PET image quality and quantitation using CT attenuation correction reconstruction techniques.[22]

PET/CT has been shown to improve accuracy, sensitivity, and specificity in the diagnosis of osteosarcoma.[23] PET/CT can also be used in tumor surveillance to assess tumor response to chemotherapy and radiation treatment, and for detection of recurrent tumor.[24] While helpful, this imaging modality does not have the spatial resolution to properly evaluate for the development of pulmonary nodules. For this reason, a dedicated CT scan of the chest is also typically obtained for completeness.[25–27] In the setting of Ewing sarcoma, a bone marrow biopsy to evaluate for bone marrow infiltration is also included as part of staging.

TUMOR CLASSIFICATION

Primary bone tumors are classified by staging guidelines released by the American Joint Committee on Cancer (AJCC). Tumors are described based on the location of the primary tumor and then staged based on the size, regional lymph node involvement, distant organ metastasis, and histologic grade (Table 2). Tumor classification influences treatment recommendations and allows for prognostication based on stage and grade. Tumor grade continues to be the most significant predictor of metastatic disease.[21]

MANAGEMENT

Historically, primary bone sarcomas were treated almost exclusively with surgical resection. Disease-specific survival was poor. The introduction of chemotherapy led to a dramatic improvement in the prognosis for patients with localized osteosarcoma and Ewing sarcoma. Long-term survival rates of less than 20% improved to 65% to 70% after the initiation of multiagent chemotherapy

Table 2
The American Joint Committee on Cancer staging system for bone sarcomas

Stage	Primary Tumor (T)	Regional Lymph Node (N)	Distant Metastasis (M)	Histologic Grade (G)
IA;	T1	N0	M0	G1 or GX
IB	T2 or T3	N0	M0	G1 or GX
IIA	T1	N0	M0	G2 or G3
IIB	T2	N0	M0	G2 or G3
III	T3	N0	M0	G2 or G3
IVA	Any T	N0	M1a	Any G
IVB	Any T	N1	Any M	Any G
	Any T	Any N	M1b	Any G

regimens.[28] The current standard of care for localized osteosarcoma and Ewing sarcoma is multiagent doxorubicin-based neoadjuvant chemotherapy followed by complete surgical resection of the primary disease and adjuvant chemotherapy.[29] Regimens differ between the 2 subtypes, but improvements in understanding of cell biology and genetics have allowed the development of novel forms of treatment, including the immunomodulation of T-cells, gene therapy trials, and angiogenesis inhibitors, allowing a more targeted approach to therapy.[30]

While there is no role for radiotherapy in the treatment of localized osteosarcoma, Ewing sarcoma is extremely radiosensitive. Definitive radiation can be used as an alternative to surgery in inoperable disease or in locations whereby surgery is felt to be extremely morbid. Radiotherapy plays an important role in the treatment of metastatic disease or, rarely, in the setting of a microscopically positive margin.

Wide resection alone is the mainstay of treatment of localized intermediate and high-grade chondrosarcoma,[31] despite significant efforts to identify novel chemotherapeutics over the years. Grade 1 extremity chondrosarcoma demonstrates low malignant potential, and can often safely be treated with intralesional curettage.[32] Grade 1 chondrosarcoma of axially-based lesions like the pelvis, on the other hand, behave more aggressively and should be treated as a higher grade tumor with wide en bloc resection. Significant overlap in imaging and histopathology characteristics makes the diagnosis and treatment of enchondromas, atypical cartilaginous tumors (ACTs), and low-grade chondrosarcomas somewhat challenging. Surveillance of ACTs is recommended, and careful attention to symptom changes, for instance, new non-activity-related pain, nocturnal discomfort, or changes in pain quality, should prompt a careful evaluation of these lesions. Growth, endosteal scalloping over 50%, development of new lucencies, or more aggressive features around a known ACT should prompt further investigation by an orthopedic oncologist. Low interrater agreement in interpreting imaging and pathology has been demonstrated in radiologists, pathologists, and orthopedic oncologists,[33] and requires additional strategies to standardize and inform the management of these lesions.

SURGICAL CONSIDERATIONS

Complete surgical excision is the definitive treatment of bone sarcoma. The goal of surgery is to remove the entire primary tumor with a cuff of normal surrounding tissue and negative margins.

Limb salvage surgery is a viable option for patients when complete tumor resection is possible with a reasonable anticipated functional outcome. Limb salvage procedures are generally indicated for patients with localized disease and no evidence of metastasis.[34]

With the development of more effective chemotherapy, limb-sparing surgery has become the mainstay of treatment of localized osteogenic and Ewing sarcoma. Patients who undergo limb salvage tend to have lower rates of distant relapse and better survival than those who require amputation to achieve local control.[35] Ninety to 95% of patients with extremity osteosarcoma avoid amputation with successful limb-sparing resections.[36]

Amputation may be necessary for patients with locally advanced tumors, joint invasion whereby an extraarticular resection is not feasible, encasement of critical structures not amenable to reconstruction, and in some patients with pathologic fractures.[35]

Rotationplasty provides an excellent option for younger children with locally advanced tumors or who are judged to be too young for or wish to avoid the complications of endoprosthetic reconstruction.[37]

Reconstruction after wide resection will depend on patient age, location, and extent of bony involvement. Tumors located in epiphyseal/metaphyseal locations are commonly managed with endoprosthetic reconstruction, which allows for noninvasive growing mechanisms in skeletally immature patients. Diaphyseal tumors will often be managed by allograft reconstructions and osteosynthesis whereby feasible (Fig. 3).

Computer-assisted tumor surgery is a relatively new concept that allows for preoperative 3D planning and image-guided bone resection.[38] This can be achieved by using preoperative CT/MR imaging or intraoperative CT with navigation. These techniques are especially helpful in difficult locations such as the pelvis, spine, and sacrum. Early results suggested that these techniques can reduce the risk of intralesional margins and may improve surgical accuracy.[39]

Custom cutting guides and 3D printing technologies have changed the landscape by improving the precision of resection and reconstruction in difficult locations.[40] These techniques allow for precise bony cuts based on preplanned resection margins and create excellent host-bone contact to promote long-term implant stability (Fig. 4).

TREATMENT OF UNPLANNED EXCISIONS

Unplanned sarcoma excision occurs when a mass is removed before proper workup and biopsy without respecting oncological principles and excising

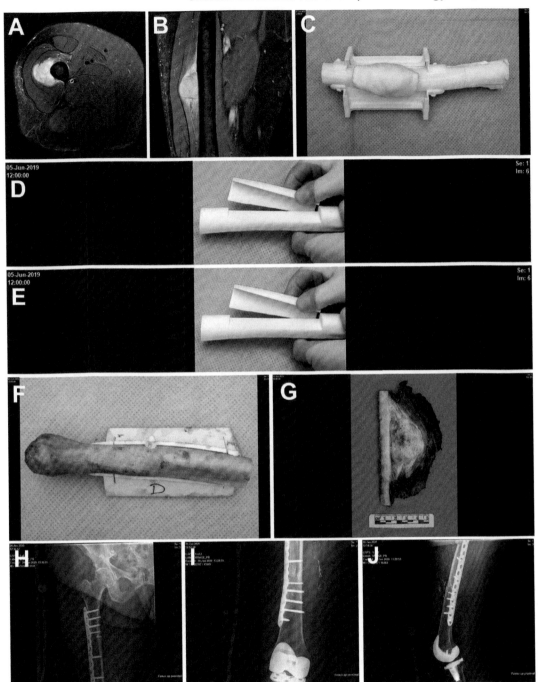

Fig. 3. Sarcoma involving the femoral diaphysis (*A, B*) that was treated with a geometric resection with the use of 3D-printed custom cutting guides for resection (*C-E*) and matched allograft reconstruction (*F*). Resection specimen (*G*) and postoperative radiographs are shown (*H–J*).

appropriate margins. Residual disease can be found in approximately 50% of these patients according to one series.[41] A second surgery is generally indicated in these cases to mitigate the possibility of residual tumor or local contamination.

While unplanned excision is more common in soft tissue sarcoma, inappropriate surgery involving bone sarcomas do occur and can have deleterious consequences for both oncological and functional outcome. Common unplanned excisions include intralesional procedures and osteosynthesis for presumed benign disease or osteomyelitis, metastatic disease, and trauma. The second operation required may be more extensive and require

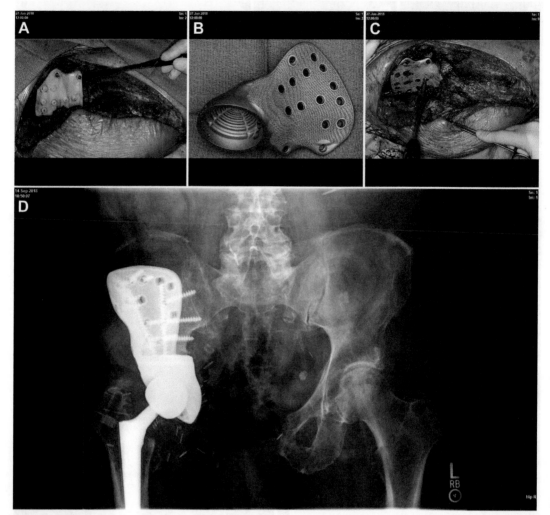

Fig. 4. Custom 3D printed hemipelvis reconstruction following an internal hemipelvectomy. Images demonstrate (*A*) custom 3D-printed cutting guide, (*B*) custom 3D printed hemipelvis showing porous coating to promote bony ongrowth, (*C*) implantation of device, and (*D*) postoperative radiographs.

significant upgrading such as a soft tissue flap reconstruction or amputation to control local disease.[42]

Local control rates of 28% have been reported after unplanned resection of bone sarcoma despite re-resection or amputation and standard neo- and adjuvant therapies. Patients who develop local recurrence in this setting have significantly worse 5-year disease-specific survival (44% vs 74% in one series).[43] Bone lesions of the unknown primary should be appropriately imaged and biopsied before definitive management to avoid such devastating complications.

COMMON POSTOPERATIVE COMPLICATIONS

Postoperative complications occur frequently after sarcoma surgery (**Fig. 5**). Common complications of limb salvage surgery are categorized into

mechanical and nonmechanical factors.[44] Mechanical modes of failure include dislocation, aseptic loosening, and structural failure of prostheses or periprosthetic fracture. Nonmechanical modes of failure include tumor recurrence in up to 10% of patients[45] and periprosthetic joint infection (PJI). PJI remains one of the most challenging problems throughout patient survivorship and is reported in up to 20% of cases.[46] PJI and aseptic loosening are the most common causes of implant failure.[44]

Allograft reconstruction is also subject to high rates of complications, including infection, fracture, and graft resorption.[47] Complications of amputation include infection, wound healing issues, neuroma, and phantom limb pain. The estimated prevalence of the phantom limb phenomenon is 49% to 83%. Various surgical techniques have been developed in conjunction with colleagues in

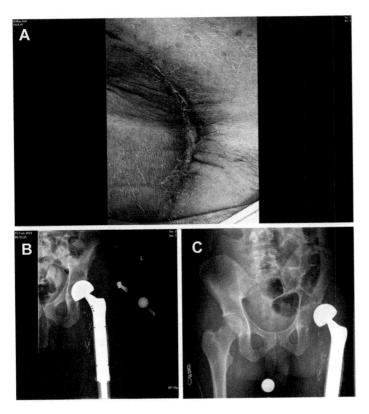

Fig. 5. Common complications after wide resection and reconstruction. Wound dehiscence in the groin after an extended iliofemoral approach for internal hemipelvectomy and proximal femoral replacement for Ewing sarcoma (*A, B*). The same patient subsequently developed metastatic disease involving the ipsilateral acetabulum with associated hip dislocation (*C*).

peripheral nerve surgery to try to minimize phantom limb pain.

POSTOPERATIVE SURVEILLANCE IMAGING

Surveillance for individuals with a bone sarcoma is typically performed for 10 years. Imaging consists of radiographs, a contrast-enhanced MR imaging of the surgical site with metal artifact reduction whereby necessary, and a CT scan of the chest and chest radiograph to evaluate for pulmonary disease.[48,49] Surveillance MR imagings have a mean sensitivity and specificity of 71.7% and 79.3%, respectively, for the detection of residual disease and 87.9% and 85.9%, respectively, for local recurrence.[5]

Interval surveillance varies based on institutional protocols and is the focus of ongoing research to identify optimal, safe, and cost-effective protocols.

DEALING WITH RECURRENT DISEASE

Local and distant relapses of bone sarcoma are both associated with decreased survival. Bone sarcomas spread hematogenously, and the lung is most often the first site of distant relapse. A multi-disciplinary approach is required to optimize patient outcome, and often involves additional chemotherapy and/or radiation. Up to 30% of patients with localized osteosarcoma at presentation will relapse.[50] Complete surgical resection of all sites of disease is essential and remains the most predictive aspect of long-term survival in osteosarcoma.[50] Radiation therapy is an alternative option for patients with Ewing sarcoma due to tumor radiosensitivity. Chemotherapy can also be considered for patients who do not achieve complete surgical remission and is favored for those who develop metastatic disease. In patients with metastatic chondrosarcoma, clinical trials targeting IDH-1 mutations, immunotherapy, and hypomethylating agents targeting HDAC inhibitors are showing promise.

SUMMARY

The management of bone sarcoma is challenging due to low disease incidence and tumor heterogeneity. Collaborative case-by-case review is critical to achieve accurate pretreatment diagnosis and ensure appropriate oncological and surgical decision-making. Image-guided biopsies should be guided by an orthopedic oncologist to avoid tissue contamination and prevent unnecessarily invasive procedures and amputation. Novel diagnostics are improving the capacity to deliver personalized medicine for individuals with sarcoma. Limb salvage surgery can be facilitated by improved imaging diagnostics. Advanced computer-assisted surgery and customized 3D printed models, cutting guides, and implants improve the precision of resection and reconstruction. A multi-disciplinary approach to the diagnosis and treatment of these malignant tumors in a specialized center is crucial to improving patient survival, enhancing function and quality of life.

CLINICS CARE POINTS

- Collaborative case-by-case review is critical to achieve accurate pretreatment diagnosis and appropriate oncological and surgical decision-making.
- Novel diagnostics are improving the capacity to deliver personalized medicine for individuals with sarcoma.
- Computer-assisted surgery and 3D printing technologies facilitates improved preoperative planning and execution.

DISCLOSURE

The authors have received research support from Summit Medical and the Desmoid Tumor Research Foundation.

REFERENCES

1. Cancer.org. Key Statistics about bone cancer | bone cancer Statistics 2021. Available at: https://www.cancer.org/cancer/bone-cancer/about/key-statistics.html. Accessed 24 July 2021.
2. de Pinieux G, Karanian M, Le Loarer F, et al. Nationwide incidence of sarcomas and connective tissue tumors of intermediate malignancy over four years using an expert pathology review network. PLoS One 2021;16(2):e0246958.
3. Siegel RL, Miller KD, Jemal A. Cancer statistics, 2020. CA Cancer J Clin 2020;70(1):7–30.
4. Pullan JE, Budh DP. Primary Bone Cancer. In: StatPearls. Treasure Island (FL): StatPearls Publishing; 2021.
5. Lozano Calderón SA, Garbutt C, Kim J, et al. Clinical and Molecular Analysis of Pathologic Fracture-associated Osteosarcoma: MicroRNA profile Is Different and Correlates with Prognosis. Clin Orthop Relat Res 2019;477(9):2114–26.
6. Zwolak P, Kühnel SP, Fuchs B. Extraarticular knee resection for sarcomas with preservation of the extensor mechanism: surgical technique and review of cases. Clin Orthop Relat Res 2011;469(1):251–6.
7. Casali PG, Bielack S, Abecassis N, et al. Bone sarcomas: ESMO-PaedCan-EURACAN Clinical Practice Guidelines for diagnosis, treatment and follow-up. Ann Oncol 2018;29(Suppl 4):iv79–95.
8. Segaran N, Saini G, Mayer JL, et al. Application of 3D Printing in Preoperative Planning. J Clin Med 2021;10(5):917.
9. Subramanian S, Viswanathan VK. Lytic Bone Lesions. StatPearls. Treasure Island (FL): StatPearls Publishing; 2021.
10. Welker JA, Henshaw RM, Jelinek J, et al. The percutaneous needle biopsy is safe and recommended in the diagnosis of musculoskeletal masses. Cancer 2000;89(12):2677–86.
11. Bickels J, Jelinek JS, Shmookler BM, et al. Biopsy of musculoskeletal tumors. Current concepts. Clin Orthop Relat Res 1999;368:212–9.
12. Liu PT, Valadez SD, Chivers FS, et al. Anatomically based guidelines for core needle biopsy of bone tumors: implications for limb-sparing surgery. Radiographics 2007;27(1):189–206.
13. MankinHJ Mankin CJ, Simon MA. The hazards of the biopsy, revisited. Members of the Musculoskeletal Tumor Society. J Bone Joint Surg Am 1996;78(5):656–63.
14. Avedian RS. Principles of musculoskeletal biopsy. Cancer Treat Res 2014;1–7. https://doi.org/10.1007/978-3-319-07323-1_1.
15. Ray-Coquard I, Thiesse P, Ranchère-Vince D, et al. Conformity to clinical practice guidelines, multidisciplinary management and outcome of treatment for soft tissue sarcomas. Ann Oncol 2004;15(2):307–15.
16. Gage MM, Nagarajan N, Ruck JM, et al. Sarcomas in the United States: Recent trends and a call for improved staging. Oncotarget 2019;10(25):2462–74.
17. Tanaka K, Ozaki T. New TNM classification (AJCC eighth edition) of bone and soft tissue sarcomas: JCOG Bone and Soft Tissue Tumor Study Group. Jpn J Clin Oncol 2019;49(2):103–7.
18. Hesla AC, Papakonstantinou A, Tsagkozis P. Current Status of Management and Outcome for Patients with Ewing Sarcoma. Cancers (Basel) 2021;13(6):1202.
19. Puri A, Jaffe N, Gelderblom H. Osteosarcoma: lessons learned and future avenues. Sarcoma 2013;2013:641687.
20. Conrad DH, Goyette J, Thomas PS. Proteomics as a method for early detection of cancer: a review of proteomics, exhaled breath condensate, and lung cancer screening. J Gen Intern Med 2008;23(supplement 1):78–84.
21. Aran V, Devalle S, Meohas W, et al. Osteosarcoma, Chondrosarcoma and ewing Sarcoma: Clinical aspects, biomarker discovery and Liquid biopsy. Crit Rev Oncology/Hematology 2021;162:103340.
22. Behzadi AH, Raza SI, Carrino JA, et al. Applications of PET/CT and PET/MR Imaging in Primary Bone Malignancies. PET Clin 2018;13(4):623–34.

23. Zhang X, Guan Z. PET/CT in the diagnosis and prognosis of osteosarcoma. Front Biosci (Landmark Ed 2018;23:2157–65.

24. Kumar R, Kumar M, Malhotra K, et al. Primary Osteosarcoma in the Elderly Revisited: Current Concepts in Diagnosis and Treatment. Curr Oncol Rep 2018; 20(2). https://doi.org/10.1007/s11912-018-0658-1.

25. Hudson TM, Schakel M 2nd, Springfield DS, et al. The comparative value of bone scintigraphy and computed tomography in determining bone involvement by soft-tissue sarcomas. J Bone Joint Surg Am 1984;66(9):1400–7.

26. Conrad EU 3rd, Morgan HD, Vernon C, et al. Fluorodeoxyglucose positron emission tomography scanning: basic principles and imaging of adult soft-tissue sarcomas. J Bone Joint Surg Am 2004;86-A-(Suppl 2):98–104.

27. Schuetze SM, Rubin BP, Vernon C, et al. Use of positron emission tomography in localized extremity soft tissue sarcoma treated with neoadjuvant chemotherapy. Cancer 2005;103(2):339–48.

28. Isakoff MS, Bielack SS, Meltzer P, et al. Osteosarcoma: Current Treatment and a Collaborative Pathway to Success. J Clin Oncol 2015;33(27): 3029–35.

29. Reed DR, Hayashi M, Wagner L, et al. Treatment pathway of bone sarcoma in children, adolescents, and young adults. Cancer 2017;123(12):2206–18.

30. Nathenson MJ, Conley AP, Sausville E. Immunotherapy: A New (and Old) Approach to Treatment of Soft Tissue and Bone Sarcomas. Oncologist 2018;23(1):71–83.

31. Leddy LR, Holmes RE. Chondrosarcoma of Bone. In: Peabody T, Attar S, editors. Orthopaedic Oncology. Cancer treatment and research, 162. Cham: Spr-inger; 2014. https://doi.org/10.1007/978-3-319-07323-1_6.

32. Dierselhuis EF, Goulding KA, Stevens M, et al. Intralesional treatment versus wide resection for central low-grade chondrosarcoma of the Long Bones. Cochrane Database Syst Rev 2019;2019(4). https://doi.org/10.1002/14651858.cd010778.pub2.

33. Zamora T, Urrutia J, Schweitzer D, et al. Do orthopaedic oncologists agree on the diagnosis and treatment of cartilage tumors of the appendicular skeleton? Clin Orthopaedics Relat Res 2017; 475(9):2176–86.

34. Yin K, Liao Q, Zhong D, et al. Meta-analysis of limb salvage versus amputation for treating high-grade and localized osteosarcoma in patients with pathological fracture. Exp Ther Med 2012;4(5):889–94.

35. Li X, Zhang Y, Wan S, et al. A comparative study between limb-salvage and amputation for treating osteosarcoma. J Bone Oncol 2016;5(1):15–21. https://doi.org/10.1016/j.jbo.2016.01.001.

36. Wittig JC, Bickels J, Priebat D, et al. Osteosarcoma: a multidisciplinary approach to diagnosis and treatment. Am Fam Physician 2002;65(6):1123–32.

37. Agarwal M, Puri A, Anchan C, et al. Rotationplasty for bone tumors. Clin Orthopaedics Relat Res 2007;459: 76–81.

38. Wong KC, Niu X, Xu H, et al. Computer Navigation in Orthopaedic Tumour Surgery. Adv Exp Med Biol 2018;1093:315–26.

39. Staats K, Panotopoulos J, Tiefenboeck TM, et al. Computer navigation-assisted surgery for musculoskeletal tumors: a closer look into the learning curve. Eur J Orthop Surg Traumatol 2017;27(6):851–8.

40. McCulloch RA, Frisoni T, Kurunskal V, et al. Computer navigation and 3D printing in the surgical management of bone sarcoma. Cells 2021;10(2):195.

41. Pretell-Mazzini J, Barton MD Jr, Conway SA, et al. Unplanned excision of soft-tissue sarcomas: current concepts for management and prognosis. J Bone Joint Surg Am 2015;97(7):597–603.

42. Charoenlap C, Imanishi J, Tanaka T, et al. Outcomes of unplanned sarcoma excision: impact of residual disease. Cancer Med 2016;5(6):980–8.

43. Nakamura T, Sugaya J, Naka N, et al. standard treatment remains the recommended approach for patients with bone sarcoma who underwent unplanned surgery: Report from the Japanese Musculoskeletal Oncology Group. Cancer Management Res 2020;12:10017–22.

44. Henderson ER, O'Connor MI, Ruggieri P, et al. Classification of failure of limb salvage after reconstructive surgery for Bone Tumours. Bone Joint J 2014; 96-B(11):1436–40.

45. Picci P, Sangiorgi L, Bahamonde L, et al. Risk factors for local recurrences after limb-salvage surgery for high-grade osteosarcoma of the extremities. Ann Oncol 1997;8(9):899–903.

46. Li X, Moretti VM, Ashana AO, et al. Perioperative infection rate in patients with osteosarcomas treated with resection and prosthetic reconstruction. Clin Orthop Relat Res 2011;469(10):2889–94.

47. Gharehdaghi M, Hassani M, Parsa A, et al. Short Term Complications and Functional Results of Sarcoma Limb Salvage Surgeries. Arch Bone Jt Surg 2019;7(2):161–7.

48. King CS, Sebro R. Linear mixed-effects models for predicting sarcoma local recurrence growth rates: Implications for optimal surveillance imaging frequency. Eur J Radiol 2020;132:109308.

49. Pennington Z, Ahmed AK, Cottrill E, et al. Systematic review on the utility of magnetic resonance imaging for operative management and follow-up for primary sarcoma-lessons from extremity sarcomas. Ann Transl Med 2019;7(10):225.

50. Meazza C, Bastoni S, Scanagatta P. What is the best clinical approach to recurrent/refractory osteosarcoma? Expert Rev Anticancer Ther 2020;20(5): 415–28.

Bone Tumors
Imaging Features of Common and Rare Benign Entities

Ali M. Naraghi, FRCR[a,b], Rakesh Mohankumar, FRCPC[a,b],
Dorota Linda, MD, FRCPC[a,c], Lawrence M. White, MD, FRCPC[a,c],*

KEYWORDS

- Benign bone tumors • Chondrogenic tumors • Osteogenic tumors • Mesenchymal tumors of bone
- Computed tomography • Magnetic resonance imaging • Radiography

KEY POINTS

- Benign bone tumors encompass a set of lesions with indolent or locally aggressive biological behavior.
- In many cases, radiological features are sufficient to make a diagnosis, and no further follow-up is required.
- Follow-up imaging, specialist referral, and ultimately biopsy will be required for lesions with indeterminate features whereby low-grade neoplasms are included in the differential diagnosis or for preoperative staging.

INTRODUCTION

Primary bone tumors are rare, and most that are encountered in clinical practice are benign. The true incidence of benign bone tumors remains unknown, as many are asymptomatic and often discovered unintentionally. Imaging plays a crucial role in determining the appropriate management of these cases, whether symptomatic or incidental. In many instances, the nonaggressive nature of the lesion can be ascertained based on the radiographic appearance, negating the need for further imaging or follow-up. In some cases, however, follow-up imaging or specialist referral is warranted.

The World Health Organization (WHO) classification of soft tissue and bone tumors, currently in its 5th edition,[1] provides a framework for standardizing diagnosis and management of tumors. The different entities are subdivided based on their biological behavior into benign, intermediate (locally aggressive), intermediate (rarely metastasizing), and malignant categories. This review discusses the imaging features of the most common entities with an emphasis on their distinguishing features.

CHONDROGENIC TUMORS
Enchondroma

Enchondromas are a relatively common benign intramedullary cartilage neoplasm representing approximately 5% of all bone tumors with a peak incidence of 10 to 30 years. They arise from rests of growth plate cartilage, which become isolated within mature bone. Thus, enchondromas may be seen in any bone formed by endochondral ossification. Common sites are the short tubular bones of the hands or feet as well as the femur, tibia, and humerus. The majority arise in the metaphysis, although diaphyseal lesions are not uncommon. Chondroid lesions located in axial skeletal

a Toronto Joint Department of Medical Imaging, University of Toronto, Toronto, Ontario, Canada;
b Department of Medical Imaging, Toronto Western Hospital, 399 Bathurst Street, Toronto, Ontario M5T 2S8, Canada; c Department of Medical Imaging, Mount Sinai Hospital, 600 University Avenue, Toronto, Ontario, M5G 1X5, Canada
* Corresponding author. Department of Medical Imaging, Mount Sinai Hospital, 600 University Avenue, Toronto, Ontario, M5G 1X5, Canada.
E-mail address: lawrence.white@uhn.ca

Radiol Clin N Am 60 (2022) 205–219
https://doi.org/10.1016/j.rcl.2021.11.002

locations, such as the pelvis and scapula, are considered compatible with chondrosarcoma until proven otherwise.[2]

Key imaging features include the following[3]:

- Radiographs/computed tomography (CT)
  - Intramedullary mixed lucent and sclerotic lesion with narrow zone of transition
  - Chondroid matrix mineralization (stipples, arcs, and rings), best demonstrated on CT
  - Possible mild endosteal scalloping, less than two-thirds of cortical thickness
- MR imaging
  - Lobular morphology with primarily T2 hyperintensity and T1 isointensity to hypointensity relative to muscle intermixed with areas of T1/T2 hypointensity corresponding to matrix mineralization
  - Septal and peripheral (multilobular rimlike) gadolinium enhancement
  - Peripheral chemical shift artifact owing to high water content
  - No surrounding marrow edema

In the hands and feet, enchondromas usually lack matrix mineralization and may be expansile with more pronounced endosteal scalloping.

Rarely, an enchondroma may extend beyond the cortex and demonstrate an exophytic growth pattern. Such lesions, termed enchondroma protuberans, may occur sporadically or as part of Ollier disease.[4]

Table 1
Differential diagnoses enchondroma

Differential Diagnosis	Distinguishing Factors
Bone infarct	Serpentine contour Internal marrow fat on CT or MR imaging
Low-grade chondrosarcoma	Unexplained pain Older age Growth after skeletal maturity Size >5 cm Endosteal scalloping >2/3 cortical thickness Endosteal scalloping >2/3 of the length of the lesion Perilesional edema Cortical destruction or soft tissue mass in higher-grade lesions

The main differential considerations include bone infarcts and low-grade chondrosarcoma[3] (**Table 1**). Distinguishing between enchondroma and low-grade chondrosarcoma is often difficult, as the lesions are histologically and radiologically very similar. Because low-grade chondrosarcomas rarely metastasize, larger enchondromas may be closely followed, and if symptomatic, treated with simple curettage.

Enchondromatosis

Ollier disease and Maffucci syndrome are both rare, nonhereditary disorders characterized by multiple enchondromas.

In Ollier disease, there is asymmetrical involvement of the extremities with multiple enchondromas in a predominantly or exclusively unilateral distribution. Significant involvement may result in leg length discrepancy or Madelung deformity.

In Maffucci syndrome, hemangiomas involving the cutaneous, subcutaneous, or visceral tissues are present in addition to multiple enchondromas.

Typical imaging criteria to determine development of chondrosarcoma may be unreliable in patients with Ollier disease and Maffucci syndrome, as some of the enchondromas can have an aggressive appearance with cortical discontinuity or soft tissue extension (**Fig. 1**).[5] Patients with enchondromatosis have an increased lifetime risk of malignant transformation of enchondromas to chondrosarcoma ranging from 15% to 46%, with a higher risk in individuals with pelvic and long bone involvement. These patients should be followed closely for early detection of malignant transformation.[5]

Osteochondroma

Solitary osteochondroma is the most common tumor of bone. These lesions constitute 10% to 15% of all bone tumors, and the majority are asymptomatic. Symptomatic lesions are usually found before the age of 20 years presenting as a nontender, painless deformity. The metaphyses of the long bones of the lower extremity are most frequently affected. The femur is the most common site (30% of cases), with distal involvement predominating. Other frequent sites include the tibia and humerus. More unusual locations are the small bones of the hands and feet, pelvis, scapula, and spine.

Key (often pathognomonic) imaging features include the following:

- Radiographs/CT
  - Mineralized surface lesion with corticomedullary continuity (best depicted on CT and MR in regions of complex anatomy)
  - Two possible patterns of corticomedullary continuity: broad continuity (sessile

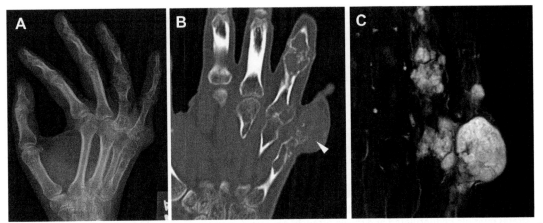

Fig. 1. Ollier disease. A 41-year-old woman presented for follow-up imaging. Radiograph (*A*) and coronal CT (*B*) of the right hand demonstrate numerous lytic lesions without matrix mineralization of the fourth digit and the fifth metacarpal and digit. The fifth proximal phalanx shows cortical discontinuity and extension into the surrounding soft tissues (*arrowhead* in *B*). Coronal T2 fat-suppressed (*C*) MR image reveals multiple T2 hyperintense masses in keeping with multiple enchondromas. All the lesions have been stable in size and appearance for many years.

osteochondroma) or narrow continuity (pedunculated osteochondroma)
  ○ Possible chondroid matrix (ring and arc calcification) within hyaline cartilage cap
- MR imaging
  ○ T1 isointense to hypointense and very T2 hyperintense cartilage cap
  ○ Septal and peripheral gadolinium enhancement of cartilage cap

Multiple osteochondromas

Hereditary multiple exostosis (HME) is an autosomal dominant disorder with incomplete penetrance in women, characterized by the development of multiple osteochondromas. Most cases are diagnosed by age 5, and virtually all are diagnosed by age 12. The distribution is variable and may be unilateral or bilateral and symmetric. Short stature occurs in 40% of cases owing to the development of exostoses during childhood and early puberty.[6] Imaging of individual osteochondromas in HME is identical to that of solitary lesions, although sessile osteochondromas predominate in HME.[7]

Possible complications related to osteochondroma include bone deformity, tendon snapping, tenosynovitis, and premature osteoarthritis. Other complications can also include restricted motion, vessel displacement, stenosis, occlusion, and pseudoaneurysm formation as well as entrapment neuropathy and overlying adventitial bursa formation (**Fig. 2**).[8] Complications of osteochondroma are more common in the setting of HME because of the multiplicity of lesions.

The grimmest complication is malignant transformation, which occurs in 1% of solitary lesions and in 3% to 5% of lesions associated with HME. The malignant transformation is usually due to chondrosarcoma arising in the cartilage cap. This type of chondrosarcoma, referred to as secondary or peripheral chondrosarcoma, is usually of a low histologic grade, although multifocal and dedifferentiated lesions may be encountered.[9] Osteochondromas in an axial location are particularly at risk. Malignant transformation occurs at an earlier age in HME.

Features suggestive of malignant transformation include the following[8,10]:

- Unexplained pain
- Growth of cartilage cap in skeletally mature patient
- Erosion or destruction of adjacent bone
- Significant soft tissue mass containing irregular mineralization
- Cartilage cap thickness of more than 1.5 cm in skeletally mature patient

Radiographically, differential considerations for osteochondromas include bizarre parosteal osteochondromatous proliferation, myositis ossificans, parosteal osteosarcoma, and fracture malunion, all of which lack corticomedullary continuity. Osteochondromas may be managed conservatively or resected in the setting of pain, neurovascular compromise, myotendinous or osteoarticular impingement, or when there is concern for malignant transformation.[11]

Chondroblastoma

Chondroblastomas are uncommon cartilaginous tumors comprising less than 1% of all primary

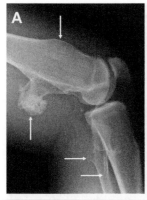
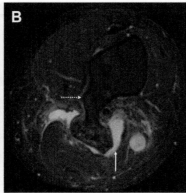
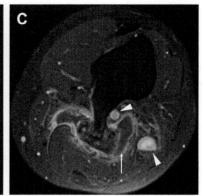

Fig. 2. Osteochondromas in HME. Lateral knee radiograph (A) in a 29-year-old woman presenting with pain demonstrates multiple pedunculated and sessile osteochondromas (*arrows* in A). Axial T2 fat-suppressed (B) and postgadolinium T1 fat-suppressed (C) MR images through the distal femur demonstrate corticomedullary continuity (*dashed arrow* in B). An irregular region of high T2 signal change overlying the osteochondroma (*arrow* in B) demonstrates peripheral rim enhancement (*arrow* in C) in keeping with adventitial bursitis. The popliteal artery and vein are displaced by the osteochondroma (*arrowheads* in C).

tumors of bone. Tumors typically arise in the epiphyses or apophyses and can be seen across a wide age range but are most frequently encountered in skeletally immature patients less than 20 years of age.[12] The most common anatomic sites are the femur, humerus, and tibia.[13,14] Bone pain is the most common presenting feature.

Key imaging features include the following (Fig. 3)[13–16]:

- Radiographs/CT
  - Small (1–4 cm) geographic oval or rounded lytic lesion
  - Epiphyseal/apophyseal location with possible metaphyseal extension

- Thin sclerotic margin
- Chondroid matrix in one-third (best depicted on CT)
- MR imaging
  Lobular morphology with heterogeneous T2 and T1 isointensity to hypointensity relative to muscle
  - Prominent perilesional marrow edema, soft tissue edema, reactive joint effusion, and synovitis
  - Periosteal new bone formation along adjacent metaphysis
  - Possible secondary aneurysmal bone cyst (ABC) formation

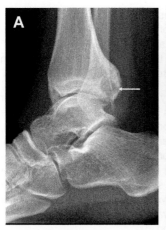
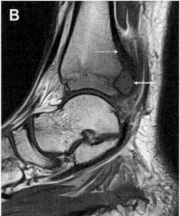
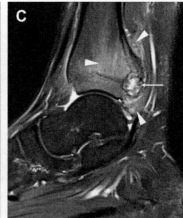

Fig. 3. Chondroblastoma. A 22-year-old man presenting with posterior medial ankle pain. Lateral radiograph (A) and corresponding sagittal T1 (B) and T2-weighted fat-suppressed (C) MR images illustrate a subarticular well-defined lytic lesion along the posterior malleolus (*white arrows*). The lesion shows a thin geographic margin with heterogeneous internal T2 signal with prominent surrounding marrow and soft tissue edema (*arrowheads* in C). Periosteal reaction and cortical thickening is seen along the posterior aspect of the tibial metaphysis (*dashed arrow* in B).

The inflammatory perilesional changes (similar to osteoid osteoma [OO] and osteoblastoma) have been proposed to be related to high levels of tumor prostaglandin, especially prostaglandin E_2.[17] Differential diagnoses include giant cell tumors, Langerhans cell histiocytosis, and Brodie abscess (Table 2), all of which can be epiphyseal in location and demonstrate associated perilesional edema.

Chondroblastomas can seldomly illustrate aggressive local biologic behavior, including cortical destruction and soft tissue extension. Metastases to lung or soft tissues are very rare.[18]

Treatment is typically surgical with intralesional curettage and bone grafting, but local disease recurrence has been reported in up to 13% to 20% of cases. The risk of recurrence can be reduced with an extended curettage and use of adjuncts, including intralesional phenol or cryotherapy.[15,18]

OSTEOGENIC TUMORS
Osteoid Osteoma

OO is a benign osteoblastic neoplasm accounting for 3% of all primary bone tumors.[19] It usually presents within the first 3 decades of life. The classic presentation is localized pain that is worse at night and is alleviated with nonsteroidal anti-inflammatory drugs.[20]

OO may be cortical (75% of cases), intramedullary, or rarely, subperiosteal. Lesions are typically within the diaphysis or metadiaphysis of the long bones, with the proximal femur and the tibia being the most common locations.[21] Other reported sites include the spine, pelvis, and hands and feet. When arising in the spine, they most frequently occur in the posterior elements, a location that can predispose the patient to scoliosis. If scoliosis is present, the lesion is typically centered along the concavity of the scoliotic curve.[22]

Key imaging features (dependent on location) (Fig. 4)[23,24]:

- Radiographs/CT
  - Lucent nidus (<1.5–2 cm) with surrounding dense reactive sclerosis
  - Thin, serpentine grooves in the surrounding sclerosis ("vascular groove")—highly specific feature of OO on CT
- MR imaging
  - Nidus demonstrates intermediate to high T2 signal intensity and T1 hypointensity relative to muscle
  - Prominent perilesional edema and enhancement; joint effusion and synovitis if intra-articular
  - Avid enhancement of nidus

Differential considerations include Brodie abscess, stress fracture, osteoblastoma, or enostosis (Table 3). Treatment options include either surgical resection, radiofrequency ablation, or cryoablation. Posttreatment follow-up is largely clinical. Posttreatment MR imaging may be considered in individuals with residual or recurrent symptoms or posttreatment complications.[25]

Osteoblastoma

Osteoblastoma is another benign osteoblastic lesion that is rarer than OO, accounting for approximately 1% of all primary bone tumors.[26] It has similar histologic characteristics to OO with woven bone trabeculae of varying mineralization, osteoblastic rimming, and a fibrovascular stroma without host bone permeation. However, osteoblastomas are less well organized and may demonstrate secondary ABC change.[27] Osteoblastomas are typically identified in the second to fourth decades of life. The spine is the most frequent site of involvement, accounting for one-third of cases. When occurring in the spine, posterior element involvement, whether in isolation or in combination with vertebral body involvement, is most common.[28] Other possible locations include the jaw or the diaphysis or metaphysis of long tubular bones, most often the femur and tibia.

Table 2	
Differential diagnosis of chondroblastoma (epiphyseal lytic lesions)	
Differential Diagnosis	**Distinguishing Factors**
Subchondral cyst	Typically older Signs of osteoarthritis Lack of chondroid matrix
Giant cell tumor of bone	Metaphyseal-epiphyseal involvement after physeal closure Typically older No chondroid matrix
Langerhans cell histiocytosis	Variable appearance depending on phase No chondroid matrix
Infection/Brodie abscess	Lacks thin sclerotic margin—may have a thick sclerotic rind
Clear cell chondrosarcoma	Older age Larger

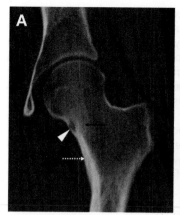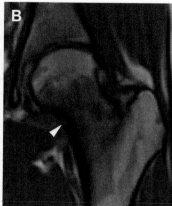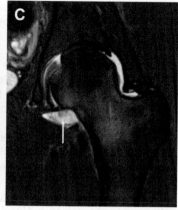

Fig. 4. OO. Coronal CT (*A*) T1-weighted (*B*) and T2 fat-suppressed (*C*) MR images in a 20-year-old woman with hip pain demonstrate a cortically based radiolucent nidus in the femoral neck (*arrowheads* in *A* and *B*), calcar thickening (*dashed arrow* in *A*), intramedullary sclerosis (*black arrow* in *A*), and reactive bone marrow changes in the femoral neck on MR imaging. There is a joint effusion with synovitis (*arrow* in *C*). The nidus is not as well appreciated on the T2 image.

Key imaging features (can be variable) include the following:

- Radiographs/CT
  - Lucent center with surrounding sclerosis— similar to OO but greater than 2 cm in size and less intense sclerosis
  - Expansile lytic lesion with foci of calcification and sclerotic periphery—most common in spine (**Fig. 5**)
- Aggressive lesions with cortical destruction, soft tissue infiltration, and periosteal reaction
  - Calcification seen in 30%
- MR imaging
  - Variable MR imaging appearances with low-intermediate T1 and variable T2 signal changes

Table 3
Differential diagnosis osteoid osteoma

Differential Diagnosis	Distinguishing Factors
Brodie abscess	Irregular margin May demonstrate a sinus tract Medullary component
Stress fracture	Cortical component linear—best demonstrated on CT
Osteoblastoma	Nidus >2 cm More expansile
Enostosis	No central lucency No surrounding reactive sclerosis

- Cystic ABC-like fluid-fluid levels

Differential diagnosis can be broad given the variability in imaging appearances and depends on location (spine vs appendicular skeleton) and imaging aggressiveness. The main differential diagnoses include OO and low-grade osteosarcoma. Treatment options include curettage and bone grafting or en bloc resection and instrumentation depending on the location.[29]

OSTEOCLASTIC GIANT CELL-RICH TUMORS
Aneurysmal Bone Cyst

Classic primary ABC is a benign lytic lesion that represents 1% to 2% of all primary bone tumors.[30] Primary ABCs are most commonly diagnosed in young adult patients, with 75% to 90% of cases occurring in patients less than 20 years of age.[31] They usually present as solitary expansile lesions, and common sites include the long bones, posterior elements of the spine, or pelvis. Primary ABC has a specific genetic translocation involving the ubiquitin-specific protease 6 oncogene on chromosome 17.[32] Conversely, secondary ABC are associated with other underlying lesions and do not illustrate a genetic translocation. They are hypothesized to arise because of intralesional hemorrhage and intraosseous venous pressure activating osteoclastic bone resorption.[31]

Key imaging features include the following[31,33]:

- Radiographs/CT
  - Geographic expansile lytic lesion with "bubbly" appearance
  - Variable degree of thin expanded neocortical ossification, depending on lesion growth rate

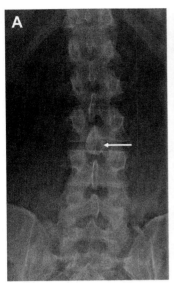 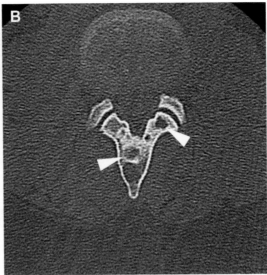

Fig. 5. Osteoblastoma. Frontal lumbar spine radiograph (A) in a 20-year-old man with back pain demonstrates expansion of the spinous process of L3 with mixed lucency and sclerosis (arrow). Axial CT (B) demonstrates expansion of the spinous process and lamina with central lucencies (arrowheads) and surrounding sclerosis.

- MR imaging
  - Multilobular fluid-fluid levels separated by thin intrinsic septae (Fig. 6)
  - Primary ABC: thin internal septal enhancement
  - Secondary ABC: solid nodular enhancing components related to the underlying bone lesion

Radiographically, differential considerations include giant cell tumor of bone, unicameral bone cyst (UBC), telangiectatic osteosarcoma, expansile metastases, and plasmacytoma depending on the age at presentation.

Treatment of ABC typically involves aggressive intralesional curettage with or without bone grafting. Unfortunately, local recurrence occurs in up to 20%.[31,34] Neoadjuvant or nonoperative therapies include preoperative arterial embolization, denosumab therapy, cryotherapy as well as intralesional sclerotherapeutic injections.[35,36] Post-treatment follow-up consists of clinical and radiographic evaluation. CT or MR imaging is indicated in cases of clinically/radiographically suspected recurrence.

Giant Cell Tumor of Bone

Giant cell tumor of bone (GCTB) represents approximately 5% of all primary bone tumors.[37] GCTB is most common in patients between the third and sixth decades of life.[38] Although GCTB usually has benign behavior, it can be locally aggressive and can metastasize to the lungs. Multifocal GCTB has also been reported.[38]

Malignant transformation of GCTB is rare but can occur as a result of tumor dedifferentiation or as a complication of prior radiation therapy.

Most GCTB arise at the end of long bones. The most common anatomic sites are the distal femur, proximal tibia (50%–65% occur at the knee), and distal radius.[38]

Key imaging features include the following[39,40]:

- Radiographs/CT
  - Geographic lytic lesion with nonsclerotic margins
  - Eccentric metaphyseal location extending to subchondral bone (Fig. 7)
  - Cortical thinning and expansion
- MR imaging
  - Intermediate to low T2 signal intensity reflective of internal cellularity, high collagen content, or intralesional hemosiderin deposition
  - Blurred margins (paint-brush border) on T1 (correlates histologically to local tumor infiltration)
  - Contrast enhancement
  - Secondary ABC change in up to 14% of cases

The differential diagnosis is dependent on the age at presentation and includes primary ABC and epiphyseal lesions (see Table 2). In a slightly older age group, clear cell chondrosarcoma and metastases would also be considerations.

Intralesional curettage and cement/bone grafting have generally been the treatment of choice.

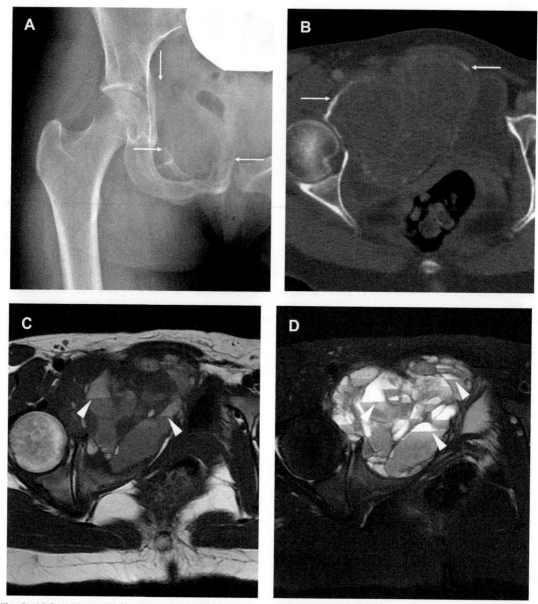

Fig. 6. ABC. A 20-year-old woman presenting with pelvic pain and fullness. Anteroposterior (AP) radiograph (*A*) and CT (*B*) show an osteolytic lesion of the superior pubic ramus with faint areas of neocortical ossification (*arrows*). Axial T1- (*C*) and T2-weighted (*D*) MR images illustrate the expansile nature of the lesion with multiple thin internal septae with fluid-fluid levels (*arrowheads*) throughout the lesion. No solid enhancing components were observed following contrast administration.

However, intralesional curettage has been associated with an incidence of locally recurrent disease ranging from 12% to 65%.[41] To reduce recurrence risk, neoadjuvant therapy with denosumab, a monoclonal antibody that prevents the activation of multinucleated osteoclasts and giant cells, has been trialed. Denosumab treatment typically results in marginal osteosclerosis and reconstitution of thin cortical bone, which may make surgical management easier.[42] However, more recent studies have shown a significantly increased incidence of locally recurrent disease in patients treated with denosumab and curettage versus curettage alone.[43] Following treatment, patients are assessed radiographically or, in the presence of symptoms or concerning radiographic features such as osteolysis, with CT or MR imaging.

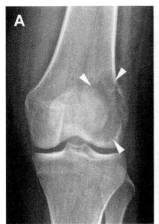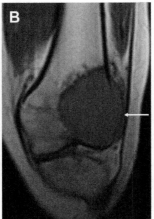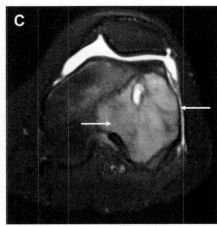

Fig. 7. Giant cell tumor of bone. AP radiograph (*A*) in a 17-year-old following an acute injury demonstrates an expansile osteolytic lesion eccentrically located within the lateral femoral metaphysis and subarticular aspect lateral femoral condyle (*arrowheads*). Coronal T1- (*B*) and T2-weighted fat-suppressed (*C*) images demonstrate the expanded and thinned cortex of the lateral femoral condyle (*arrows*) and the intermediate to low T2 signal intensity commonly observed with giant cell tumors of bone (*dashed arrow* in *C*).

OTHER MESENCHYMAL TUMORS OF BONE
Unicameral (Simple) Bone Cysts

UBC (simple) is a fluid-filled unilocular intramedullary lesion that accounts for approximately 3% to 5% of primary bone tumors. The majority present in the first and second decades of life.[44] More than 50% arise in the humerus, but the femur and proximal tibia are also common sites of involvement. The lesion develops in the metaphysis, but with growth of the host bone, it can extend into the diaphysis.[45] In adults, UBC has a predilection for the anterior calcaneus but can also occur in the posterior ilium adjacent to the sacroiliac joints. They are typically asymptomatic unless complicated by a pathologic fracture.[45]

Pathologic fracture is the most common complication of this lesion in children. Radiographically, a fracture fragment may be visualized in the dependent part of the cyst (fallen fragment sign), reflecting the true cystic unilocular nature of the lesion. Alternatively, gas locules may collect within the nondependent portion of the cyst (rising bubble sign).[46] On MR imaging, T1 and T2 heterogeneity, fluid-fluid levels, and heterogeneous nodular enhancement can be seen after pathologic fracture (**Fig. 8**).[47]

Key imaging features include the following[45]:

- Radiographs/CT
  - Children: Geographic lytic lesion with thin sclerotic margin abutting open physis of long bone (humerus >50%)
  - Adults: Geographic lytic lesion inferior to the critical angle of Gissane (similar location to calcaneal intraosseous lipoma)
    - No periosteal reaction (unless complicated by fracture)
    - Fluid attenuation on CT
    - Fallen fragment sign when complicated by fracture
- MR imaging
  - Homogenous T2 hyperintensity and T1 iso-intensity hypointensity relative to muscle; T1 hyperintensity when contain high protein levels
  - Thin peripheral rim enhancement

Differential considerations consist primarily of ABC or cystic fibrous dysplasia (FD) in the long bones and calcaneal lipoma in the calcaneus (**Table 4**). As lesions can heal either spontaneously or after fractures, asymptomatic lesions and those with a low risk of pathologic fracturing may be treated conservatively. Symptomatic lesions and those at risk of fracturing are treated by curettage with either bone grafting or application of bone substitutes, although injection therapy with steroids or sclerosing agents has also been used.[48]

Intraosseous Lipomas

Intraosseous lipoma is a rare benign neoplasm typically seen in adults that represents less than 0.1% of bone tumors.[49] They can be intramedullary, intracortical, or parosteal in location, with intramedullary being most common of the three. More than 70% involve the lower limb, particularly the calcaneus and the intertrochanteric and subtrochanteric regions of the femur.[49] Long bone involvement is usually metaphyseal but may extend into the diaphysis. Isolated epiphyseal involvement is unusual.

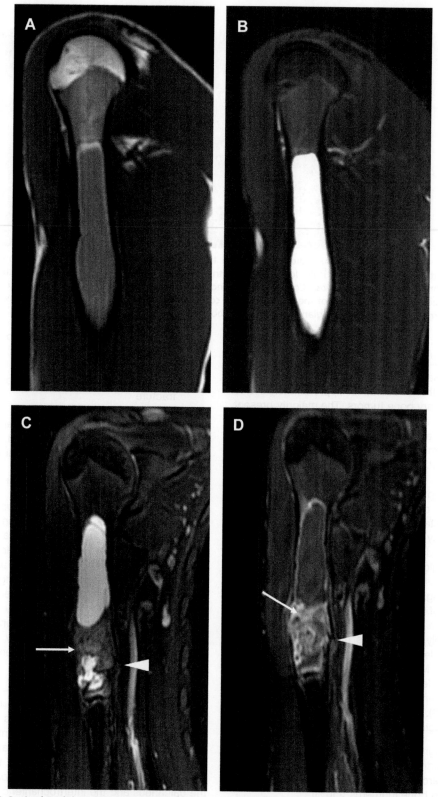

Fig. 8. UBC. Sagittal T1 (*A*) and T2 fat-suppressed (*B*) MR images in an 18-year-old woman demonstrate a well-defined intermediate T1 and homogeneous high T2 signal lesions in the humeral diaphysis. Coronal T2 fat-suppressed (*C*) and postgadolinium T1 fat-suppressed (*D*) MR images in the same patient obtained 2 years later following a subacute pathologic fracture (*arrowheads* in *C* and *D*) demonstrate complex T2 signal change (*arrow* in *C*) and heterogeneous enhancement (*arrow* in *D*).

Table 4 Differential diagnosis of solitary bone cysts	
Differential Diagnosis	**Distinguishing Features**
ABC	More expansile, cortical destruction, periosteal reaction, fluid levels on CT and MR imaging
Cystic fibrous dysplasia	Areas of ground glass Sclerotic rind
Calcaneus lipoma	Central calcification Intralesional fat on MR imaging

The cause of intraosseous lipomas is controversial. Various histopathological stages have been described, including viable mature fat cells, partial ischemic necrosis of fat cells with associated calcification, and finally, more diffuse necrosis, cystic degeneration, and calcification.[50] The relationship between UBC and intraosseous lipoma has also been debated.[51] A recent study of 6 patients reported that there was partial to complete fill-in of UBC with fat, which supports the theory that at least some intraosseous lipomas represent healed UBCs.[51,52]

Key imaging features (dependent on stage) include the following (**Fig. 9**)[53]:

- Radiographs/CT/MR imaging
  - Well-defined mildly expansile lytic lesions with peripheral sclerotic rim (70%)
  - Homogeneous fatty attenuation/signal intensity
  - Cystic areas and peripheral or central calcification (bull's-eye appearance) when involuting

Radiographic differential considerations include UBC and osteonecrosis (**Table 5**). When macroscopic fat is recognized within the lesion, additional workup, follow-up, and unnecessary treatment can be avoided.

Fibrous Dysplasia

FD is a congenital nonhereditary lesion that accounts for 5% of benign bone tumors. In most cases it is characterized by a mutation in the GNAS1 gene on chromosome 20. It may be monostotic or polyostotic and may present clinically at any age. The polyostotic form accounts for 20% of cases but is more likely to be symptomatic

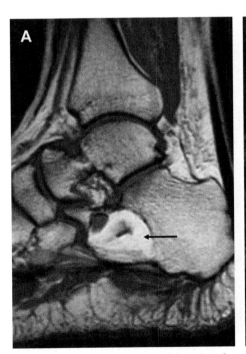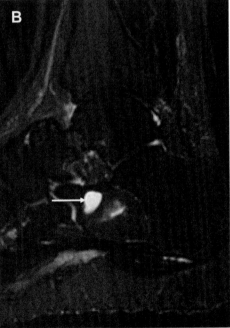

Fig. 9. Intraosseous lipoma. Sagittal T1 (*A*) and T2 fat-suppressed (*B*) MR images obtained in a 40-year-old man for a suspected peroneal tendon tear demonstrate an incidental calcaneal lipoma with intralesional fat (*black arrow* in *A*) and involutional cystic changes (*white arrow* in *B*).

Table 5
Differential diagnosis of intraosseous lipomas

Differential Diagnosis	Distinguishing Factors
Solitary bone cyst	No calcification No intralesional fat on CT or MR imaging
Osteonecrosis	Mixed lucency and sclerosis on radiography Serpentine contour High T2 signal intensity rim No expansion

and presents at a younger age. The polyostotic form can be of variable extent but tends to have a unilateral distribution with lower extremity and craniofacial predominance. Any bone may be affected, but the monostotic form most commonly affects the femur and tibia. Lesions are intramedullary and arise centrally within the diaphysis or metadiaphysis, usually sparing the epiphysis. Spinal involvement is rare but most commonly involves the vertebral body, either in isolation or in combination with the posterior elements.[54]

Polyostotic disease may be associated with McCune-Albright syndrome, which manifests as a triad of polyostotic FD, café-au-lait spots, and precocious puberty (or other endocrine abnormalities).[55]

FD may also be associated with Mazabraud syndrome, which manifests with FD (monostotic or polyostotic) and soft tissue myxomas. Myxomas tend to be multiple and located in the same anatomic region as the FD (Fig. 10). FD typically develops before the myxoma or myxomas.[56]

FD may be discovered incidentally or may present with pain, swelling, deformity, leg length discrepancy, or pathologic fracture. Intralesional chondroid change is uncommon, seen in approximately 10%, most often in the proximal femur.[57,58] ABC change is also uncommon, seen in approximately 6% and usually in monostotic or craniofacial disease.[54]

Key imaging features (may be variable) include the following[57,58]:

- Radiographs/CT
  - Elongated, mildly expansile lesion in long bone
  - Variable internal matrix depending on the underlying constituents
    - Ground glass (Fig. 11)
    - Lytic
    - Purely sclerotic (uncommon)

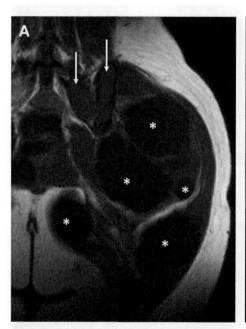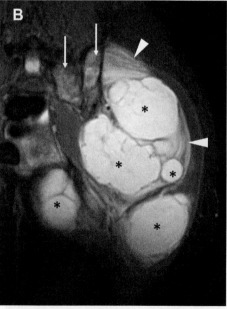

Fig. 10. Mazabraud syndrome. Coronal T1 (*A*) and T2 fat-suppressed MR images (*B*) in a 41-year-old woman demonstrate intraosseous lesions within the posterior ilium and sacrum (*arrows* in *A* and *B*) and multiple low T1 and very high T2 signal intensity soft tissue masses (*asterisks*) with perilesional high T2 (*arrowheads* in *B*) in keeping with FD and multiple intramuscular myxomas.

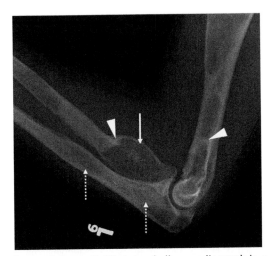

Fig. 11. Polyostotic FD. Lateral elbow radiograph in a 21-year-old woman with numerous intramedullary lesions of varying densities ranging from lytic lesions within the proximal radius (*white arrow*) to ground glass change within the proximal ulna (*dashed arrows*). The lesions demonstrate variable expansion and sclerotic margins (*arrowheads*).

  ○ Limb deformities: tibial bowing, acetabular protrusion, Shepherd's crook of proximal femur
- MR imaging
  ○ Variable T2 signal changes ranging from hypointense regions to areas of hyperintense signal, including chondroid elements and areas of cystic change

Although cortical destruction and soft tissue extension have been described in locally aggressive forms of FD, biopsy is warranted in these cases to exclude malignant transformation. Malignant transformation is rare but may be seen with either monostotic or polyostotic variants. Osteosarcoma is the most common type of malignancy in these cases and will usually present with an extraosseous soft tissue mass (75% of cases).[57]

SUMMARY

The lesions described above account for most benign bone tumors encountered in clinical practice. In many instances, the combination of patient age, skeletal location, and radiographic appearance is sufficient in identifying the nonaggressive nature of the lesion and allowing for a specific or limited differential diagnosis without the need for additional imaging. Cross-sectional imaging with CT or MR imaging is warranted in lesions with indeterminate features with more aggressive radiographic appearances or for treatment planning of lesions in close proximity to an articular surface or other critical

structure. In some cases, however, malignant neoplasms remain as a differential consideration even after cross-sectional imaging, and biopsy is necessary to plan optimal patient management.

CLINICS CARE POINTS

- Typical imaging features used to distinguish between enchondromas and chondrosarcomas may be unreliable in patients with enchondromatosis as some enchondromas can have an aggressive appearance. Given the increased risk of malignant transformation, these lesions require close follow-up.

- The risk of malignant transformation of osteochondromas is higher in patients with HME, particularly when there is involvement of the axial skeleton.

- Unicameral bone cysts can have a complex appearance on MRI, simulating a more aggressive lesion, following a pathological fracture.

- Some benign lesions can exhibit locally aggressive features on imaging including cortical destruction. These lesions typically require biopsy to exclude a malignant neoplasm.

DISCLOSURE

The authors have nothing to disclose.

REFERENCES

1. WHO classification of tumors editorial board WHO classification of tumours: soft tissue and bone tumors. 5th editionvol. 3. IARC Press; 2020.
2. Murphey MD, Walker EA, Wilson AJ, et al. From the archives of the AFIP: imaging of primary chondrosarcoma: radiologic-pathologic correlation. Radiographics 2003;23(5):1245–78.
3. Murphey MD, Flemming DJ, Boyea SR, et al. Enchondroma versus chondrosarcoma in the appendicular skeleton: differentiating features. Radiographics 1998;18(5):1213–37.
4. An YY, Kim JY, Ahn MI, et al. Enchondroma protuberans of the hand. AJR Am J Roentgenol 2008;190(1):40–4.
5. Verdegaal SH, Bovee JV, Pansuriya TC, et al. Incidence, predictive factors, and prognosis of chondrosarcoma in patients with Ollier disease and Maffucci syndrome: an international multicenter study of 161 patients. Oncologist 2011;16(12):1771–9.

6. McCormick C, Duncan G, Tufaro F. New perspectives on the molecular basis of hereditary bone tumours. Mol Med Today 1999;5(11):481–6.

7. Taniguchi K. A practical classification system for multiple cartilaginous exostosis in children. J Pediatr Orthop 1995;15(5):585–91.

8. Murphey MD, Choi JJ, Kransdorf MJ, et al. Imaging of osteochondroma: variants and complications with radiologic-pathologic correlation. Radiographics 2000;20(5):1407–34.

9. Park YK, Yang MH, Ryu KN, et al. Dedifferentiated chondrosarcoma arising in an osteochondroma. Skeletal Radiol 1995;24(8):617–9.

10. Norman A, Sissons HA. Radiographic hallmarks of peripheral chondrosarcoma. Radiology 1984; 151(3):589–96.

11. Ellatif M, Sharif B, Lindsay D, et al. An update on the imaging of diaphyseal aclasis. Skeletal Radiol 2021; 50(10):1941–62.

12. Qasem SA, DeYoung BR. Cartilage-forming tumors. Semin Diagn Pathol 2014;31(1):10–20.

13. Douis H, Saifuddin A. The imaging of cartilaginous bone tumours. I. Benign lesions. Skeletal Radiol 2012;41(10):1195–212.

14. Robbin MR, Murphey MD. Benign chondroid neoplasms of bone. Semin Musculoskelet Radiol 2000; 4(1):45–58.

15. Bloem JL, Mulder JD. Chondroblastoma: a clinical and radiological study of 104 cases. Skeletal Radiol 1985;14(1):1–9.

16. Weatherall PT, Maale GE, Mendelsohn DB, et al. Chondroblastoma: classic and confusing appearance at MR imaging. Radiology 1994;190(2): 467–74.

17. Yamamura S, Sato K, Sugiura H, et al. Prostaglandin levels of primary bone tumor tissues correlate with peritumoral edema demonstrated by magnetic resonance imaging. Cancer 15 1997;79(2):255–61.

18. Suneja R, Grimer RJ, Belthur M, et al. Chondroblastoma of bone: long-term results and functional outcome after intralesional curettage. J Bone Joint Surg Br. Jul 2005;87(7):974–8.

19. French J, Epelman M, Johnson CM, et al. MR imaging of osteoid osteoma: pearls and pitfalls. Semin Ultrasound CT MRI 2020;41(5):488–97.

20. Greco F, Tamburrelli F, Ciabattoni G. Prostaglandins in osteoid osteoma. Int Orthop 1991;15(1):35–7.

21. Cerase A, Priolo F. Skeletal benign bone-forming lesions. Eur J Radiol 1998;27(Suppl 1):S91–7.

22. Saifuddin A, White J, Sherazi Z, et al. Osteoid osteoma and osteoblastoma of the spine. Factors associated with the presence of scoliosis. Spine (Phila Pa 1976) 1998;23(1):47–53.

23. Liu PT, Kujak JL, Roberts CC, et al. The vascular groove sign: a new CT finding associated with osteoid osteomas. Am J Roentgenology 2011; 196(1):168–73.

24. Liu PT, Chivers FS, Roberts CC, et al. Imaging of osteoid osteoma with dynamic gadolinium-enhanced MR imaging. Radiology 2003;227(3): 691–700.

25. Mahnken AH, Bruners P, Delbruck H, et al. Contrast-enhanced MRI predicts local recurrence of osteoid osteoma after radiofrequency ablation. J Med Imaging Radiat Oncol 2012;56(6):617–21.

26. Greenspan A. Benign bone-forming lesions: osteoma, osteoid osteoma, and osteoblastoma: clinical, imaging, pathologic, and differential considerations. Skeletal Radiol 1993;22(7). https://doi.org/10.1007/BF00209095.

27. Franceschini N, Lam SW, Cleton-Jansen AM, et al. What's new in bone forming tumours of the skeleton? Virchows Arch 2020;476(1):147–57.

28. Liu J, Han S, Li J, et al. Spinal osteoblastoma: a retrospective study of 35 patients' imaging findings with an emphasis on MRI. Insights Imaging 2020; 11(1):122.

29. Atesok KI, Alman BA, Schemitsch EH, et al. Osteoid osteoma and osteoblastoma. J Am Acad Orthop Surg 2011;19(11):678–89.

30. Mendenhall WM, Zlotecki RA, Gibbs CP, et al. Aneurysmal bone cyst. Am J Clin Oncol 2006;29(3): 311–5.

31. Mascard E, Gomez-Brouchet A, Lambot K. Bone cysts: unicameral and aneurysmal bone cyst. Orthop Traumatol Surg Res 2015;101(1 Suppl): S119–27.

32. Baumhoer D, Amary F, Flanagan AM. An update of molecular pathology of bone tumors. Lessons learned from investigating samples by next generation sequencing. Genes Chromosomes Cancer 2019;58(2):88–99.

33. Kransdorf MJ, Sweet DE. Aneurysmal bone cyst: concept, controversy, clinical presentation, and imaging. AJR Am J Roentgenol 1995;164(3):573–80.

34. Mankin HJ, Hornicek FJ, Ortiz-Cruz E, et al. Aneurysmal bone cyst: a review of 150 patients. J Clin Oncol 2005;23(27):6756–62.

35. Reddy KI, Sinnaeve F, Gaston CL, et al. Aneurysmal bone cysts: do simple treatments work? Clin Orthop Relat Res 2014;472(6):1901–10.

36. Batisse F, Schmitt A, Vendeuvre T, et al. Aneurysmal bone cyst: a 19-case series managed by percutaneous sclerotherapy. Orthop Traumatol Surg Res 2016;102(2):213–6.

37. Chakarun CJ, Forrester DM, Gottsegen CJ, et al. Giant cell tumor of bone: review, mimics, and new developments in treatment. Radiographics 2013;33(1): 197–211.

38. Murphey MD, Nomikos GC, Flemming DJ, et al. From the archives of AFIP. Imaging of giant cell tumor and giant cell reparative granuloma of bone: radiologic-pathologic correlation. Radiographics 2001;21(5):1283–309.

39. Chen L, Shi XL, Zhou ZM, et al. Clinical significance of MRI and pathological features of giant cell tumor of bone boundary. Orthop Surg 2019;11(4):628–34.

40. He Y, Wang J, Du L, et al. MRI assessment of the bone adjacent to giant cell tumours and its association with local recurrence after intralesional curettage. Clin Radiol 2018;73(11):984 e19–28.

41. Klenke FM, Wenger DE, Inwards CY, et al. Recurrent giant cell tumor of long bones: analysis of surgical management. Clin Orthop Relat Res 2011;469(4):1181–7.

42. Rutkowski P, Ferrari S, Grimer RJ, et al. Surgical downstaging in an open-label phase II trial of denosumab in patients with giant cell tumor of bone. Ann Surg Oncol 2015;22(9):2860–8.

43. Errani C, Tsukamoto S, Leone G, et al. Denosumab may increase the risk of local recurrence in patients with giant-cell tumor of bone treated with curettage. J Bone Joint Surg Am 2018;100(6):496–504.

44. Baig R, Eady JL. Unicameral (simple) bone cysts. South Med J 2006;99(9):966–76.

45. Noordin S, Allana S, Umer M, et al. Unicameral bone cysts: current concepts. Ann Med Surg (Lond) 2018; 34:43–9.

46. Jordanov MI. The "rising bubble" sign: a new aid in the diagnosis of unicameral bone cysts. Skeletal Radiol 2009;38(6):597–600.

47. Margau R, Babyn P, Cole W, et al. MR imaging of simple bone cysts in children: not so simple. Pediatr Radiol 2000;30(8):551–7.

48. Kadhim M, Thacker M, Kadhim A, et al. Treatment of unicameral bone cyst: systematic review and meta analysis. J Child Orthop 2014;8(2):171–91.

49. Kang HS, Kim T, Oh S, et al. Intraosseous lipoma: 18 years of experience at a single institution. Clin Orthop Surg 2018;10(2):234–9.

50. Milgram JW. Intraosseous lipomas: radiologic and pathologic manifestations. Radiology 1988;167(1): 155–60.

51. Malghem J, Lecouvet F, Vande Berg B. Calcaneal cysts and lipomas: a common pathogenesis? Skeletal Radiol 2017;46(12):1635–42.

52. Tins BJ, Berkowitz YJ, Konala P, et al. Intraosseous lipomas originating from simple bone cysts. Skeletal Radiol 2021;50(4):801–6.

53. Campbell RS, Grainger AJ, Mangham DC, et al. Intraosseous lipoma: report of 35 new cases and a review of the literature. Skeletal Radiol 2003;32(4): 209–22.

54. Kinnunen AR, Sironen R, Sipola P. Magnetic resonance imaging characteristics in patients with histopathologically proven fibrous dysplasia—a systematic review. Skeletal Radiol 2020;49(6): 837–45.

55. Dumitrescu CE, Collins MT. McCune-Albright syndrome. Orphanet J Rare Dis 2008;3:12.

56. Cabral CE, Guedes P, Fonseca T, et al. Polyostotic fibrous dysplasia associated with intramuscular myxomas: Mazabraud's syndrome. Skeletal Radiol 1998;27(5):278–82.

57. Bousson V, Rey-Jouvin C, Laredo JD, et al. Fibrous dysplasia and McCune-Albright syndrome: imaging for positive and differential diagnoses, prognosis, and follow-up guidelines. Eur J Radiol 2014;83(10): 1828–42.

58. Kransdorf MJ, Moser RP Jr, Gilkey FW. Fibrous dysplasia. Radiographics 1990;10(3):519–37.

Bone Tumors
Imaging Features of the Most Common Primary Osseous Malignancies

Aline Serfaty, MD, PhD[a,b,*], Mohammad Samim, MD[c]

KEYWORDS

- Primary osseous malignancy • Bone tumor • Radiographs • Computed tomography
- Magnetic resonance imaging

KEY POINTS

- Radiographs are the most appropriate initial imaging modality for the characterization of primary bone tumors.
- Advanced imaging with magnetic resonance provides additional essential information on lesion characterization and local staging. Computed tomography can also play an important role in this regard.
- Comprehensive reporting of imaging findings that affect local staging is important for prognostication and treatment planning purposes.

INTRODUCTION

Primary malignant bone tumors are rare, accounting for less than 1% of all new cancers.[1] Clinical symptoms, patient age, skeletal location, and tumor imaging characteristics often allow for a narrow differential diagnosis. In this review, the authors discuss the clinical characteristics and the radiographic, computed tomography (CT), and MR imaging features of the most common primary bone malignancies.

GENERAL IMAGING CONSIDERATIONS

Radiographs are the most appropriate initial imaging modality for the characterization of primary bone tumors. The margin of the tumor, presence of intratumoral matrix, and the status of the adjacent periosteum and cortex are key radiographic features to consider when attempting to differentiate benignity from malignancy.[2,3] Of these features, the tumor margin, which is a reflection of the tumor growth rate, is the most cogent differentiator between malignant and benign.[2] Tumors that are well-defined and round or oval are generally the least aggressive, whereas those with ill-defined margins and a wide zone of transition are generally more aggressive. The response of the periosteum and cortex to the tumor is also a reflection of the tumor growth rate. Aggressive periosteal reaction and cortical destruction raise concern for malignancy, whereas smooth periosteal reaction and cortical expansion indicate slower growth and support benignity. Intratumoral matrix helps to distinguish osteoid, chondroid, or fibrous tumor types.[2,4]

If an aggressive bone tumor is suspected radiographically, additional imaging of the area of concern with MR imaging is usually appropriate. MR imaging can provide further information regarding the nature of the matrix, the presence of fat or blood products, and the presence of soft tissue involvement. MR imaging has become

[a] Department of Radiology, Faculty of Medicine, Universidade Federal do Rio de Janeiro, Rio de Janeiro, Rio de Janeiro, Brazil; [b] Medscanlagos Radiology, Rua Manoel Francisco Valentim, 57, Cabo Frio, Rio de Janeiro 28906220, Brazil; [c] NYU Langone Medical Center, New York University, NYU Orthopedic Hospital, 301 East 17th Street, 6th Floor, Radiology, New York, NY 10003, USA
* Corresponding author. Medscanlagos Radiology, Rua Manoel Francisco Valentim, 57, Cabo Frio, Rio de Janeiro 28906220, Brazil.
E-mail address: alineserfaty@gmail.com

Radiol Clin N Am 60 (2022) 221–238
https://doi.org/10.1016/j.rcl.2021.11.003

the diagnostic method of choice for preoperative local staging and posttreatment evaluation because of its ability to accurately assess tumor extent and evaluate the surrounding structures. CT may also be indicated, as it can characterize tumor matrix and demonstrate cortical destruction and periosteal reaction to better advantage.[5,6] Of note, evaluation of a bone tumor on advanced imaging without comparison radiographs should be avoided whenever possible.

BONE TUMOR SUBTYPES

In the most recent edition[7] of the World Health Organization (WHO) classification of tumors of soft tissue and bone, [7]tumors of bone are categorized by cell lineage and include osteogenic, chondrogenic, fibrogenic, vascular, osteoclastic giant-cell rich, notochordal, other mesenchymal, hematopoietic, and new in the current edition, undifferentiated small round cell sarcomas of bone and soft tissue, which includes Ewing sarcoma (ES). Each of these lineages contains malignant variants, some with several subtypes. In this review, the authors include only the primary bone malignancies and/or malignant subtypes most frequently encountered in clinical practice (**Table 1**).

OSTEOGENIC TUMORS

Osteosarcoma (OS) is the term used to denote malignancy within the osteogenic tumor family. The 2020 WHO classification of OS includes 6 subtypes (**Box 1**).[7,8] The peak incidence is in the second decade with a worldwide incidence of 3.4 per million people per year.[9,10] It most commonly develops in the distal femur, proximal tibia, and humerus. It is classified as primary when the underlying bone is normal and secondary when there is a primary underlying bone abnormality, such as infarction, Paget disease, or previous radiation.

Conventional Osteosarcoma

Conventional OS is the most common primary bone sarcoma of the skeleton (80% of all OS) and typically originates in the intramedullary cavity.[9,10] There is a bimodal age distribution with greatest incidence in the first and second decades and in those older than 65 years of age. The cause is still not fully understood, with unusual chromosomal instability leading to cytogenetic heterogeneity.[11] Although most cases are sporadic, conventional OS can be seen with several genetic disorders, such as Li-Fraumeni, Rothmund-Thomson, and Bloom syndromes as well as hereditary retinoblastoma.[12,13]The overall 5-year survival rate for conventional OS is approximately 60%.[14]

Most conventional OS originate from the metaphyses (90%) of long bones followed by the diaphyses. Although conventional OS with metaphyseal involvement often extends to the epiphysis, origin within the epiphysis is rarely observed.[15] On radiographs, the vast majority (90%) of conventional OS presents as a mixed lytic-sclerotic destructive mass with a fluffy, cloudlike osteoid matrix. Occasionally, a completely lytic or blastic lesion is observed. Ill-defined margins with a wide zone of transition are often present. Periosteal reaction is frequent and can demonstrate various aggressive patterns, including (1) Codman triangle, where the periosteum is lifted off of the cortex by the tumor; (2) laminated or onion skin, where multiple layers of new bone are formed concentrically around the cortex; (3) hair on end, where spicules of bone form perpendicular to the periosteal surface; and (4) sunburst, where spicules of new bone radiate divergently[2,4,13,15] (**Fig. 1**). On CT, assessment of the presence and extent of osteoid matrix and assessment of cortical integrity, including detection of a possible pathologic fracture, can be achieved to better advantage. In addition, CT is the preferred modality for biopsy guidance and detection of lung metastases. CT can also be valuable for detection or further evaluation of recurrence.[13,15]

MR imaging has become the preferred imaging modality for preoperative evaluation and staging of OS because of its ability to accurately discern the intraosseous and extraosseous soft tissue extent of the tumor (**Fig. 2**). The proximity of extraosseous tumor extension with the neurovascular structures can determine whether the patient is eligible for limb salvage surgery.[15] The MR imaging examination should be protocoled to include at least 1 sequence of the entire length of the bone of origin, including the proximal and distal joints, to assess for possible skip lesions, physeal/epiphyseal involvement, or joint involvement.[13] Conventional OS typically demonstrates low T1 and heterogeneous high T2 signal and enhancement. Both ossified matrix, which manifests as areas of low T1 and T2 signal, and hemorrhage, which manifests as areas of high T1 and T2 signal, are frequently observed. When present, necrosis will manifest as areas of low T1 and high T2 signal without enhancement.[5,13,15–17]

Dynamic contrast-enhanced (DCE) MR imaging provides information on tissue vascularization and perfusion, capillary permeability, and the volume of interstitial space.[6] This technique may be helpful in identifying areas of viable tumor to guide biopsy, monitoring of response to preoperative

Table 1
Histology, treatment, and prognosis of primary osseous malignancies

	Histology	Percent in Regard to All Primary Malignant Bone tumors[7,36,66]	Treatment	5-y Survival Rate (%)
Osteogenic tumors				
Conventional osteosarcoma	Three histologic subtypes: osteoblastic (the most common), fibroblastic, and chondroblastic	28	Neoadjuvant chemotherapy, surgical resection	60
Telangiectatic osteosarcoma	Multiple dilated blood-filled cavities and high-grade sarcomatous cells within the peripheral rim and the septa	1.4	Similar to conventional OS	67
Parosteal osteosarcoma	Long bone trabeculae or ill-defined islands of osteoid and woven bone separated by a fibrous stroma with minimal fibroblastic atypia	1.8	Surgical resection, chemotherapy	90
Periosteal osteosarcoma	Intermediate grade tumor that contains a predominant cartilaginous matrix with small amount of osteoid matrix	0.5	Surgical resection	89
Chondrogenic tumors				
Conventional central chondrosarcoma grades 2–3 and grade 1/atypical cartilaginous tumor	Depends primarily on the nuclear size, nuclear staining, cellularity, and mitosis	20–27	Intralesional curettage and local adjuvant therapy (low grade); surgical resection (high grade)	Variable

(continued on next page)

Table 1
(continued)

	Histology	Percent in Regard to All Primary Malignant Bone tumors[7,36,66]	Treatment	5-y Survival Rate (%)
Secondary peripheral chondrosarcoma grades 2–3 and grade 1/atypical cartilaginous tumor	Criteria for histologic grading are similar to those for central chondrosarcoma	1	Surgical resection (all grades)	Variable
Dedifferentiated chondrosarcoma	There is an abrupt transition between the low-grade chondrosarcoma and the high-grade spindle cell sarcoma	2.2	Surgical resection	25
Fibrogenic tumors				
Fibrosarcoma	Herringbone or fascicular disposition of atypical, monomorphic fibroblasts, without malignant osteoid and cartilage	5	Surgical resection, chemotherapy	30
Undifferentiated small round cell sarcomas of bone and soft tissue				
Ewing sarcoma	Small round cell sarcoma with pathognomonic molecular findings and varying degrees of neuroectodermal differentiation	6–8	Surgical resection, chemotherapy, radiation therapy	25
Notochordal tumors				
Chordoma	Large cells with clear to eosinophilic cytoplasm separated into lobules by fibrous septae	2–4	Surgical resection, radiation therapy	50

than those of necrotic tissue, which is a helpful distinguishing feature to assess treatment response.[6,16,18] In fact, a direct relation has been observed between treatment-induced increase of ADC and the extent of necrosis.[19] Furthermore, a significant difference in minimum ADC values of solid tumor components has also been observed between patients with good and poor response to treatment.[6,20] ADC differences between conventional OS subtypes are also observed, with osteoblastic OS showing lower mean ADC values than chondroblastic OS owing to the high ADC values of the chondroblastic tissues.[16,17]

Key imaging features of conventional OS include the following:
- Radiographs/CT
  - Osteoid matrix
  - Wide zone of transition
  - Aggressive periosteal reaction
  - Cortical destruction
  - Soft tissue mass
- MR imaging
  - Need at least one long-axis sequence of entire host bone (including joints)
  - Heterogeneous low T1, high T2 signal
  - Heterogeneous enhancement
  - Other components
    - Osteoid matrix (low T1, low T2, no enhancement)

chemotherapy, and detection of residual or recurrent tumor. Of note, when used for the assessment of treatment response, DCE is best performed 3 months after the first round of chemotherapy because perfusion of the tumor-replacing granulation tissue is reduced and residual tumor tissue is still highly vascularized.[6,17]

Diffusion-weighted imaging (DWI) is a useful technique, as it allows quantitative and qualitative analyses of tissue cellularity. Apparent diffusion coefficient (ADC) values of viable tumor are lower

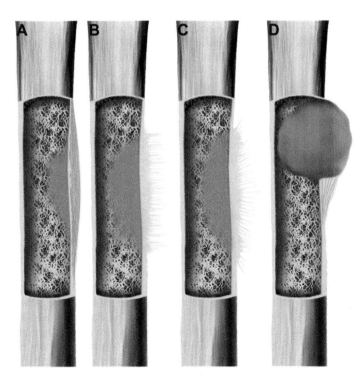

Fig. 1. Different types of periosteal reaction: (*A*) laminated; (*B*) hair on end; (*C*) sunburst; and (*D*) Codman triangle.

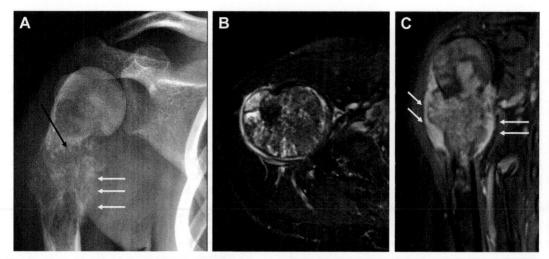

Fig. 2. Conventional OS in an 18-year-old girl with shoulder pain. (*A*) Anteroposterior (AP) radiograph of the shoulder shows an osseous lesion centered within the proximal right humeral diaphysis associated with cortical destruction, sunburst periosteal reaction (*white arrows*), and pathologic fracture (*black arrow*). (*B, C*) Axial fat-suppressed T2-weighted (T2W) and coronal fat-suppressed T1-weighted (T1W) postcontrast MR images show an expansile and heterogeneously enhancing intraosseous mass with cortical destruction, aggressive periosteal reaction, and enhancing soft tissue component (*arrows* in *C*).

- Hemorrhage (high T1, variable T2, no enhancement)
- Necrosis (low T1, high T2, no enhancement)

Telangiectatic Osteosarcoma

Telangiectatic osteosarcoma (TOS) represents 2% to 12% of all OS. The mean age at presentation is 17.5 years with a male-to-female (M:F) ratio of 2:1. The metaphysis of long bones, including distal femur and proximal tibia, is the most common affected site.[21–23] It can be a secondary lesion associated with fibrous dysplasia or Paget disease or may follow radiation. The main differential diagnosis is aneurysmal bone cyst.[15] The estimated 5-year overall survival rate is 66.8%.[24]

The most common radiographic appearance is of a purely lytic lesion with a wide zone of transition, often with associated bone expansion and cortical destruction. Moth-eaten or permeative destruction, osteoid matrix, and aggressive periosteal reaction can be seen.[15,21,25–27] On CT, TOS will replace the normal fatty marrow with heterogeneous attenuation that is predominantly lower than that of muscle. However, the tumor tissue will demonstrate higher attenuation similar to muscle at the periphery and along the septations. CT may also frequently demonstrate an infiltrative tumor margin and cortical destruction with associated soft tissue extension. CT is the best imaging modality to demonstrate osteoid matrix, seen in up to 85% of TOS cases.[27] Pathologic fractures are frequent and more common in TOS than in aneurysmal bone cyst.[25–27] On MR imaging, the tumor replaces the normal fatty marrow with predominantly intermediate to high T1 and high T2 signal. The areas of high T1 signal are consistent with hemorrhagic blood products and are usually seen in association with fluid-fluid levels (**Fig. 3**). Fluid-fluid levels with blood products are frequent findings in both TOS and aneurysmal bone cyst, so careful assessment is key. There are 3 findings that favor the diagnosis of TOS over aneurysmal bone cyst: (1) thick peripheral, septal, and nodular enhancement; (2) matrix mineralization; and (3) aggressive growth with cortical destruction and soft tissue component.[22,24–27] Of note, TOS shows higher mean ADC values in comparison to other OS subtypes because of the predominance of hemorrhage and necrosis.[16]

Parosteal Osteosarcoma

Parosteal osteosarcoma (PAOS) is the most common type of juxtacortical OS (65%) and accounts for approximately 5% of all OS. It is a slow-growing tumor that originates from the outer fibrous layer of the periosteum and most often involves the metaphysis of long bones (80%–90%), especially the posterior aspect of the distal femur (50%–65%).[10,15,28] PAOS typically manifests in the second to fourth decades with a slight female predominance. Occasionally, dedifferentiation of low-grade PAOS to high-grade malignancy, such as a higher-grade OS or a sarcoma of different

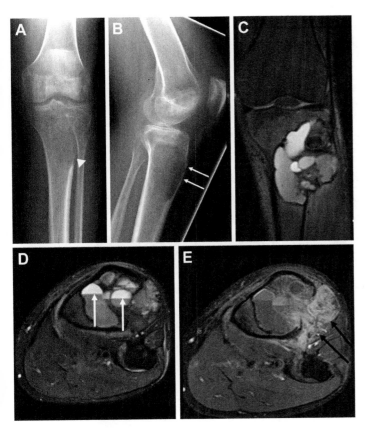

Fig. 3. TOS in a 41-year-old man with knee pain. (*A, B*) AP and lateral radiographs of the knee show a large expansile lytic lesion centered in the proximal tibial metaphysis (*arrows* in *B*), with wide narrow zone of transition along its posterior and inferior margin, and lateral cortical destruction (*arrowhead* in *A*). (*C*) Coronal fat-suppressed T2W. (*D, E*) Axial fat-suppressed T2W and fat-suppressed T1 postcontrast MR images show a lobulated mass within the proximal tibial metadiaphysis, with internal cystic regions, fluid-fluid levels (*white arrows*), and solid enhancing soft tissue components along the anterior and lateral margins of the lesion (*black arrows* in *E*).

histologic type, may occur. Tumors that have undergone differentiation or invade the underlying bone are more aggressive and carry a greater risk of metastasis.[15,28–30] The 5-year disease-free survival of PAOS is approximately 90%.[29]

Radiographically, PAOS appears as a lobulated, exophytic mass with central dense ossification adjacent to the bone. Cortical thickening without aggressive periosteal reaction is a frequent finding. A cleavage plane can be observed in areas where the tumor does not directly attach to the cortex. Of note, the presence of this plane does not help distinguish low- from high-grade tumor[2,10] (**Fig. 4**). CT and MR imaging are useful to demonstrate soft tissue extension and invasion of the medullary canal. On MR imaging, PAOS has predominantly low T1 and T2 signal because of the predominance of an ossified matrix. Occasionally, a high T2 cartilaginous peripheral rim can be seen, which could potentially mimic the cartilage cap of an osteochondroma. When an associated unmineralized high T2 signal soft tissue mass is observed, the tumor is more likely to be high grade.[15,28] Other poor prognostic features are size greater than 10 cm, the presence of satellite lesions, and metastasis. MR imaging and CT

can also be helpful in identifying the optimal site for biopsy and in determining the most appropriate surgical strategy.[30,31] Differential considerations include benign entities, such as osteochondroma, myositis ossificans, and periosteal chondroma, as well as malignant entities, such as chondrosarcoma (CS) and other subtypes of juxtacortical OS.[28]

Periosteal Osteosarcoma

Periosteal osteosarcoma (PEOS) accounts for 25% of all juxtacortical OS and 1% to 2% of all OS. Most cases present in the second and third decades. PEOS originates from the deep layer of the periosteum along the diaphysis of long bones, most often the anteromedial aspect of the tibia or distal femur (85%–95%), and ulna or humerus (5%–10%).[9,15,28] Histologically, PEOS predominantly demonstrates a cartilaginous matrix and a small amount of osteoid matrix.[32] The 5-year overall survival rate is 89.0%.[7]

Typical radiographic findings include a juxtacortical mass that often shows extensive osteoid and chondroid mineralization associated with cortical thickening and erosion. Aggressive

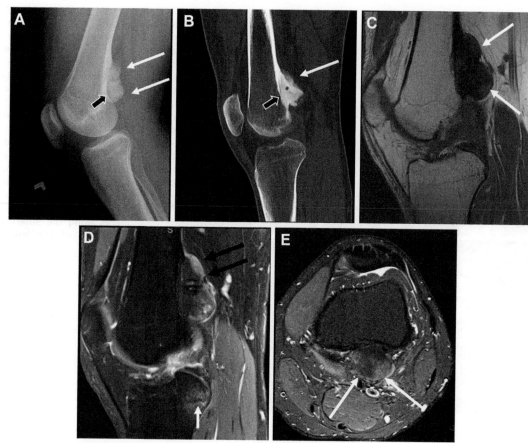

Fig. 4. PAOS in a 42-year-old man with knee pain. (*A*) Lateral radiograph of the knee shows a surface ossific mass along the posterior aspect of the distal femoral metadiaphysis with subjacent cortical thickening (*arrows*) and a fine radiolucent cleft between the thickened cortex and the surface tumor (*cleft sign; black arrow*). (*B*) CT sagittal image shows a lobulated, juxtacortical, cauliflower-like mass with central sclerotic stalk arising from the periosteum of the posterior aspect of the distal femoral metadiaphysis, associated with cortical thickening (*white arrow*) and the cleft sign (*black arrow*). (*C, D*) Sagittal T1W and postcontrast fat-suppressed T1W and (*E*) axial short tau inversion recovery (STIR) MR images show a lobular mass (*long white arrows* in *C* and *E*) that is predominantly low in signal secondary to its ossified matrix, with an enhancing solid component at its posterior aspect (*black arrows* in *D*). There is stress fracture of the posterior and lateral tibia (*short white arrow* in *D*).

Codman triangle or hair-on-end periosteal reaction is frequently observed.[9,15,33]

PEOS often involves 50% of the bone circumference, which is best recognized on CT or MR imaging. The chondroblastic nature of PEOS manifests as lower attenuation compared with muscle on CT and as low T1 and high T2 signal on MR imaging. Any calcified chondroid matrix will manifest as low T1 and T2 signal, as will the hair-on-end periosteal reaction.[28] Areas of marrow invasion or marrow reaction will demonstrate low T1 and high T2 signal. Marrow invasion is favored over marrow reaction if there is continuity between a soft tissue component and the medullary signal abnormality[15] and if the intervening cortex is not completely intact.[33] PEOS typically demonstrates variable enhancement depending on the proportion of intermixed fibrous and osteoid components and the presence of a soft tissue component. Differential diagnosis includes other types of juxtacortical OS and periosteal chondroid tumors.[15,28,33]

CHONDROGENIC TUMORS

CS is the term used to denote malignancy within the chondrogenic tumor family. According to the 2020 WHO classification, there are 8 subtypes of CS (**Box 2**), of which 4 are considered conventional CS and are subclassified according to the following: (1) histologic grade 1, 2, or 3; and (2) site of origin, either central (intramedullary) or peripheral, of which 100% secondarily arises from the cartilage cap of an osteochondroma.[7]

Approximately 75% of CS is conventional central CS and only approximately 9% is conventional peripheral CS arising from osteochondroma. The remaining 4 nonconventional CS subtypes are less common and include dedifferentiated (~10%), mesenchymal (~2%), clear cell (~2%), and periosteal (~2%) types. In general, the most common anatomic sites of CS origin are the pelvis, femur, and humerus.[7,34] Here, the 3 most common subtypes of CS that one is most likely to encounter in clinical practice are reviewed, central CS, secondary peripheral CS, and dedifferentiated CS.

Central Chondrosarcoma

Central chondrosarcoma (CCS) is an intramedullary neoplasm accounting for approximately 20% to 27% of all malignant bone neoplasms and the second most common primary bone malignancy, after OS.[7,35] Most affected patients are older than 50 years. The most common sites are the bones of the pelvis (especially the ilium), followed by the proximal femur, proximal humerus, distal femur, and ribs. It rarely involves the spine and craniofacial bones.[36,37] They are usually large tumors that originate from the metaphysis and diaphysis when affecting long bones. Higher-grade CS show larger noncalcified areas with high water content, varying from mature hyaline cartilage to a more myxoid stroma.[38,39]

In the 5th edition[7] of the WHO classification of tumors of soft tissue and bone, the conventional CS are classified as central atypical cartilaginous tumor (ACT)/CS grade 1 (CS1), secondary peripheral ACT/CS1, central CS grade 2 and 3, and secondary peripheral CS grades 2 and 3. The term ACT was first introduced in the 2013 WHO classification, synonymous for CS1, and was classified as intermediate to reflect the clinical behavior of well-differentiated or low-grade lesions.[40] These lesions, especially in the long bones, can be locally aggressive but do not metastasize. The appropriate application of the terms ACT and CS1 is analogous to that of atypical lipomatous tumor and well-differentiated liposarcoma. The use of the term ACT should be reserved for tumors in the appendicular skeleton, and CS1 should be used for tumors in the axial skeleton, including the pelvis, scapula, and skull base, because of the poorer clinical outcome of tumor in these sites.[7,37,41] CCS and secondary peripheral CS grades 2 and 3 are intermediate- and high-grade malignant cartilaginous neoplasms with a more aggressive clinical behavior and can metastasize.[8] The 5-year overall survival rate for central ACT/CS1 is 87% to 99%, 74% to 99% for CS grade 2, and 31% to 77% for CS grade 3. The 5-year local recurrence rate for secondary peripheral ACT/CS1 is 15.9%.[7]

On radiographs, a lobular lytic lesion with chondroid matrix and endosteal scalloping is usually present. Endosteal scalloping of greater than two-thirds the normal thickness of the cortex is more suggestive of CS than enchondroma.[34,36] Permeative appearance is observed in higher-grade tumors.[34,42] CT can show subtle matrix mineralization, endosteal scalloping, and cortical breach. The evaluation of the depth and extension of endosteal scalloping on multiplanar CT images is useful to distinguish between enchondroma and CS.[34,36]

On MR imaging, CCS typically presents as a lobulated high T2 and low-intermediate T1 mass. There is often septal enhancement in low-grade lesions and more diffuse and heterogeneous enhancement in higher-grade tumors (Fig. 5). Medullary involvement and soft tissue extension are usually well delineated. Because of the chondroid matrix, CS commonly demonstrates high ADC values.[34,43]

Differentiation between enchondroma and low-grade CS is sometimes challenging, especially in the long tubular bones. Maximum dimension greater than 5 cm, endosteal scalloping greater than two-thirds of the cortical thickness, cortical destruction, and early enhancement on DCE imaging favor diagnosis of CS over enchondroma[6,38,44] (Fig. 6).

Secondary Peripheral Chondrosarcoma

Secondary peripheral chondrosarcoma (SPC) is a CS originating from a preexisting osteochondroma.[7,45] It constitutes 1% of all malignant bone tumors. The risk of malignant transformation of an osteochondroma to SPC is approximately 0.4% to 2% in patients with solitary

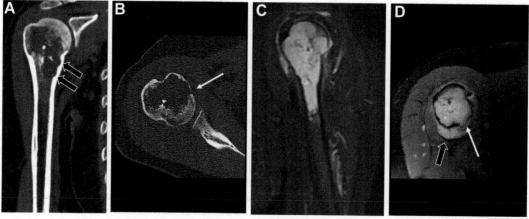

Fig. 5. Conventional CCS grade 3 in a 56-year-old man with shoulder pain. (*A, B*) Coronal and axial CT images show a proximal humeral mass with endosteal scalloping (*black arrows*), permeation, and cortical disruption (*white arrow*). (*C, D*) Sagittal and axial fat-suppressed T2W MR images show a lobular T2W hyperintense mass with cortical disruption (*white arrow*) and extraosseous soft tissue component along the posteromedial shaft of the humerus (*black arrow*).

osteochondroma and 5% to 25% in those with hereditary multiple exostoses.[46,47] SPC is more frequently observed in the pelvis and osseous structures of the shoulder girdle. The 5-year survival rate is approximately 90%.[45]

On radiographs, irregularity and indistinct margins of the osteochondroma with areas of lucency and inhomogeneous mineralization along with a soft tissue mass containing foci of scattered, punctate calcifications may be observed. On MR imaging, a large inhomogeneous mass with low T1 and high T2 signal intensity is the most common presentation. An osteochondroma with a cartilaginous cap greater than 1.5 to 2.0 cm in an adult patient should raise suspicion for malignant transformation.[46,47] Other aggressive features similar to CCS can be observed if the lesion has intramedullary extension (**Fig. 7**).

Dedifferentiated Chondrosarcoma

Dedifferentiated CS is a highly malignant variant of CS that accounts for approximately 9% to 10% of all CS.[42,48,49] It is characterized by the presence of a low- or intermediate-grade CS with a higher-grade noncartilaginous spindle cell sarcoma, most frequently OS, fibrosarcoma, or malignant fibrous histiocytoma.[36,48] It affects patients between 50 and 70 years old, with a 5-year survival rate of 11%.[50]

Radiographic characteristics vary according to the proportion of the low- to high-grade components. Usually, radiographic findings are that of a high-grade cartilaginous tumor with a multilobulated chondroid lesion along with aggressive osteolytic component.[42]

CT and MR imaging may depict mild septal and peripheral enhancement with more diffuse enhancement in the high-grade noncartilaginous areas.[36] MR imaging can guide the biopsy target by showing the bimorphic feature of this tumor characterized by usually nonmineralized intraosseous chondroid component and the dedifferentiated soft tissue component with variable T2 signal[36,51] (**Fig. 8**).

Key imaging features of CCS include the following:
- Radiographs/CT
  - Chondroid matrix
  - Endosteal scalloping greater than two-thirds of the cortical thickness
  - Cortical destruction
  - Permeative appearance
  - Soft tissue mass
- MR imaging
  - Lobulated high T2 and low-intermediate T1
  - Septal enhancement in low-grade lesions
  - Diffuse and heterogeneous enhancement in higher-grade tumors
  - Extraosseous soft tissue component with or without calcified matrix
  - High ADC values

FIBROGENIC TUMORS
Fibrosarcoma

Fibrosarcoma is a rare primary malignant spindle cell bone tumor characterized by a herringbone or fascicular disposition of atypical, monomorphic fibroblasts, without malignant osteoid and cartilage. It is a diagnosis of exclusion that requires a

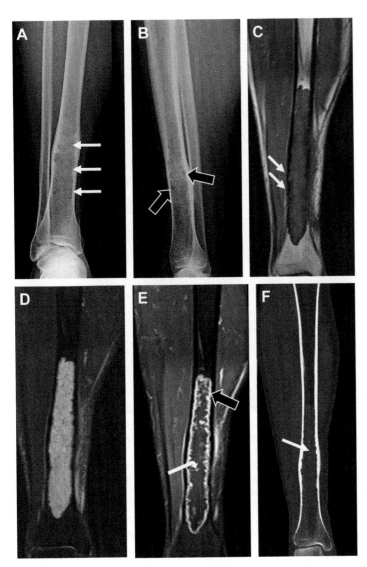

Fig. 6. Conventional CCS grade 1/ACT in a 41-year-old woman with right leg pain for a few weeks. (*A*, *B*) AP and lateral radiographs of the leg show an ill-defined intramedullary mass within the distal tibial diaphysis (*white arrows*), with scattered areas of lucency (*black arrows*), resulting in cortical expansion as well as endosteal scalloping and thinning. (*C–E*) Coronal T1W, STIR, and fat-suppressed postcontrast T1W MR images show a well-circumscribed predominantly T1 isointense and STIR hyperintense, mildly expansile intramedullary lesion with a rind of peripheral enhancement (*black arrow in E*) and scattered areas of internal nodular (*curved white arrow in E*) and septal enhancement associated with endosteal scalloping and slight cortical thinning (*arrows* in *C*). (*F*) Coronal CT image shows subtle ring and arch calcifications within the lesion (*arrow*).

generous biopsy sample to make the correct diagnosis.[52] Fibrosarcoma comprises 5% of all primary malignant bone sarcomas, has equal sex distribution, and occurs primarily in patients between 30 and 60 years of age. Long tubular bones are involved in 70% of fibrosarcomas with distal femur being the most common location.[53] The 5-year survival rate is approximately 30%.

Radiographs show an eccentric purely lytic lesion with a wide zone of transition and thinning and widening of the adjacent cortex. There may be little or no periosteal reaction.[53] CT is more accurate in detecting cortical thinning or destruction and internal septation. The lytic lesion may contain sequestered bone fragments.[54] On MR imaging, fibrosarcoma has nonspecific aggressive features,

including low T1 and heterogeneous low and high T2 signal with variable enhancement and perilesional edema. Intrinsic fibrous elements of the tumor show low T1 and T2 signal intensity. Soft tissue extension may be observed[20] (**Fig. 9**).

Key imaging features of fibrosarcoma include the following:
- Radiographs/CT
  - Purely lytic lesion
  - Thinning and widening of the adjacent cortex
  - Indistinct contour
  - Little or no periosteal reaction
  - Sequestered internal bone fragment
- MR imaging

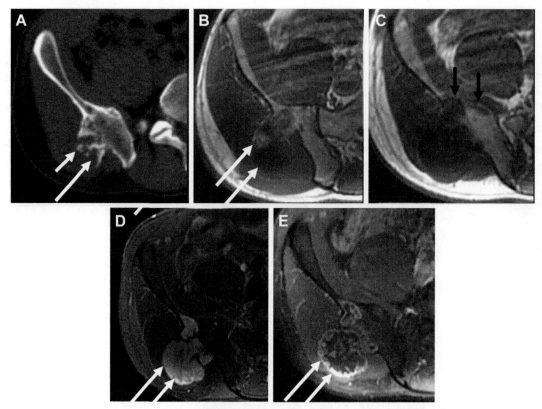

Fig. 7. SPC in a 38-year-old man with vague buttock pain. (*A*) CT axial image shows an osteochondroma arising from the right ilium with erosions of the osteochondroma (*long arrow*) and some overlying calcific matrix (*short arrow*). (*B, C*) Two axial T1W MR images depict a heterogeneous soft tissue mass with both high and low T1 signal (*arrows* in *B*) and areas of marrow replacement in the ilium (*arrows* in *C*) indicative of medullary involvement. (*D, E*) Axial fat-suppressed T2W and T1W postcontrast MR images show lobular T2 hyperintense predominantly peripherally enhancing mass (*arrows*) arising from the osteochondroma.

○ Low T1 and heterogeneous low and high T2 signal
○ Intrinsic fibrous elements with low T1 and T2 signal intensity
○ Variable enhancement
○ Soft tissue extension

UNDIFFERENTIATED SMALL ROUND CELL SARCOMAS OF BONE AND SOFT TISSUE
Ewing Sarcoma

ES is a small, round cell sarcoma with pathognomonic molecular findings and varying degrees of neuroectodermal differentiation.[55] It accounts for 6% to 8% of all primary malignant bone tumors,[7] overall third after OS and CS, and the second most common malignant tumor in children and young adults, accounting for 3% of all pediatric cancers.[56,57] It mainly affects patients in the first 3 decades of life with a slight male predominance (1.4 M:1 F). The femur, ilium, tibia, and humerus are the most commonly affected locations.[57]

Most of the ES that involves the long bones are metadiaphyseal associated with a large extraosseous mass. Epiphyseal extension may be seen in up to 10% of tumors; however, tumors centered in the epiphysis are rare.[58,59] The 5-year survival rate has been recently described as less than 25%.[58]

On radiographs, this tumor shows aggressive features, such as a moth-eaten destructive appearance with a wide zone of transition (**Fig. 10**). Cortical destruction with an associated soft tissue mass and aggressive periosteal reaction is usually seen.[57] Sclerosis in the intraosseous component of the tumor may also be visualized. Cortical thickening, pathologic fracture, and expansile bone remodeling are less common.[60] The tumor appearance on CT is similar to the appearance on radiographs. On MR imaging, the tumor has homogeneous intermediate T1 and T2 signal with diffuse or peripheral nodular enhancement, likely related to the high cellularity of the tumor. Tumor heterogeneity, hemorrhage, and

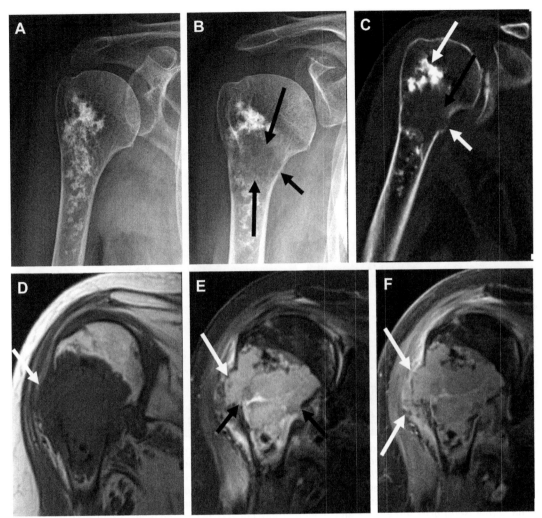

Fig. 8. Dedifferentiated CS arising from prior enchondroma/ACT in a 76-year-old woman with arm pain. (*A, B*) Frontal radiographs of the shoulder from 2018 and 2021 show loss of calcific matrix of the lesion with medullary lucency (*long arrows*) and cortical thinning (*short arrow*). (*C*) Coronal CT image shows partial chondroid matrix (*long white arrow*) with an aggressive lytic area (*black arrow*) causing cortical thinning (*short white arrow*). (*D–F*) Coronal T1W, fat-suppressed T2W, and T1 postcontrast MR images depict aggressive high T2 enhancing mass with cortical destruction (*short black arrows* in *E*) and soft tissue component (*white arrows* in *D–F*).

necrosis are more common in larger lesions. Cortical involvement in ES manifests as focal destruction and permeation of the cortical haversian canal system and neurovascular channels with small nests of tumor cells. This feature may be characterized by channels of intermediate signal intensity extending through the low-signal-intensity cortex[56,57,60] (see **Fig. 10**).

Key imaging features of sarcomas include the following:
- Radiographs/CT
  - Moth-eaten destructive appearance
  - Wide zone of transition
  - Aggressive periosteal reaction
  - Cortical destruction
  - Soft tissue mass
- MR imaging
  - Homogeneous intermediate T1 and T2 signal
  - Diffuse or peripheral nodular enhancement
  - Channels of intermediate signal intensity extending through the low signal intensity cortex
  - Other components
    - Hemorrhage (high T1, variable T2, no enhancement)
    - Necrosis (low T1, high T2, no enhancement)

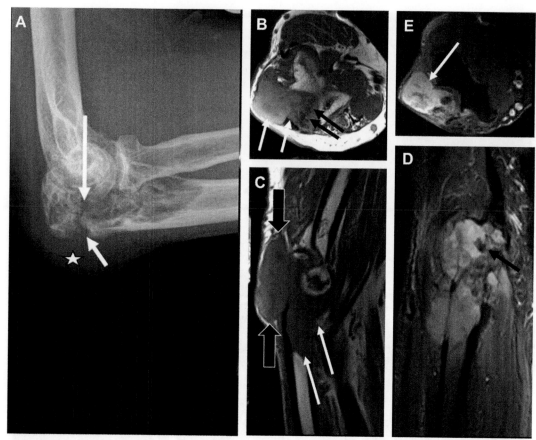

Fig. 9. Fibrosarcoma in a 78-year-old man with a palpable mass and pain of the right elbow. (A) Lateral radiograph shows lytic mass with no internal matrix and aggressive features, including cortical destruction (*short arrow*) and a pathologic fracture line (*long arrow*) associated with soft tissue mass in the posterior elbow (*star*). (B–E) Axial and sagittal T1W, fat-suppressed coronal T2W and axial T1W postcontrast MR images show a destructive mass (*white arrows*) with an extraosseous component (*black arrows* in C) and areas of internal low signal representing fibrosis (*short black arrows* in B and D) with diffuse enhancement (*long white arrow* in E).

Notochordal Tumors

Chordoma

Chordoma is a slow-growing malignant tumor derived from notochordal remnants that occurs predominantly in the sacrococcyx (50%–60%), clivus, and spheno-occipital synchondrosis (30%–35%). When affecting the spine, the cervical segment is most commonly involved, followed by the lumbar and thoracic segments.[61] Chordoma accounts for 2% to 4% of all malignant bone tumors and is the most common malignant sacral tumor.[62] They have a broad age distribution, from the fourth to seventh decades, with a peak incidence in the fifth decade. Men are more commonly affected (2–3 M:1 F).[63] The 5-year survival rate is approximately 50%.[62]

Chordoma frequently presents as a destructive lytic tumor associated with a large, well-circumscribed, locally aggressive soft tissue mass[62,64] (Fig. 11). On CT, these tumors are osteolytic with a low-attenuation soft tissue component reflecting mucoid content. When calcifications are present, they are usually distributed in an amorphous or punctate pattern.[62] On MR imaging, a lobulated low-intermediate T1 and a distinctly high T2 enhancing mass is seen (see Fig. 11). Foci of hemorrhage and calcifications and low T2 internal septations can be present.[62,65]

Key imaging features of chordoma include the following:
- Radiographs/CT
  - Predominantly in the sacrococcyx, clivus, and the spheno-occipital synchondrosis
  - Destructive lytic tumor
  - Calcifications may be present (amorphous or punctate pattern)
  - Soft tissue mass

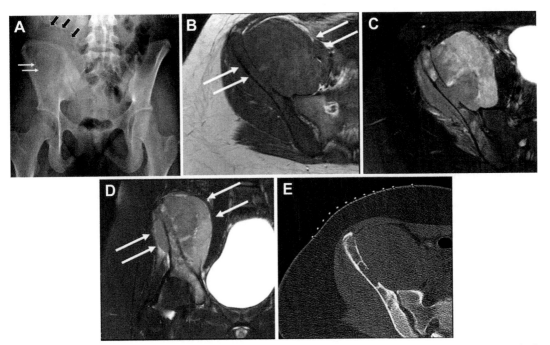

Fig. 10. ES in a 14-year-old girl with right hip pain. (*A*) AP radiograph of the pelvis shows mixed lucent and sclerotic lesion involving the right iliac bone (*white arrows*) with suggestion of soft tissue component (*black arrows*). (*B, C*) Axial fat-suppressed T1W and T2W and (*D*) coronal fat-suppressed T2W MR images show a large destructive osseous mass arising from the right iliac bone invading into the iliopsoas and gluteal muscles (*arrows*). Notice the significantly larger extraosseous soft tissue component in relation to the intraosseous component. (*E*) Axial CT image at the time of biopsy shows the mass with no mineralized matrix.

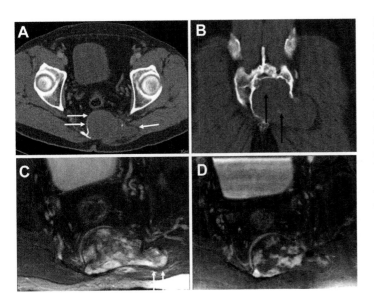

Fig. 11. Chordoma in an 86-year-old man with low back pain. (*A, B*) CT axial and coronal images after contrast show a large lobulated mass (*white arrows*) with internal foci of enhancement (*black arrows*) arising from the sacrum extending from the midline laterally through the left greater sciatic foramen, with bone expansion, and cortical destruction. (*C, D*) Axial fat-suppressed T2W and T1W postcontrast MR images show a predominantly T2 hyperintense mass with heterogeneous enhancement, with extraosseous soft tissue component (*arrows*) impressing upon the left gluteus maximus muscle.

- MR imaging
  - Lobulated low-intermediate T1 and a distinctly high T2 mass
  - Low T2 internal septations
  - Heterogeneous enhancement

SUMMARY

Primary malignant bone tumors are a diverse group of tumors with varying treatment algorithms and prognoses. Several of the most common primary malignant bone tumors have characteristic imaging features, which can suggest the diagnosis and allow for more confident radiologic-pathologic correlation. Radiographs are an essential component of the imaging evaluation, and interpretation of a bone tumor on MR imaging without the comparison radiographs should be avoided. Imaging also provides key information for local staging. An understanding of the findings that impact local staging and accurate reporting of those findings are important for prognostication and treatment planning.

CLINICS CARE POINTS

- Although clinical history and physical examination are important in the initial evaluation of a patient with a potential primary osseous malignancy, they are often nonspecific. Adequate imaging exams of a primary osseous malignancy are essential for its appropriate management.

- Radiographs are recommended as the initial imaging modality for the evaluation of bone pain, a frequent complaint in patients with a primary osseous tumor. The key radiographic features that help to differentiate benign from malignant tumors are the tumor margins, the presence and characteristics of intratumoral matrix and the status of the adjacent periosteum and cortex.

- CT plays an important role in the setting of a primary osseous malignancy as it better demonstrates tumor mineralization, and cortical bone involvement including pathologic fractures.

- MRI provides additional information on a primary osseous malignancy characterization including tumor extension, integrity of the cortex, soft-tissue components, involvement of the subjacent joint or neurovascular bundle, and local staging.

DISCLOSURE

The authors have nothing to disclose.

REFERENCES

1. Hui JY. Epidemiology and etiology of sarcomas. Surg Clin North Am 2016;96(5):901–14.
2. Costelloe CM, Madewell JE. Radiography in the initial diagnosis of primary bone tumors. AJR Am J Roentgenol 2013;200(1):3–7.
3. Gemescu IN, Thierfelder KM, Rehnitz C, et al. Imaging features of bone tumors: conventional radiographs and MR imaging correlation. Magn Reson Imaging Clin N Am 2019;27(4):753–67.
4. Rana RS, Wu JS, Eisenberg RL. Periosteal reaction. AJR Am J Roentgenol 2009;193(4):W259–72.
5. Lalam R, Bloem JL, Noebauer-Huhmann IM, et al. ESSR consensus document for detection, characterization, and referral pathway for tumors and tumor-like lesions of bone. Semin Musculoskelet Radiol 2017;21(5):630–47.
6. Costa FM, Canella C, Gasparetto E. Advanced magnetic resonance imaging techniques in the evaluation of musculoskeletal tumors. Radiol Clin North Am 2011;49(6):1325–58. vii-viii.
7. WHO classification of tumours editorial board. Soft tissue and bone tumours. 5th edition.vol. 3 IARC Press; 2020.
8. Choi JH, Ro JY. The 2020 WHO classification of tumors of bone: an updated review. Adv Anat Pathol 2021;28(3):119–38.
9. Messerschmitt PJ, Garcia RM, Abdul-Karim FW, et al. Osteosarcoma. J Am Acad Orthop Surg 2009;17(8):515–27.
10. Misaghi A, Goldin A, Awad M, et al. Osteosarcoma: a comprehensive review. SICOT J 2018;4:12.
11. Martin JW, Squire JA, Zielenska M. The genetics of osteosarcoma. Sarcoma 2012;2012:627254.
12. Lindsey BA, Markel JE, Kleinerman ES. Osteosarcoma overview. Rheumatol Ther 2017;4(1):25–43.
13. Kundu ZS. Classification, imaging, biopsy and staging of osteosarcoma. Indian J Orthop 2014;48(3):238–46.
14. Xin S, Wei G. Prognostic factors in osteosarcoma: a study level meta-analysis and systematic review of current practice. J Bone Oncol 2020;21:100281.
15. Murphey MD, Robbin MR, McRae GA, et al. The many faces of osteosarcoma. Radiographics 1997;17(5):1205–31.
16. Zeitoun R, Shokry AM, Ahmed Khaleel S, et al. Osteosarcoma subtypes: magnetic resonance and quantitative diffusion weighted imaging criteria. J Egypt Natl Canc Inst 2018;30(1):39–44.
17. Saifuddin A, Sharif B, Gerrand C, et al. The current status of MRI in the pre-operative assessment of

intramedullary conventional appendicular osteosarcoma. Skeletal Radiol 2019;48(4):503–16.

18. Kubo T, Furuta T, Johan MP, et al. Value of diffusion-weighted imaging for evaluating chemotherapy response in osteosarcoma: a meta-analysis. Mol Clin Oncol 2017;7(1):88–92.

19. Costa FM, Ferreira EC, Vianna EM. Diffusion-weighted magnetic resonance imaging for the evaluation of musculoskeletal tumors. Magn Reson Imaging Clin N Am 2011;19(1):159–80.

20. Ahlawat S, Fayad LM. Revisiting the WHO classification system of bone tumours: emphasis on advanced magnetic resonance imaging sequences. Part 2. Pol J Radiol 2020;85:e409–19.

21. Sangle NA, Layfield LJ. Telangiectatic osteosarcoma. Arch Pathol Lab Med 2012;136(5):572–6.

22. Yin JQ, Fu YW, Xie XB, et al. Telangiectatic osteosarcoma: outcome analyses and a diagnostic model for differentiation from aneurysmal bone cyst. J Bone Oncol 2018;11:10–6.

23. Vanel D, Tcheng S, Contesso G, et al. The radiological appearances of telangiectatic osteosarcoma. A study of 14 cases. Skeletal Radiol 1987;16(3):196–200.

24. Liu JJ, Liu S, Wang JG, et al. Telangiectatic osteosarcoma: a review of literature. Onco Targets Ther 2013;6:593–602.

25. Murphey MD, wan Jaovisidha S, Temple HT, et al. Telangiectatic osteosarcoma: radiologic-pathologic comparison. Radiology 2003;229(2):545–53.

26. Zishan US, Pressney I, Khoo M, et al. The differentiation between aneurysmal bone cyst and telangiectatic osteosarcoma: a clinical, radiographic and MRI study. Skeletal Radiol 2020;49(9):1375–86.

27. Discepola F, Powell TI, Nahal A. Telangiectatic osteosarcoma: radiologic and pathologic findings. Radiographics 2009;29(2):380–3.

28. Yarmish G, Klein MJ, Landa J, et al. Imaging characteristics of primary osteosarcoma: nonconventional subtypes. Radiographics 2010;30(6):1653–72.

29. Prabowo Y, Kamal AF, Kodrat E, et al. Parosteal osteosarcoma: a benign-looking tumour, amenable to a variety of surgical reconstruction. Int J Surg Oncol 2020;2020:4807612.

30. Donmez FY, Tuzun U, Basaran C, et al. MRI findings in parosteal osteosarcoma: correlation with histopathology. Diagn Interv Radiol 2008;14(3):147–52.

31. Jelinek JS, Murphey MD, Kransdorf MJ, et al. Parosteal osteosarcoma: value of MR imaging and CT in the prediction of histologic grade. Radiology 1996;201(3):837–42.

32. Cesari M, Alberghini M, Vanel D, et al. Periosteal osteosarcoma: a single-institution experience. Cancer 2011;117(8):1731–5.

33. Murphey MD, Jelinek JS, Temple HT, et al. Imaging of periosteal osteosarcoma: radiologic-pathologic comparison. Radiology 2004;233(1):129–38.

34. Ollivier L, Vanel D, Leclere J. Imaging of chondrosarcomas. Cancer Imaging 2003;4(1):36–8.

35. Nota SP, Braun Y, Schwab JH, et al. The identification of prognostic factors and survival statistics of conventional central chondrosarcoma. Sarcoma 2015;2015:623746.

36. Murphey MD, Walker EA, Wilson AJ, et al. From the archives of the AFIP: imaging of primary chondrosarcoma: radiologic-pathologic correlation. Radiographics 2003;23(5):1245–78.

37. van Praag Veroniek VM, Rueten-Budde AJ, Ho V, et al. Incidence, outcomes and prognostic factors during 25 years of treatment of chondrosarcomas. Surg Oncol 2018;27(3):402–8.

38. Douis H, Parry M, Vaiyapuri S, et al. What are the differentiating clinical and MRI-features of enchondromas from low-grade chondrosarcomas? Eur Radiol 2018;28(1):398–409.

39. Douis H, Singh L, Saifuddin A. MRI differentiation of low-grade from high-grade appendicular chondrosarcoma. Eur Radiol 2014;24(1):232–40.

40. Hogendoorn PCWB, Bovée JVMG, Nielsen GP. Chondrosarcoma (grade I-III), including primary and secondary variants and periosteal chondrosarcoma. In: Fletcher CDB, A.J., Hogendoorn CW, Mertens F, editors. WHO classification of tumours of soft tissue and bone. 4th edition. IARC; 2013.

41. Bus MPA, Campanacci DA, Albergo JI, et al. Conventional primary central chondrosarcoma of the pelvis: prognostic factors and outcome of surgical treatment in 162 patients. J Bone Joint Surg Am 2018;100(4):316–25.

42. Soldatos T, McCarthy EF, Attar S, et al. Imaging features of chondrosarcoma. J Comput Assist Tomogr 2011;35(4):504–11.

43. Deckers C, Steyvers MJ, Hannink G, et al. Can MRI differentiate between atypical cartilaginous tumors and high-grade chondrosarcoma? A systematic review. Acta Orthop 2020;91(4):471–8.

44. Campanacci DA, Scoccianti G, Franchi A, et al. Surgical treatment of central grade 1 chondrosarcoma of the appendicular skeleton. J Orthop Traumatol 2013;14(2):101–7.

45. Zang J, Guo W, Yang R, et al. Differences in clinical characteristics and tumor prognosis between primary and secondary conventional pelvic chondrosarcoma. BMC Cancer 2020;20(1):1054.

46. Ahmed AR, Tan TS, Unni KK, et al. Secondary chondrosarcoma in osteochondroma: report of 107 patients. Clin Orthop Relat Res 2003;(411):193–206.

47. Cho HS, Han I, Kim HS. Secondary chondrosarcoma from an osteochondroma of the proximal tibia involving the fibula. Clin Orthop Surg 2017;9(2):249–54.

48. Weber KL, Raymond AK. Low-grade/dedifferentiated/high-grade chondrosarcoma: a case of

histological and biological progression. Iowa Orthop J 2002;22:75–80.

49. Miao R, Choy E, Raskin KA, et al. Prognostic factors in dedifferentiated chondrosarcoma: a retrospective analysis of a large series treated at a single institution. Sarcoma 2019;2019:9069272.

50. Amer KM, Munn M, Congiusta D, et al. Survival and prognosis of chondrosarcoma subtypes: SEER database analysis. J Orthop Res 2020;38(2):311–9.

51. Littrell LA, Wenger DE, Wold LE, et al. Radiographic, CT, and MR imaging features of dedifferentiated chondrosarcomas: a retrospective review of 174 de novo cases. Radiographics 2004;24(5):1397–409.

52. Huvos AG, Higinbotham NL. Primary fibrosarcoma of bone. A clinicopathologic study of 130 patients. Cancer 1975;35(3):837–47.

53. Cunningham MP, Arlen M. Medullary fibrosarcoma of bone. Cancer 1968;21(1):31–7.

54. Qu N, Yao W, Cui X, et al. Malignant transformation in monostotic fibrous dysplasia: clinical features, imaging features, outcomes in 10 patients, and review. Medicine (Baltimore) 2015;94(3):e369.

55. Bishop MW, Somerville JM, Bahrami A, et al. Mesenchymal chondrosarcoma in children and young adults: a single institution retrospective review. Sarcoma 2015;2015:608279.

56. McCarville MB, Chen JY, Coleman JL, et al. Distinguishing osteomyelitis from Ewing sarcoma on radiography and MRI. AJR Am J Roentgenol 2015;205(3):640–50. quiz: 651].

57. Murphey MD, Senchak LT, Mambalam PK, et al. From the radiologic pathology archives: Ewing sarcoma family of tumors: radiologic-pathologic correlation. Radiographics 2013;33(3):803–31.

58. Ross KA, Smyth NA, Murawski CD, et al. The biology of Ewing sarcoma. ISRN Oncol 2013;2013:759725.

59. Kaste SC. Imaging pediatric bone sarcomas. Radiol Clin North Am 2011;49(4):749–65. vi-vii.

60. Patnaik S, Yarlagadda J, Susarla R. Imaging features of Ewing's sarcoma: special reference to uncommon features and rare sites of presentation. J Cancer Res Ther 2018;14(5):1014–22.

61. Wippold FJ 2nd, Koeller KK, Smirniotopoulos JG. Clinical and imaging features of cervical chordoma. AJR Am J Roentgenol 1999;172(5):1423–6.

62. Farsad K, Kattapuram SV, Sacknoff R, et al. Sacral chordoma. Radiographics 2009;29(5):1525–30.

63. Young VA, Curtis KM, Temple HT, et al. Characteristics and patterns of metastatic disease from chordoma. Sarcoma 2015;2015:517657.

64. Chang C, Chebib I, Torriani M, et al. Osseous metastases of chordoma: imaging and clinical findings. Skeletal Radiol 2017;46(3):351–8.

65. Aivazoglou LU, Zotti OR, Pinheiro MM, et al. Topographic MRI evaluation of the sacroiliac joints in patients with axial spondyloarthritis. Rev Bras Reumatol Engl Ed 2017;57(5):378–84.

66. Evola FR, Costarella L, Pavone V, et al. Biomarkers of osteosarcoma, chondrosarcoma, and Ewing sarcoma. Front Pharmacol 2017;8:150.

Bone Tumors
Common Mimickers

Stephen M. Broski, MD*, Laurel A. Littrell, MD, Benjamin M. Howe, MD,
Doris E. Wenger, MD

KEYWORDS

- Bone tumor • Pseudolesion • Mimics • CT • Radiographs • MR imaging • PET/CT

KEY POINTS

- Numerous nonneoplastic processes may cause bone lesions that are confused for primary or metastatic bone tumors.
- Most nonneoplastic lesions exhibit pathognomonic imaging features that can allow for confident distinction from neoplastic bone disease.
- In some cases, distinguishing benign nonneoplastic lesions from bone tumors may be difficult on radiographs, but usually cross-sectional imaging with CT, MR imaging, or PET/CT allows for accurate diagnosis. However, when these lesions possess atypical imaging features, or are particularly exuberant, biopsy may be needed to differentiate.

INTRODUCTION

A wide variety of benign nonneoplastic bone lesions may mimic benign and malignant bone tumors. These lesions are often incidentally discovered, but may also be symptomatic and diagnosed after focused imaging evaluation for pain or other symptoms. Some of these lesions (eg, normal variants or developmental abnormalities) require no further work-up once recognized. Other skeletal processes, such stress fractures or osteomyelitis, may require semiurgent management to prevent complication. Some osseous abnormalities, such as brown tumors of hyperparathyroidism or bone lesions of sarcoidosis, may be the first indication of a more serious systemic process that warrants further evaluation and treatment. Familiarity with the spectrum of imaging features of these lesions is necessary to direct appropriate work-up and management, and importantly, to avoid unnecessary tests and procedures that might result in patient morbidity.

CALCANEAL PSEUDOCYST

A relative radiolucency may be outlined by the major trabecular groups within the midportion of the calcaneus, caused by a triangular area lacking normal spongy bone.[1] This area is visible on up to 70% of radiographs, and has a "pseudocystic" appearance in 7% of cases.[2] This pseudolesion is characterized by ill-defined margins (Fig. 1), which distinguishes it from other lesions that may occur in this region, including simple bone cyst and intraosseous lipoma. Simple bone cyst and intraosseous lipoma present with a peripheral sclerotic rim, which is not present with the normal trabecular rarefaction in this area. Intraosseous lipomas also may develop central dystrophic calcification, which is absent in the calcaneal pseudolesion. More recently, there has been imaging evidence that anterior calcaneal intraosseous lipomas and cysts represent a spectrum of the same process, with several reports detailing intraosseous cystic lesions that fill in with fat over time.[3–5]

RHOMBOID FOSSA

A normal variant oval concavity or osteolytic defect may occur along the undersurface of the medial clavicle at the insertion of the costoclavicular ligament, termed the rhomboid fossa (Fig. 2).[6,7] In a 2014 study, Koudela and colleagues[8] analyzed

Department of Radiology, Mayo Clinic, 200 First Street Southwest, Rochester, MN 55905, USA
* Corresponding author. Mayo Clinic, Charlton Building North, 1st Floor, 200 First Street Southwest, Rochester, MN 55905.
E-mail address: Broski.stephen@mayo.edu

Radiol Clin N Am 60 (2022) 239–252
https://doi.org/10.1016/j.rcl.2021.11.004
0033-8389/22/© 2021 Elsevier Inc. All rights reserved.

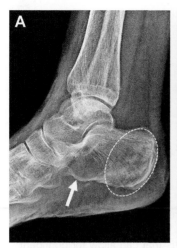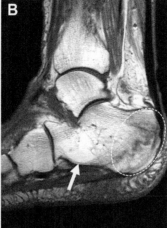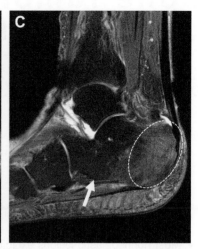

Fig. 1. Calcaneal pseudocyst. Lateral radiograph (*A*) demonstrates an ill-defined lucency in the anterior calcaneus (*arrow*) and patchy sclerosis in the posterior calcaneus (*oval*) consistent with a stress fracture. Corresponding sagittal T1-weighted (*B*) and T2-weighted fat-saturated MR images (*C*) demonstrate decreased trabeculation and fat in the anterior calcaneus, confirming a pseudolesion (*arrows*). MR imaging also confirms a stress fracture with surrounding bone marrow edema (*ovals*).

1017 radiographs in patients aged 2 to 90 who experienced clavicle fractures. In this cohort, they found that 21% had a concave costoclavicular ligament insertion, consistent with a rhomboid fossa, which ranged between 2 and 10 mm in depth. Asymmetry was invariably present in patients with bilateral rhomboid fossae, and this variant was much more commonly seen in males.[8] It has also been noted that the rhomboid fossa occurs more commonly on the side of the dominant hand, supporting a mechanical theory of fossa formation from applied pressure by the costoclavicular ligament.[9]

RED BONE MARROW

Fat and hematopoietic cells are the primary components of normal bone marrow. Hematopoietic cells are unevenly distributed throughout the bone marrow, and most of the hematopoietic elements in adults are present in the axial skeleton and proximal long bone metaphyses. Children and young adults have an increased ratio of hematopoietic elements to marrow fat compared with adults. A normal regression of hematopoietic cells occurs with maturation and the adult pattern of red marrow is established by the early 20s.[10]

Expansion of red marrow in adults may result from a variety of nonneoplastic conditions, including medications, smoking, anemia, and exercise. Red marrow expansion occurs in the reverse pattern of normal regression, with increased marrow elements most often occurring first in the axial skeleton and metaphyses of long bones.[11]

Red marrow expansion is most notable on positron emission tomography/computed tomography (PET/CT) and MR imaging. On PET/CT this typically manifests as increased bone marrow metabolic activity. On MR imaging, red marrow demonstrates decreased T1-weighted signal in relation to fatty marrow, although this typically does not reach the same level of T1 hypointensity as adjacent skeletal muscle. Chemical shift imaging with in-phase and opposed-phase sequences is helpful to confirm red marrow because even the most prominent red marrow typically demonstrates signal drop out in the opposed-phase because of the presence of intravoxel fat (Fig. 3). Quantitative signal intensity ratios between in-phase and out-of-phase sequences between 0.65 and 0.8 have been suggested to differentiate red marrow from neoplastic lesions.[12–14] Red marrow most often demonstrates mild increased T2-weighted signal on fluid-sensitive sequences and mild postgadolinium enhancement. Recognizing red marrow may pose a challenge in cases where there is marked diffuse red marrow hyperplasia, or where there is focal heterogeneity mimicking an osseous neoplasm. In both cases, T1-weighted and chemical shift sequences are useful in the differentiation.

Key imaging features:

- Common locations: axial skeleton, long bone metaphyses
- MR imaging:
  - T1 signal > skeletal muscle

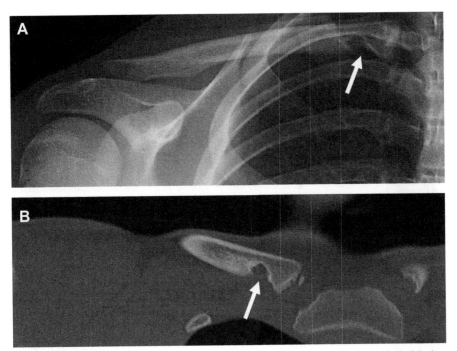

Fig. 2. Rhomboid fossa. Frontal radiograph (*A*) and coronal computed tomography (CT) (*B*) demonstrate a normal variant concave defect along the inferior aspect of the medial clavicle (*arrows*) at the attachment of the costoclavicular ligament.

- Chemical shift opposed phase signal drop out

ISCHIOPUBIC SYNCHONDROSIS

The ischiopubic synchondroses enlarge during normal early childhood growth, but in older children and adolescents, this enlargement is commonly unilateral, particularly on the side of the nondominant limb.[15] Although often encountered incidentally, some patients develop pain in the area of the synchondrosis, which has been referred to as ischiopubic synchondrosis syndrome or van Neck-Odelberg disease.[16,17] It has been hypothesized that the asymmetric closure may be secondary to mechanical strain produced by the hamstring muscles.[18,19] This may result in an expansile appearance with irregular central lucency on radiographs and CT (**Fig. 4**). On MR imaging, T2-hyperintense edema and enhancement can be present in the surrounding bone marrow and soft tissues, which may mimic a tumor or infection. A linear band of MR hypointense signal within the center of the synchondrosis

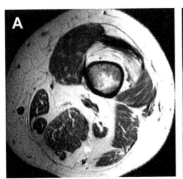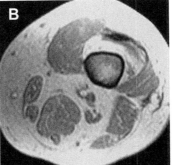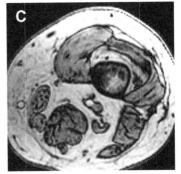

Fig. 3. Red marrow hyperplasia. Axial T1-weighted MR image of the femur (*A*) demonstrates heterogeneous marrow signal. Note the areas of decreased marrow show T1-weighted signal greater than the adjacent skeletal muscle. In-phase (*B*) and opposed-phase (*C*) images of the distal femur show marked signal drop out, confirming the presence of intravoxel fat and the diagnosis of red marrow hyperplasia.

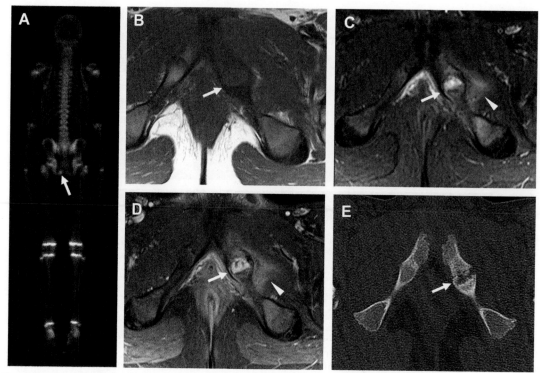

Fig. 4. Prominent ischiopubic synchondrosis. Posterior planar bone scan image demonstrates increased uptake in the left inferior pubic ramus (*A, arrow*). Axial T1-weighted (*B*), T2-weighted (*C*), and postgadolinium (*D*) fat-suppressed MR images demonstrate an expansile lesion with heterogeneous signal and enhancement at the left ischiopubic synchondrosis (*arrows*) with surrounding soft tissue edema and enhancement (*arrowheads*). Note the central linear hypointense band. Axial CT (*E*) demonstrates an expansile lesion with central irregular lucency with predominantly transverse morphology (*arrow*).

corresponds to fibrous bridging, and can help distinguish this developmental lesion from neoplastic etiologies (**Fig. 5**).[18] Asymmetric increased uptake has been noted at the ischiopubic synchondroses on fluorodeoxyglucose (FDG) PET/CT[16,20] and bone scintigraphy[17] (see **Fig. 4**), which may also mimic neoplasm or infection. Therefore, awareness of the classic location, age demographic, and imaging features of ischiopubic synchondrosis is important to avoid misdiagnosis.

BONE ISLAND (ENOSTOSIS)

A bone island is a benign osseous lesion that consists of a focal area of mature cortical bone within an area of trabecular bone. These are considered to be developmental hamartomatous lesions that are generally stable over time. They can occur anywhere but are most frequently found in the pelvis, spine, ribs, and distal aspects of the femora. Bone islands generally range in size from 1 to 20 mm but can be larger. When measuring greater than 20 mm, they are referred to as giant bone islands.[21] The radiographic and CT appearance

is often characteristic, consisting of a circular or oval sclerotic lesion with irregular, spiculated margins. These bony spicules tend to blend in with the trabeculae in the surrounding cancellous bone, and the margin has been described as a "brush border."[22] This morphology is helpful in differentiating a bone island from osteoblastic metastases or primary bone-forming tumors. The CT attenuation can also be helpful in distinguishing enostoses from untreated osteoblastic metastases, because enostoses tend to be denser. In a study by Ulano and colleagues,[23] a mean attenuation of 885 HU and maximum attenuation of 1060 HU provided reliable thresholds below which metastatic lesion would be favored, and a follow-up study showed overall good accuracy, but slightly decreased sensitivity and specificity when applied to differentiating enostoses from treated metastases.[24] However, these thresholds are intended solely for distinguishing bone islands from osteoblastic metastases and should not be extrapolated to other sclerotic bone lesions.[25] On MR imaging, bone islands demonstrate very low signal intensity on all sequences and the surrounding bone

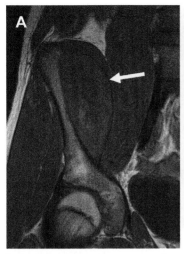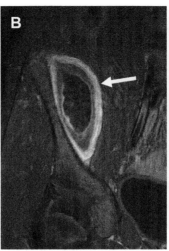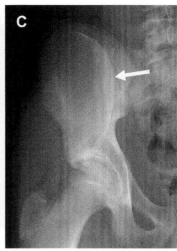

Fig. 5. Subperiosteal hematoma. Coronal T1 (*A*) and postgadolinium fat-saturated (*B*) MR images of a 14-year-old demonstrate a subperiosteal mass along the inner table of the right ilium (*arrows*) with heterogeneous signal suggesting evolving blood products. A subsequent pelvic radiograph (*C*) shows peripheral ossification (*arrow*).

marrow is normal.[21,22] Bone islands are generally not radiotracer-avid on bone scintigraphy or FDG PET/CT and therefore, molecular imaging may be helpful to differentiate from metastatic disease. These imaging features and stability over time can usually allow for confident diagnosis. However, bone islands can demonstrate growth[26] and can occasionally exhibit uptake on bone scan[27] and FDG PET,[28] which may warrant follow-up or biopsy for further evaluation.

Key imaging features:

- Radiographs/CT
  - Homogeneously sclerotic with density equivalent to cortical bone
  - Circular or oval with spiculated margins
- MR imaging
  - Low signal on all sequences
  - Normal surrounding marrow signal
- Bone scan and PET/CT
  - Most demonstrate no uptake

SUBPERIOSTEAL HEMATOMA

Subperiosteal hematoma occurs when traction on the periosteum results in separation/elevation from the underlying bone with accumulation of blood products in the subperiosteal space and is most common in children or adolescents.[29] It is usually post-traumatic in nature but may also occur without a history of injury or in patients with hemophilia.

The imaging appearance of subperiosteal hematoma evolves with the age of the lesion. Radiographs and CT show periosteal elevation or reaction early in the presentation. Over time, the

hematoma undergoes ossification, which can mimic a bone malignancy. The MR imaging signal characteristics depend on the stage of blood products and the degree of inflammation and healing bone formation. The key features that can facilitate the diagnosis include the subperiosteal location, lenticular shape (see **Fig. 5**), and temporal evolution with healing. In adults, this may be encountered incidentally on CT or MR imaging, manifesting as apparently expansile osseous lesions containing bone marrow fat and mature cortical bone at the site of injury.

SUBCHONDRAL CYSTIC LESIONS

Intraosseous ganglia are cystlike lucent lesions of variable size that contain gelatinous material, have a fibrous lining, and are generally surrounded by a rim of sclerosis. They are usually eccentric within the subchondral bone and the most common sites include the femoral head, distal radius/ulna, proximal tibia, medial malleolus (**Fig. 6**), and bones of the hands and feet.[30] Larger lesions may extend into the metaphysis. Although their exact pathogenesis is not clear, there is debate as to whether they are distinct from degenerative or post-traumatic cysts. Unlike degenerative cysts (subchondral geodes), ganglia usually develop without significant degenerative arthritis. On radiographs and CT, ganglia have a narrow zone of transition with a thin peripheral rim of sclerosis. They are unilocular or multilocular.[31] On radiographs, the differential diagnosis may include other epiphyseal lesions, such as chondroblastoma, clear cell chondrosarcoma, and giant cell

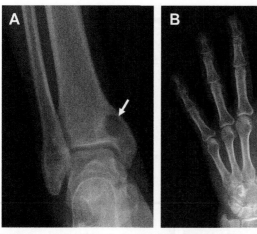
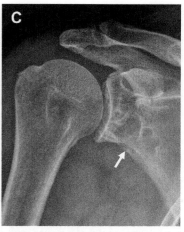

Fig. 6. Spectrum of benign subchondral cystic lesions. (*A*) Frontal radiograph of the left ankle in a 50-year-old man demonstrates a well-circumscribed lucency in the medial malleolus (*arrow*) without significant degenerative arthritis consistent with an intraosseous ganglion cyst. (*B*) Frontal radiograph of the left hand in a 57-year-old woman demonstrates advanced osteoarthritis of the first carpometacarpal joint with a large subchondral geode (*arrow*). (*C*) Frontal radiograph of the right shoulder in a 61-year-old man with shoulder pain demonstrates an intraosseous paralabral cyst in the right glenoid (*arrow*), confirmed on subsequent MR imaging.

tumor. On MR imaging, intraosseous ganglia are well-circumscribed and demonstrate T1 hypointensity, T2 hyperintensity, and peripheral enhancement within the rim of fibrous tissue. Some may contain fluid-fluid levels and be associated with surrounding reactive marrow edema.[32] These MR imaging features allow differentiation of ganglia from primary bone tumors, but there is significant overlap in the imaging appearance of ganglia and subchondral geodes and intraosseous paralabral cysts (see **Fig. 6**). There is also feature overlap of these lesions on bone scan, where all three can demonstrate uptake. Identification of secondary findings are the most helpful in discrimination of these entities. For instance, the presence of osteoarthritic change with marginal osteophytes and joint space narrowing strongly favors a degenerative cyst over a ganglion. Similarly, identification of a labral tear can distinguish an intraosseous ganglion from intraosseous extension of a paralabral cyst.

OSTEOMYELITIS

There have been multiple reports and small series illustrating how osteomyelitis can mimic several types of bone tumors, including Ewing sarcoma, metastatic disease, and leukemia.[33–35] For example, McCarville and coworkers[33] assessed a variety of radiographic and MR imaging features in 32 subjects with osteomyelitis, and 31 with Ewing sarcoma. They found that such features as a wide transition zone, permeative cortical involvement, Codman triangle, periosteal reaction,

and soft tissue mass were more common in Ewing sarcoma, and also found that serpiginous tracts were more likely to be seen on MR imaging in subjects with osteomyelitis. However, on multiple regression analysis, many of the features were associated with both entities, and only patient ethnicity and presence of a soft tissue mass were statistically significant predictive variables. For Ewing sarcoma, only 70% of cases were correctly predicted by radiography, and 76% by MR imaging.[33] Another study analyzing 21 cases of osteomyelitis presenting as a bone tumor reported preoperative diagnoses of osteoid osteoma, osteosarcoma, chondroblastoma, Ewing sarcoma, giant cell tumor, and fibrosarcoma.[36]

Osseous infection is divided by clinical course into acute, subacute, and chronic osteomyelitis, and any stage of infection may mimic neoplasm. Changes on radiographs may not develop for days to weeks after the onset of infection.[37] The earliest findings on radiographs are trabecular destruction and localized osteopenia, which can progress to geographic permeative lucencies. Lamellated periosteal reaction is a frequent finding, and a Codman triangle may occur, although this is more often seen in osseous malignancy than osteomyelitis. MR imaging is more sensitive and detects marrow changes earlier than radiographs. On MR imaging, infection may manifest as high signal on T2 and low signal relative to muscle on T1, although these findings are not specific, and are also seen with tumors.[38] The presence of reactive edema in the bone marrow and surrounding soft tissues is an

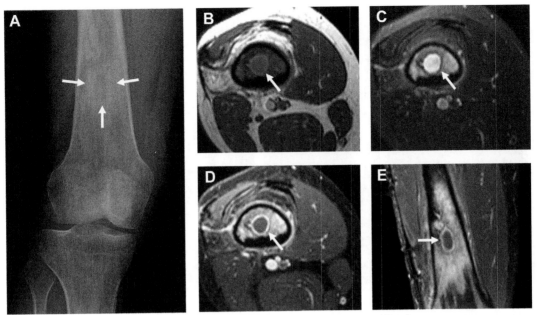

Fig. 7. Subacute osteomyelitis. Frontal radiograph of the right femur in a 25-year-old man (A) shows subtle lytic lesion with surrounding sclerosis in the distal femoral diametaphysis (*arrows*). Axial T1-weighted (B) and T2-weighted (C) and axial (D) and coronal postgadolinium (E) MR images demonstrate an intraosseous abscess with central T2 hyperintensity, a T1-hyperintense rim consistent with the "penumbra sign" (B), and peripheral enhancement (*arrows*) with a halo of reactive edema and enhancement.

important clue, as is the formation of an intraosseous abscess, which manifests as a central focus of nonenhancement with a peripheral rim of enhancement.[38] Cortical permeation adjacent to areas of soft tissue abscess can also point to the diagnosis of osteomyelitis. However, all of these findings, including cortical permeation, areas of nonenhancement, and reactive edema in the bone marrow and soft tissues, can also be seen with some tumors.

When infection is contained to a localized area in the medullary space, the process may evolve to subacute osteomyelitis, which is characterized on radiographs and CT as a mixture of bone destruction and reactive sclerosis, and in some cases, formation of a Brodie abscess. A Brodie abscess is characterized by a well-defined lytic lesion, usually 1 to 5 cm in size, which is surrounded by thick reactive sclerosis, and may be accompanied by periostitis. If small and eccentric, these can mimic osteoid osteoma, and when larger, these can mimic other primary bone tumors. On MR imaging, a Brodie abscess is usually T2 hyperintense and centrally nonenhancing. In long bones, a targetoid appearance is created by central pus, which demonstrates low T1 and high T2 signal intensity without enhancement, surrounded by an inner ring of high signal intensity on T1- and T2-weighted sequences, and an outer ring of low signal intensity, all of which is surrounded by a halo of edema.[39] The T1 hyperintense inner ring has been termed the "penumbra sign" (Fig. 7). This has been found to have variable sensitivity for osteomyelitis, but most studies have shown a specificity of greater than 90%.[34,40] If present, this is a critical feature for diagnosis.

Chronic osteomyelitis is characterized by irregular sclerosis, hyperostosis, and solid periosteal reaction (Fig. 8). Areas of sclerosis may contain lytic foci that represent sites of active infection, pus, or granulation tissue.[38] Development of a sequestrum, which represents a fragment of necrotic bone within the area of infection, can occur. However, sequestra can also be seen in undifferentiated pleomorphic sarcoma, lymphoma, and eosinophilic granuloma.[41] Osteoid osteoma may also simulate a bone sequestrum.[41] In chronic osteomyelitis, a direct communication between the area of medullary infection and the surrounding soft tissue may form, termed a cloaca, which is well-seen by cross-sectional imaging,[38] and can also be an important clue indicating the diagnosis if present.

The imaging features of osteomyelitis may overlap with those of bone tumors on molecular imaging. Multiphase bone scintigraphy is highly sensitive in the detection of osteomyelitis but is not specific in isolation. Hypervascular tumors,

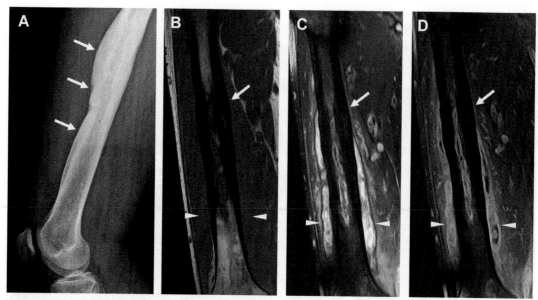

Fig. 8. Chronic osteomyelitis. Lateral radiograph of the right femur in a 23-year-old man (*A*) demonstrates prominent cortical thickening, hyperostosis, and benign periosteal reaction in the right femoral shaft (*arrows*). Corresponding coronal T1-weighted (*B*), T2-weighted (*C*), and postgadolinium (*D*) MR images demonstrate cortical thickening and periosteal new bone formation with intramedullary T1-hypointensity, T2-hyperintensity, and enhancement (*arrows*). There is extensive abscess formation in the medullary canal and in the surrounding soft tissues (*arrowheads*).

fractures, and advanced arthritis can also show three-phase positivity. Specificity may be increased by using bone scan with single-photon emission CT (SPECT)/CT or by combining bone scan with radiolabeled leukocyte scintigraphy. Osteomyelitis is also usually positive on FDG PET/CT, which has been shown to have higher sensitivity, specificity, and summary receiver operating characteristic for diagnosing osteomyelitis than bone scan or leukocyte scintigraphy.[42] Regardless, osteomyelitis can still mimic metastatic disease or primary bone tumor on FDG PET/CT.[43]

Key imaging features:

- Findings depend on stage: acute, subacute, chronic
- Radiographs: trabecular destruction/permeative lucency → periosteal reaction → irregular sclerosis/hyperosteosis
- MR imaging:
  ○ Reactive bone marrow and soft tissue edema are helpful clues
  ○ Intraosseous abscess: central nonenhancement, T1 hyperintense rim (penumbra sign)
  ○ Sequestrum and cloaca in chronic osteomyelitis
- Bone scan and PET/CT
  ○ Increased uptake, high sensitivity

  ○ Bone scan specificity is increased by SPECT and/or SPECT/CT

SARCOIDOSIS

Sarcoidosis is an inflammatory disorder characterized by development of noncaseating granulomas that can affect multiple organ systems, most commonly the lungs and skin, but may also manifest in bone. Osseous involvement by sarcoidosis occurs in approximately 5% of patients (range between 1% and 13%).[44] Osseous involvement by sarcoidosis has been well-described in the hands and feet, where there can be bilateral but asymmetric osteolytic destruction with a latticework or honeycomb pattern in the small bones. Radiographically, these lesions usually involve the middle and distal phalanges to a greater extent than the proximal phalanges or metacarpal bones, and usually appear as lytic lesions with well-defined margins, narrow zone of transition, and periosteal reaction.[45]

Involvement of the hands and feet is not likely to be mistaken for neoplastic disease. However, the distinction is more difficult when lesions occur in the axial skeleton or long bones. Up to 50% of axial sarcoid lesions are asymptomatic[46] and can have overlapping imaging features with metastatic disease.[47–49] On radiographs and CT, the lesions may be lytic (**Fig. 9**), sclerotic, or mixed, but can

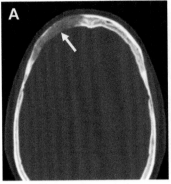 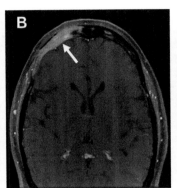 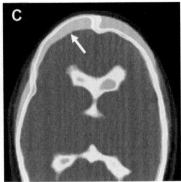

Fig. 9. Osseous sarcoidosis. Axial CT (*A*), T1-weighted postgadolinium MR imaging (*B*), and fused FDG PET/CT (*C*) images in a 50-year-old woman who initially presented with headache demonstrate an ill-defined lytic lesion in the right frontal calvarium, with avid enhancement, and intense FDG activity (*arrows*). The differential diagnosis included metastatic disease and primary bone sarcoma. Biopsy revealed noncaseating granulomas consistent with sarcoidosis.

occasionally be undetectable. In a study comparing MR imaging with radiographs, 45% of patients had lesions visible on MR imaging that were either less conspicuous or occult on radiographs.[47]

Mostard and colleagues[50] reviewed 122 patients with sarcoidosis who underwent FDG PET/CT and found that more than one-third had bone involvement (see **Fig. 9**), and that most of the lesions were multifocal and without underlying morphologic change on CT. Similar findings were reported in a separate cohort of nearly 100 patients with sarcoidosis, in which 22% showed bone involvement, but only 5% showed CT bone abnormalities.[51]

On MR imaging, osseous lesions typically demonstrate T1 hypointensity relative to muscle, T2 hyperintensity, and variable enhancement.[47] These nonspecific MR imaging features can simulate metastases, multiple myeloma, lymphoproliferative disorders, and even primary bone tumors when solitary (see **Fig. 9**). Moore and colleagues[52] examined MR imaging features that might help to differentiate osseous sarcoidosis from metastatic disease on MR imaging in 34 patients and found that this distinction was not possible, even by experienced musculoskeletal readers.

Importantly, bone involvement in sarcoidosis rarely occurs without concomitant clinical or radiologic manifestations in other organ systems. Awareness of the clinical history and recognition of other imaging features, such as involving the reticuloendothelial system in addition to the skeleton, are important for more confident diagnosis.

Key imaging features:

- Radiographs and CT: lesions may be lytic, sclerotic, or mixed but are frequently occult

- MR imaging and FDG/PET CT are most sensitive
- Recognizing involvement of other organ systems is key to diagnosis

CALCIFIC TENDONITIS (HYDROXYAPATITE DEPOSITION DISEASE)

Calcific tendinitis/ hydroxyapatite deposition disease (HADD) is typically limited to tendons, bursae, and ligaments, but can erode into the underlying bone. Cortical erosion most often occurs in the proximal humerus at the insertion of the rotator cuff, pectoralis major, or latissimus dorsi, and in the proximal femur at the insertion of the gluteus maximus muscle.[53,54] The deposits can also penetrate and focally accumulate within the bone, which may result in a focal region of sclerosis (**Fig. 10**).[53–57] Although not well understood, the mechanism of HADD bone involvement is theorized to occur through enzymatic osteolysis of cortical bone with subsequent subcortical migration and eventual intramedullary diffusion.[54]

The resorptive phase of HADD is characterized by extensive abnormal signal in the surrounding soft tissues that can mimic soft tissue sarcoma. It can also be confused with juxtacortical lesions, such as osteoid osteoma, juxtacortical chondroma/chondrosarcoma, and periosteal osteosarcoma.[58] Intraosseous deposition is typically associated with prominent reactive marrow edema, which can mimic a bone tumor or infection (see **Fig. 10**). Correlation of T1 and fluid-sensitive sequences is critical for distinguishing between marrow edema and neoplasm. CT can also be helpful for problem solving in difficult cases by depicting the characteristic mineralization pattern and providing a better assessment of cortical erosion at tendinous attachments.

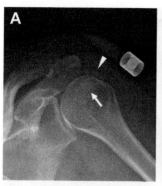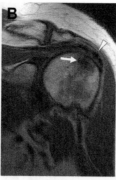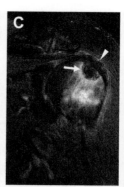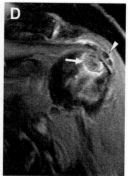

Fig. 10. Calcific tendonitis/hydroxyapatite deposition disease. Frontal radiograph (*A*) in a 47-year-old woman with shoulder pain demonstrates amorphous mineralization along the distal left rotator cuff tendons (*arrowhead*) with an area of sclerosis in the humeral head (*arrow*). Coronal T1-weighted (*B*), T2-weighted (*C*), and post-gadolinium images (*D*) demonstrate low signal calcium hydroxyapatite within the distal rotator cuff tendons (*arrowheads*), and also within the humeral head (*arrows*) with surrounding bone marrow edema and enhancement.

GOUT

Gout is characterized by the deposition of monosodium urate crystals in the joints and periarticular soft tissues. Although the radiographic features of joint involvement are well-recognized, tophaceous gout can lead to destructive osteolytic lesions that may mimic malignancy when occurring in isolation, uncommon locations, or when particularly robust.[38] If there is a gouty osteolytic lesion, radiographs and CT typically show mineralized soft tissue tophi and juxta-articular erosions (**Fig. 11**). On MR imaging, intraosseous gout demonstrates low T1 signal. Variable but typically low T2 signal corresponding to mineralization allows for differentiation from alternative diagnoses (see **Fig. 11**). Reactive marrow edema surrounding the intraosseous gout is common and there is also usually some degree of post-gadolinium enhancement.[59–61] Dual-energy CT is valuable to confirm monosodium urate deposition when the diagnosis is suspected (see **Fig. 11**).[62]

BONE INFARCT

The term "bone infarct" refers to osteonecrosis that occurs in the metaphysis or diaphysis of a bone, as opposed to avascular necrosis, which is osteonecrosis that occurs in the subarticular region, most commonly the femoral head. Osteonecrosis may result from a variety of etiologies, including trauma, steroid use, alcoholism, radiotherapy, and chemotherapy.[63] The classic radiographic appearance of bone infarct is a serpiginous sclerotic band separating a central necrotic area with variable lucency from the surrounding normal bone.[38] Multiple bilateral lesions are not uncommon, and may be symmetric. However, in the acute phase osteonecrosis may present as a vague area of intramedullary lucency, sometimes with accompanying periosteal reaction.[38,64]

On MR imaging, the acute phase of osteonecrosis is characterized by a circumscribed lesion with high T2 signal caused by marrow edema. It may

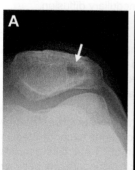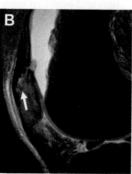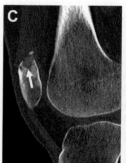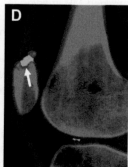

Fig. 11. Intraosseous gout. Sunrise view radiograph of the left knee (*A*) demonstrates a lytic lesion in the patella (*arrow*). Sagittal T2-weighted MR image (*B*) demonstrates intermediate and low signal within the lesion (*arrow*) and bone marrow edema throughout the patella. Sagittal CT (*C*) and post-processed dual-energy CT (*D*) images demonstrate a lytic lesion with internal mineralization, confirmed to be caused by monosodium urate deposition (*arrows*).

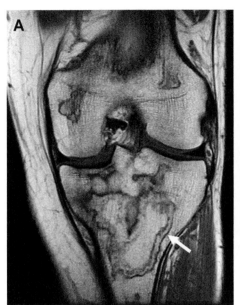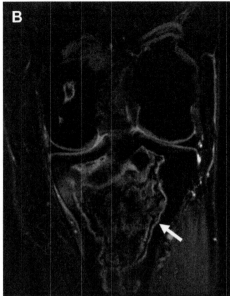

Fig. 12. Bone infarcts. Coronal T1-weighted (*A*) and T2-weighted (*B*) MR images of the left knee in a 28-year-old man with Crohn disease treated with steroids demonstrate multiple bone infarcts about the knee, the largest in the proximal tibia (*arrows*). The internal marrow fat is maintained, and there is a peripheral "double line" sign.

also be associated with increased T2 signal in the periosteum and adjacent soft tissues.[31] With further evolution, the lesion border becomes well-defined, appearing as a serpentine rim of low T1 signal, and low or high T2 signal. When the rim is comprised of parallel bands of high and low T2 signal ("double line sign"), which corresponds to a hyperintense inner ring of granulation tissue and hypointense outer rim of sclerosis (**Fig. 12**), this is pathognomonic for osteonecrosis.[38,65,66] However, the most common MR imaging pattern is that of an area of yellow marrow that is surrounded by a low signal intensity rim on all pulse sequences (see **Fig. 12**). This is a critical discriminator from enchondroma or other bone neoplasms, in which marrow fat will be replaced centrally.[67] In a minority of patients, osteonecrosis can have more variable MR imaging signal characteristics in the center, including cystic areas (low T1/high T2 signal), hemorrhage (high T1/high T2 signal, but variable depending on age), or fibrous tissue (low T1/low T2 signal). This is also more common when osteonecrosis occurs in epiphyseal rather than metadiaphyseal locations.[67]

Bone scintigraphy has also been used to evaluate bone infarcts. In the early stages, osteonecrosis may be characterized by decreased or absent uptake on blood flow, blood pool, and delayed phase images, which may be better delineated by pinhole-collimated images that offer higher resolution. During subsequent stages, there is usually increased radionuclide uptake at the periphery of the lesion as reparative processes take place, and new sclerosis and healing occur, whereas central photopenia usually persists.[67,68] Several studies have shown increased sensitivity with SPECT/CT for detection compared with planar or stand-alone SPECT imaging.[69,70]

Key imaging features:

- Bilateral and/or symmetric lesions is an important clue
- Radiographs: serpiginous sclerosis with central lucency
- MR imaging:
  - Double line sign is pathognomonic
  - Most commonly normal yellow bone marrow surrounded by low signal intensity rim on all sequences

SUMMARY

Several benign nonneoplastic bone lesions may mimic benign and malignant bone tumors. These include a broad spectrum of normal variants, developmental abnormalities, post-traumatic lesions, degenerative findings, infectious/inflammatory processes, and primary disorders of bone. It is important for radiologists to recognize these lesions because being able to provide a specific diagnosis can limit unnecessary work-up, prevent unwarranted biopsies, and minimize patient anxiety and potential morbidity.

CLINICS CARE POINTS

- A variety of benign, nonneoplastic bone lesions may mimic benign and malignant bone tumors. Usually, a combination of lesion location, patient demographics, and imaging features allows distinction from neoplastic bone disease.

- Red bone marrow is characterized by T1 signal intensity greater than skeletal muscle and significant signal dropout on opposed-phase imaging.

- Bone islands are characterized by spiculated margins and similar density to cortical bone on CT. On MR imaging, bone islands usually exhibit normal surrounding bone marrow signal.

- Sarcoid bone lesions detected by MRI and FDG PET are often occult on CT. Recognizing involvement of other organ systems can be key to diagnosing osseous sarcoid.

- Osteomyelitis can mimick bone tumors at any stage of infection. The presence of a T1 hyperintense rim (penumbra sign) can be critical to diagnosing intraosseous abscess.

DISCLOSURE

The authors have no relevant financial disclosures or conflicts of interest.

REFERENCES

1. Diard F, Hauger O, Moinard M, et al. Pseudo-cysts, lipomas, infarcts and simple cysts of the calcaneus: are there different or related lesions? JBR-BTR. 2007;90(5):315–24.
2. Sirry A. The pseudo-cystic triangle in the normal os calcis. Acta Radiol 1951;36(6):516–20.
3. Malghem J, Lecouvet F, Vande Berg B. Calcaneal cysts and lipomas: a common pathogenesis? Skeletal Radiol 2017;46(12):1635–42.
4. Powell GM, Turner NS 3rd, Broski SM, et al. Intraosseous "lipoma" of the calcaneus developing in an intraosseous ganglion cyst. J Radiol Case Rep 2018; 12(12):16–24.
5. Tins BJ, Berkowitz YJ, Konala P, et al. Intraosseous lipomas originating from simple bone cysts. Skeletal Radiol 2021;50(4):801–6.
6. Kumar R, Madewell JE, Swischuk LE, et al. The clavicle: normal and abnormal. Radiographics 1989;9(4): 677–706.
7. Shauffer IA, Collins WV. The deep clavicular rhomboid fossa. Clinical significance and incidence in 10,000 routine chest photofluorograms. Jama 1966;195(9): 778–9.
8. Koudela K Jr, Koudelova J, Koudela K, et al. Concave impressio ligamenti costoclavicularis ("rhomboid fossa") and its prevalence and relevance to clinical practice. Surg Radiol Anat 2015;37(3):239–45.
9. Paraskevas G, Natsis K, Spanidou S, et al. Excavated-type of rhomboid fossa of the clavicle: a radiological study. Folia Morphol (Warsz) 2009;68(3):163–6.
10. Vogler JB 3rd, Murphy WA. Bone marrow imaging. Radiology 1988;168(3):679–93.
11. Taccone A, Oddone M, Dell'Acqua AD, et al. MRI "road-map" of normal age-related bone marrow. II. Thorax, pelvis and extremities. Pediatr Radiol 1995;25(8):596–606.
12. Disler DG, McCauley TR, Ratner LM, et al. In-phase and out-of-phase MR imaging of bone marrow: prediction of neoplasia based on the detection of coexistent fat and water. AJR Am J Roentgenol 1997;169(5): 1439–47.
13. Ragab Y, Emad Y, Gheita T, et al. Differentiation of osteoporotic and neoplastic vertebral fractures by chemical shift {in-phase and out-of-phase} MR imaging. Eur J Radiol 2009;72(1):125–33.
14. Zajick DC Jr, Morrison WB, Schweitzer ME, et al. Benign and malignant processes: normal values and differentiation with chemical shift MR imaging in vertebral marrow. Radiology 2005;237(2):590–6.
15. Herneth AM, Philipp MO, Pretterklieber ML, et al. Asymmetric closure of ischiopubic synchondrosis in pediatric patients: correlation with foot dominance. Am J Roentgenol 2004;182(2):361–5.
16. Tsuji K, Tsuchida T, Kosaka N, et al. Serial changes of (18)F-FDG PET/CT findings in ischiopubic synchondrosis: comparison with contrast-enhanced MRI. Hell J Nucl Med 2015;18(1):66–7.
17. Hardoff R, Gips S. Ischiopubic synchondrosis. Normal finding, increased pubic uptake on bone scintigraphy. Clin Nucl Med 1992;17(2):139.
18. Herneth AM, Trattnig S, Bader TR, et al. MR imaging of the ischiopubic synchondrosis. Magn Reson Imaging 2000;18(5):519–24.
19. Wait A, Gaskill T, Sarwar Z, et al. Van neck disease: osteochondrosis of the ischiopubic synchondrosis. J Pediatr Orthopaedics 2011;31(5).
20. Drubach LA, Voss SD, Kourmouzi V, et al. The ischiopubic synchondrosis: changing appearance on PET/CT as a mimic of disease. Clin Nucl Med 2006;31(7):414–7.
21. White LM, Kandel R. Osteoid-producing tumors of bone. Semin Musculoskelet Radiol 2000;4(1):25–43.
22. Murphey MD, Andrews CL, Flemming DJ, et al. From the archives of the AFIP. Primary tumors of the spine: radiologic pathologic correlation. Radiographics 1996;16(5):1131–58.

23. Ulano A, Bredella MA, Burke P, et al. Distinguishing untreated osteoblastic metastases from enostoses using CT attenuation measurements. AJR Am J Roentgenol 2016;207(2):362–8.

24. Elangovan SM, Sebro R. Accuracy of CT attenuation measurement for differentiating treated osteoblastic metastases from enostoses. AJR Am J Roentgenol 2018;210(3):615–20.

25. Azar A, Garner HW, Rhodes NG, et al. CT attenuation values do not reliably distinguish benign sclerotic lesions from osteoblastic metastases in patients undergoing bone biopsy. AJR Am J Roentgenol 2021;216(4):1022–30.

26. Onitsuka H. Roentgenologic aspects of bone islands. Radiology 1977;123(3):607–12.

27. Greenspan A, Steiner G, Knutzon R. Bone island (enostosis): clinical significance and radiologic and pathologic correlations. Skeletal Radiol 1991;20(2): 85–90.

28. Ran P, Dong A, Wang Y, et al. Increased FDG uptake in a giant bone island mimicking malignancy. Clin Nucl Med 2018;43(6):e209–11.

29. Guillin R, Moser T, Koob M, et al. Subperiosteal hematoma of the iliac bone: imaging features of acute and chronic stages with emphasis on pathophysiology. Skeletal Radiol 2012;41(6):667–75.

30. Schajowicz F, Clavel Sainz M, Slullitel JA. Juxtaarticular bone cysts (intra-osseous ganglia): a clinicopathological study of eighty-eight cases. J Bone Joint Surg Br 1979;61(1):107–16.

31. Gould CF, Ly JQ, Lattin GE Jr, et al. Bone tumor mimics: avoiding misdiagnosis. Curr Probl Diagn Radiol 2007;36(3):124–41.

32. Williams HJ, Davies AM, Allen G, et al. Imaging features of intraosseous ganglia: a report of 45 cases. Eur Radiol 2004;14(10):1761–9.

33. McCarville MB, Chen JY, Coleman JL, et al. Distinguishing osteomyelitis from Ewing sarcoma on radiography and MRI. AJR Am J Roentgenol 2015; 205(3):640–50. quiz 651.

34. Shimose S, Sugita T, Kubo T, et al. Differential diagnosis between osteomyelitis and bone tumors. Acta Radiol 2008;49(8):928–33.

35. Huang PY, Wu PK, Chen CF, et al. Osteomyelitis of the femur mimicking bone tumors: a review of 10 cases. World J Surg Oncol 2013;11:283.

36. Cottias P, Tomeno B, Anract P, et al. Subacute osteomyelitis presenting as a bone tumour. A review of 21 cases. Int Orthop 1997;21(4):243–8.

37. Bohndorf K. Infection of the appendicular skeleton. Eur Radiol 2004;14(Suppl 3):E53–63.

38. Stacy GS, Kapur A. Mimics of bone and soft tissue neoplasms. Radiol Clin North Am 2011;49(6): 1261–86.

39. Marti-Bonmati L, Aparisi F, Poyatos C, et al. Brodie abscess: MR imaging appearance in 10 patients. J Magn Reson Imaging 1993;3(3):543–6.

40. McGuinness B, Wilson N, Doyle AJ. The "penumbra sign" on T1-weighted MRI for differentiating musculoskeletal infection from tumour. Skeletal Radiol 2007;36(5):417–21.

41. Jennin F, Bousson V, Parlier C, et al. Bony sequestrum: a radiologic review. Skeletal Radiol 2011; 40(8):963–75.

42. Wang GL, Zhao K, Liu ZF, et al. A meta-analysis of fluorodeoxyglucose-positron emission tomography versus scintigraphy in the evaluation of suspected osteomyelitis. Nucl Med Commun 2011;32(12): 1134–42.

43. Kwee TC, de Klerk JMH, Nix M, et al. Benign bone conditions that may be FDG-avid and mimic malignancy. Semin Nucl Med 2017;47(4):322–51.

44. James DG, Neville E, Carstairs LS. Bone and joint sarcoidosis. Semin Arthritis Rheum 1976;6(1):53–81.

45. Sartoris DJ, Resnick D, Resnik C, et al. Musculoskeletal manifestations of sarcoidosis. Semin Roentgenol 1985;20(4):376–86.

46. Sparks JA, McSparron JI, Shah N, et al. Osseous sarcoidosis: clinical characteristics, treatment, and outcomes: experience from a large, academic hospital. Semin Arthritis Rheum 2014;44(3):371–9.

47. Moore SL, Teirstein A, Golimbu C. MRI of sarcoidosis patients with musculoskeletal symptoms. AJR Am J Roentgenol 2005;185(1):154–9.

48. Moore SL, Teirstein AE. Musculoskeletal sarcoidosis: spectrum of appearances at MR imaging. Radiographics 2003;23(6):1389–99.

49. Talmi D, Smith S, Mulligan ME. Central skeletal sarcoidosis mimicking metastatic disease. Skeletal Radiol 2008;37(8):757–61.

50. Mostard RL, Prompers L, Weijers RE, et al. F-18 FDG PET/CT for detecting bone and bone marrow involvement in sarcoidosis patients. Clin Nucl Med 2012;37(1):21–5.

51. Grozdic Milojevic I, Sobic-Saranovic D, Videnovic-Ivanov J, et al. FDG PET/CT in bone sarcoidosis. Sarcoidosis Vasc Diffuse Lung Dis 2016;33(1):66–74.

52. Moore SL, Kransdorf MJ, Schweitzer ME, et al. Can sarcoidosis and metastatic bone lesions be reliably differentiated on routine MRI? AJR Am J Roentgenol 2012;198(6):1387–93.

53. Flemming DJ, Murphey MD, Shekitka KM, et al. Osseous involvement in calcific tendinitis: a retrospective review of 50 cases. AJR Am J Roentgenol 2003;181(4):965–72.

54. Malghem J, Omoumi P, Lecouvet F, et al. Intraosseous migration of tendinous calcifications: cortical erosions, subcortical migration and extensive intramedullary diffusion, a SIMS series. Skeletal Radiol 2015;44(10):1403–12.

55. Durr HR, Lienemann A, Silbernagl H, et al. Acute calcific tendinitis of the pectoralis major insertion associated with cortical bone erosion. Eur Radiol 1997;7(8):1215–7.

56. Kachewar SG, Kulkarni DS. Calcific tendinitis of the rotator cuff: a review. J Clin Diagn Res 2013;7(7): 1482–5.

57. Klontzas ME, Vassalou EE, Karantanas AH. Calcific tendinopathy of the shoulder with intraosseous extension: outcomes of ultrasound-guided percutaneous irrigation. Skeletal Radiol 2017;46(2):201–8.

58. Kalayci CB, Kizilkaya E. Calcific tendinitis: intramuscular and intraosseous migration. Diagn Interv Radiol 2019;25(6):480–4.

59. Hsu CY, Shih TT, Huang KM, et al. Tophaceous gout of the spine: MR imaging features. Clin Radiol 2002; 57(10):919–25.

60. Khoo JN, Tan SC. MR imaging of tophaceous gout revisited. Singapore Med J 2011;52(11):840–6. quiz 847.

61. Yu JS, Chung C, Recht M, et al. MR imaging of tophaceous gout. AJR Am J Roentgenol 1997; 168(2):523–7.

62. Chou H, Chin TY, Peh WC. Dual-energy CT in gout: a review of current concepts and applications. J Med Radiat Sci 2017;64(1):41–51.

63. Shah KN, Racine J, Jones LC, et al. Pathophysiology and risk factors for osteonecrosis. Curr Rev Musculoske 2015;8(3):201–9.

64. Munk PL, Helms CA, Holt RG. Immature bone infarcts: findings on plain radiographs and MR scans. AJR Am J Roentgenol 1989;152(3):547–9.

65. Vande Berg BE, Malghem JJ, Labaisse MA, et al. MR imaging of avascular necrosis and transient marrow edema of the femoral head. Radiographics 1993;13(3):501–20.

66. Duda SH, Laniado M, Schick F, et al. The double-line sign of osteonecrosis: evaluation on chemical shift MR images. Eur J Radiol 1993;16(3):233–8.

67. Murphey MD, Foreman KL, Klassen-Fischer MK, et al. From the radiologic pathology archives imaging of osteonecrosis: radiologic-pathologic correlation. Radiographics 2014;34(4):1003–28.

68. Love C, Din AS, Tomas MB, et al. Radionuclide bone imaging: an illustrative review. Radiographics 2003; 23(2):341–58.

69. Luk WH, Au-Yeung AW, Yang MK. Diagnostic value of SPECT versus SPECT/CT in femoral avascular necrosis: preliminary results. Nucl Med Commun 2010; 31(11):958–61.

70. Ryu JS, Kim JS, Moon DH, et al. Bone SPECT is more sensitive than MRI in the detection of early osteonecrosis of the femoral head after renal transplantation. J Nucl Med 2002;43(8):1006–11.

Soft Tissue Tumors
Diagnosis, Treatment, and Follow-up from the Orthopedic Oncologist Perspective

Benjamin K. Wilke, MD[a,*], Krista A. Goulding, MD, MPH[b],
Courtney E. Sherman, MD[a], Matthew T. Houdek, MD[c]

KEYWORDS

• Musculoskeletal • Sarcoma • Orthopedic • Surgery

KEY POINTS

- Imaging should be obtained on all masses greater than 5 cm or deep to fascia to avoid a delay in the diagnosis of a soft tissue sarcoma.
- Biopsy approach is critical and should be guided by the treating orthopedic oncologist to ensure the inclusion of the biopsy tract in the resection.
- Preoperative staging studies should comment on tissue planes or tumor encasement of nearby critical structures to assist with surgical planning.
- Routine postoperative surveillance imaging is necessary to diagnose a recurrent tumor in a timely fashion.

BACKGROUND

Soft tissue masses in the extremities are a relatively common presenting complaint observed in both primary care and orthopedic practices. Often these "tumors" are of benign origin and do not require expensive work-up or treatment. Sarcomas are much rarer. It has been estimated that benign tumors outnumber sarcomas 150:1. Most orthopedic surgeons will only see 1 to 2 soft tissue sarcomas during their career.[1] There were an estimated 13,000 new soft tissue sarcomas in the United States in 2020. This is compared with 230,000 new cases of lung cancer and 280,000 new cases of breast cancer.[2]

Clinicians need to have a heightened awareness of soft tissue sarcomas during the workup of an unknown mass when the initial evaluation does not clearly identify the mass as benign. Often this requires a multidisciplinary approach and potential referral to a center specialized in treating soft tissue sarcomas to avoid a delay in diagnosis or complications from errant biopsy placement or nononcologic resection.

This article will provide information on the basic workup of an unknown soft tissue mass, including staging studies and treatment options for soft tissue sarcomas. The information is presented from an orthopedic oncologists' viewpoint and is meant to help facilitate the multidisciplinary approach to the treatment of these rare tumors to continue to improve our patients' outcomes.

CLINICAL PRESENTATION

The first requirement in the evaluation of a new soft tissue mass is to perform a focused history and physical examination. Pertinent questions involve when the mass was first noticed as well as the growth pattern of the mass as initially perceived. While it is important to note pain, including pain at night, it has been shown that both benign and malignant lesions may present as a painless growing mass.[3] The presence or absence of pain does not help further differentiate unknown tumors.

Trauma additionally is important to consider. While acute trauma may lead to the development

[a] Mayo Clinic Florida, 4500 San Pablo Road, Jacksonville, FL 32224, USA; [b] Mayo Clinic Arizona, 5777 East Mayo Boulevard, Phoenix, AZ 85054, USA; [c] Mayo Clinic, 200 1st Street Southwest, Rochester, MN 55905, USA
* Corresponding author.
E-mail address: Wilke.benjamin@mayo.edu

Radiol Clin N Am 60 (2022) 253–262
https://doi.org/10.1016/j.rcl.2021.11.005

of a mass by the way of a hematoma, often patients will recount a remote history of trauma to the affected area. Usually, this has no relevance to the development of the mass.

A history of cancer, including prior radiation to the affected site, is important to ascertain. While rare, radiation-induced sarcomas will often present years following prior radiation therapy. Radiation-induced sarcomas portend a poor prognosis.[4]

There are several physical examination characteristics that are important for the clinician to review. Soft tissue sarcomas have a generally firm consistency. This is compared with a benign lipoma, which is typically very soft on palpation. Additionally, the presence of a Tinel sign will indicate nerve irritation either due to local compression or a tumor of nerve origin. Mobility of the tumor relative to surrounding structures is important for preoperative planning; if the tumor is nonmobile this indicates adherence to the surrounding tissues and therefore portends greater difficulty in tumor removal. Finally, an examination of regional lymph nodes is important to assess for lymphadenopathy.

DIFFERENTIAL DIAGNOSIS

There is a large differential diagnosis for soft-tissue masses. This differential includes the following:

- Lipoma
- Hematoma
- Vascular malformations
- Infection (abscess)
- Cyst
- Myositis Ossificans
- Desmoid tumor
- Nodular fasciitis
- Sarcoma

Often a proper history and physical examination can lead to the correct diagnosis with little additional workup. However, all masses superficial to fascia that are greater than 5 cm in diameter and all masses that are deep to fascia should undergo

further investigation with advanced imaging and possible biopsy. A golf ball has been identified as a surrogate for sizing. If a superficial mass is larger than a golf ball, then it requires further evaluation.[5]

TUMOR CLASSIFICATION

Lichtenstein first classified musculoskeletal tumors based on histology. While this classification was useful for diagnostic purposes, it did not provide treatment recommendations and was of limited benefit for surgical guidance.[6] In 1980, Enneking introduced a classification system that assisted surgeons with both treatment and prognosis.[7] This classification system was then adapted by the Musculoskeletal Tumor Society, and subsequently by the National Institutes of Health Sarcoma Consensus Study Group.[8] The Enneking classification separated benign and malignant lesions. It emphasized tumor grade (low vs high), extension of the tumor (intracompartmental vs extracompartmental), and presence of metastases. This classification was helpful to orthopedic surgeons for preoperative planning but was not widely used across specialties.

The American Joint Committee on Cancer (AJCC) staging system for soft tissue sarcomas of the extremity is most commonly used today for interdisciplinary communication. This system classifies tumors by size, lymph node involvement, presence of metastases, and grade of the tumor (**Fig. 1**).

PREOPERATIVE IMAGING

Proper imaging of unknown tumors remains a critical component of the evaluation. Radiographic evaluation of the affected extremity is an appropriate initial imaging strategy. These are inexpensive and may demonstrate disruption of the tissue planes, changes in the underlying bone, and/or the presence of internal mineralization in the soft tissue mass (**Fig. 2**). Even negative radiographs are very helpful in narrowing the differential diagnosis.

Following radiographs the soft tissues are often further evaluated with an MR imaging of the extremity (with and without contrast) (**Fig. 3**).[9] A CT

AJCC Staging System for Sarcomas of the Extremity				
Stage	Size	Lymph Node Involvement	Metastasis	Grade
IA	<5 cm	none	No	low
IB	>5 cm	none	No	low
II	<5 cm	none	No	intermediate / high
IIIA	5–10 cm	none	No	intermediate / high
IIIB	>10 cm	none	No	intermediate / high
IVA	any	regional	No	any
IVB	any	any	Yes	any

Fig. 1. The American Joint Committee on Cancer staging system for soft tissue sarcomas.

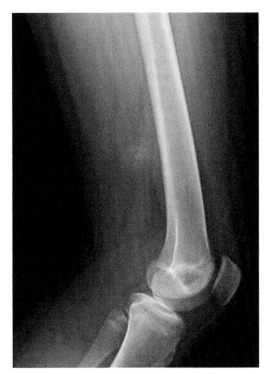

Fig. 2. An extraskeletal osteosarcoma with internal mineralization.

scan can also be useful to further evaluate associated mineralization or the relationship of the soft tissue tumor with the underlying bone.[10] Advanced imaging obtained in 3 planes (axial, sagittal, and coronal) is ideal to assist the surgical team with preoperative planning.

For tumors that are near neurovascular structures, it is important to report if there is a tissue plane between these critical structures and the tumor. If such a plane exists, then it is possible to obtain a close margin and spare the critical structure during the surgical resection. Alternatively, if the tumor encases the structure, then the nerve or vessel must be resected with the tumor.

Furthermore, evaluation for vascular invasion and tumor thrombus is essential. The presence of vascular invasion is an independent prognostic factor for the development of metastatic disease and portends a worse prognosis. If present, a more aggressive resection should be undertaken.[11]

Of note, the advanced imaging should always be completed before the biopsy to allow for the evaluation of the tumor in its most natural state without being confounded by postbiopsy inflammation or alteration of tissue planes.

STAGING STUDIES

Once a tumor is determined to be malignant, staging studies are obtained before proceeding with surgical resection. Staging involves determining both local tumor extension as well as the extent of tumoral spread into regional lymph nodes or distant organs.

A positron emission tomography/computed tomography (PET/CT) scan is commonly used to evaluate for regional and metastatic spread of disease. While helpful, this imaging modality does not have the spatial resolution to properly evaluate the development of pulmonary nodules. For this reason, a dedicated CT scan of the chest is also typically obtained for completeness.[10,12,13]

PERCUTANEOUS VERSUS OPEN BIOPSY

While imaging findings may provide a differential diagnosis, a biopsy is often necessary for the workup of lesions that are indeterminate on imaging. The biopsy specimen can also allow for histologic grading of the tumor, which may affect recommendations for adjuvant treatment.

Percutaneous biopsy with a core coaxial needle system is the preferred biopsy method due to lower risk and cost. This can be performed either in the clinic or under image guidance depending on tumor accessibility and institutional protocols. With this method, several cores of tissue are obtained from the tumor through the same coaxial introducer needle. An accurate pathologic diagnosis is provided in approximately 84% of cases with core needle biopsy.[14]

If a core needle biopsy is nondiagnostic, the patient may be offered a repeat core biopsy or an open biopsy. Open biopsy is performed in the operating room and involves a limited incision

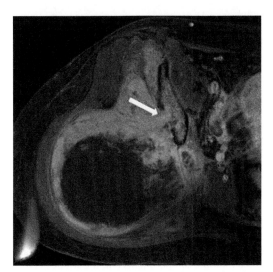

Fig. 3. A large malignant peripheral nerve sheath tumor with intraosseous extension (*arrow*).

with the removal of a wedge-shaped piece of tissue from the tumor. The primary advantage of open biopsy over core needle biopsy is that a much larger and therefore more representative specimen is provided for pathologic analysis.

Regardless of technique, careful planning of the biopsy path is critical to ensure the inclusion of the biopsy tract with the tumor resection. Therefore, the treating surgeon should provide guidance on the most desirable needle approach for percutaneous core biopsies. Likewise, the treating surgeon should be the one to perform the open biopsy if percutaneous biopsy is not successful.

When performing an open incisional biopsy there are several principles that the surgeon must follow, including placement of the biopsy incision along the same incision line planned for the eventual tumor resection. The incision should also be oriented parallel to the long axis of the extremity. Transverse incisions require much larger soft tissue resections and often necessitate a myocutaneous flap for wound coverage and closure.

The open biopsy incision should be limited in length to avoid excess contamination and should not be placed between intermuscular planes. Avoiding intermuscular planes decreases the potential for the spread of a contaminated postoperative hematoma. Expert opinion recommends against the exsanguination of the extremity (other than gravity exsanguination) to avoid potential tumoral seeding into the bloodstream. Finally, if a drain is used it must be placed in close proximity and in line with the skin incision so that the drain tract can be resected during the eventual tumor resection.

Principles of Open Biopsy

- Incision for biopsy placed along same planned incision line for tumor resection
- Incision in line with long axis of extremity
- Limit the length of the incision
- Avoid intermuscular planes
- Avoid exsanguination of the extremity
- Obtain adequate tissue specimen
- Obtain hemostasis
- Place drain close to and in line with the biopsy incision

THE HAZARDS OF THE BIOPSY

Improper biopsy placement can impact surgical options. Mankin reported a 19% rate of complications when biopsies were performed by the referring institution rather than the treating hospital. These complications included nondiagnostic tissue, wound complications resulting in increased contamination, and treatment alterations due to

errant biopsy placement. This rate of complications was 12x higher than when the biopsies were performed at the treating hospital and included 18 unnecessary amputations.[15,16]

To reduce complications, it is imperative to work closely with the surgeon when planning the location of the biopsy. Even a needle biopsy should be placed in line with the planned surgical incision to facilitate the removal of the biopsy tract. Additionally, the same principles used for open biopsies, such as the avoidance of intermuscular planes and the crossing of multiple compartments, must be followed. Avoidance of critical structures such as nerves and blood vessels is also essential to prevent contamination. Examples of inappropriate image-guided biopsy approaches are shown in **Figs. 4** and **5**.

GENERAL DIAGNOSTIC CONSIDERATIONS FOR COMMON SOFT TISSUE MASSES

Often a focused history, physical examination, and initial imaging are adequate for the diagnosis of many benign lesions. In these cases, a biopsy is often not necessary before proceeding with treatment recommendations. For example, a lipoma is often very soft on physical examination and is nontender to palpation. The MR imaging will demonstrate a homogenous mass with little internal stranding and signal characteristics matching the subcutaneous fat (**Fig. 6**).[17] This is diagnostic and marginal excision can proceed without a biopsy.

Vascular malformations represent additional soft tissue masses which are often diagnosed

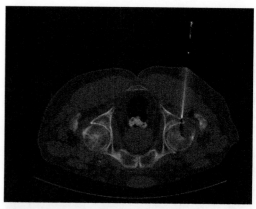

Fig. 4. This image-guided core needle biopsy was performed for a presumed metastatic lesion in the femoral head of a 70-year-old patient. The lesion represented a primary sarcoma. The biopsy tract contaminated multiple compartments and the sciatic nerve. It was ignored during tumor resection and will be closely followed for local recurrence.

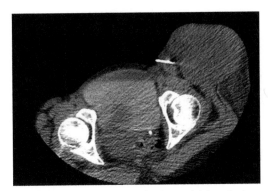

Fig. 5. This needle biopsy of a large thigh soft tissue sarcoma was performed adjacent to the neurovascular structures, causing potential contamination. A more appropriate biopsy would have been performed laterally, avoiding critical structures.

based on physical examination and imaging alone. Clinically they may be painful and often will change size. They may have a blue discoloration if located superficially. Hemangiomas may demonstrate internal phleboliths. On advanced imaging, often adipose tissue is observed within the mass in between the small vessels (**Fig. 7**). Treatment is often unnecessary, and patients are followed with clinical observation only. For recalcitrant lesions, sclerotherapy or surgical excision may be performed.[18,19]

For lesions that are indeterminate on imaging, a biopsy is warranted. Indeterminate lesions are often of a mixed, heterogenous signal intensity on MR imaging. They demonstrate low to intermediate signal intensity on T1 imaging relative to muscle and high signal intensity on T2 sequences. Both benign and malignant tumors can present in this way. Often, additional imaging features can help further identify the lesion. For example, the presence of peripheral mineralization on radiographs may help to differentiate the early phase of myositis ossificans (fibrodysplasia ossificans progressiva) from malignant lesions (**Fig. 8**).[20]

There are greater than 50 types of sarcomas[21] and an in-depth review is beyond the scope of this article. The grade and anatomic location of the primary tumor are the most significant factors determining prognosis and treatment. Malignant tumors have a worse prognosis when high grade, greater than 5 cm, and deep to the fascia.[11,22] Most sarcomas develop in adulthood, but a few, such as synovial sarcoma and rhabdomyosarcoma have predilections for younger patients.[23] Undifferentiated pleomorphic sarcoma is the most common soft tissue sarcoma in adults. It often occurs in patients greater than 50 years of age, and often in a subfascial location.

While many histologic types of soft tissue sarcomas present clinically and are treated in a similar fashion, some have distinctive features. For example, synovial sarcoma is unique in that it can remain indolent for many years before enlarging, and may contain intralesional mineralization.[24] As previously stated, synovial sarcoma often occurs in younger patients. For this reason, and for its relative chemosensitivity, synovial

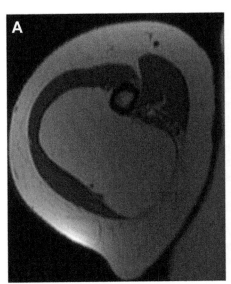
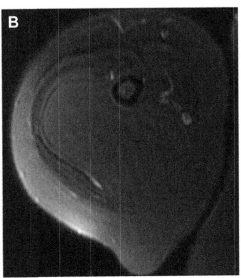

Fig. 6. An example of a large intramuscular lipoma on a T1 (*A*) and fat saturated (*B*) sequence. Note the homogenous appearance with signal characteristics identical to those of the subcutaneous adipose tissue. No biopsy is needed in this case, and the surgeon will proceed to excision.

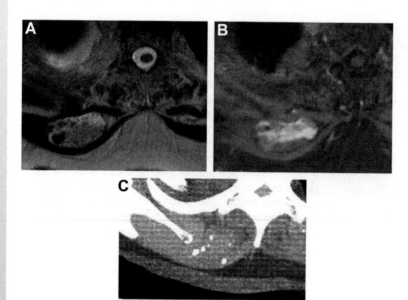

Fig. 7. Axial MR imaging (*A, B*) and CT (*C*) demonstrating a hemangioma in the paraspinal musculature. The mass demonstrates internal signal characteristics identical to the subcutaneous adipose tissue (*A, B*). Phleboliths are observed on the CT scan (*C*).

sarcoma is often treated with chemotherapy in addition to radiation.[25]

HISTORICAL TREATMENT

Treatment of soft tissue sarcomas has dramatically improved over the last half century. Early surgical management of soft tissue sarcomas often consisted of amputative procedures, attempting to favor life over limb. Unfortunately, even with a radical surgical approach, patients often succumbed to metastatic disease.[26]

In the 1970s and 1980s, chemotherapy and radiation began to be used as adjuvant therapy. These treatments improved local control and overall survival, allowing surgeons to begin to focus on less-aggressive surgical resections, now attempting to save both life and limb.[27]

In recent years, improvements in understanding of cell biology and genetics have allowed the development of novel forms of treatment, including immunomodulation of T-cells, gene therapy trials, and angiogenesis inhibitors, allowing a more targeted approach to therapy.[28]

SURGICAL CONSIDERATIONS

In the 1980s, Enneking defined surgical margins. This was instrumental in facilitating communication and allowing comparisons across institutions. At that time, it was noted that soft tissue sarcomas grew in a centrifugal pattern with the development of a reactive "pseudocapsule" around the tumor. This pseudocapsule contains inflammatory cells, cell debris, and viable tumor cells.[3,22] Enneking

defined these margins as intralesional (through gross tumor), marginal (through the reactive pseudocapsule), wide (outside of the reactive pseudocapsule), and radical (resection of the entire compartment) (**Fig. 9**).[7]

Obtaining appropriate margins is of the utmost importance to reduce the risk for local recurrence. For malignant tumors, this means obtaining a wide margin, defined by Enneking as a cuff of normal histologic tissue surrounding the specimen. This will help to ensure that the resection is outside of the reactive zone, which may contain viable tumor cells.

Anatomic barriers such as fascia can prevent tumoral spread and are often used as a margin, allowing the surgeon to get closer to the tumor than would be possible in free tissue. Similarly, a fat plane may allow the dissection and salvage of neurovascular structures that are in close proximity to the tumor. It is important to recognize these features on the preoperative imaging to appropriately plan the surgical resection and have resources available to reconstruct the vessels or perform nerve grafting at the time of surgery.

TREATMENT OF UNPLANNED EXCISIONS

An unplanned or inadvertent excision is one in which a surgical excision was performed in a non-oncologic fashion with inadequate margins around the tumor.[29] Often these procedures are performed without adequate preoperative imaging or tissue sampling, and by surgeons without specialized oncology training. In one report,

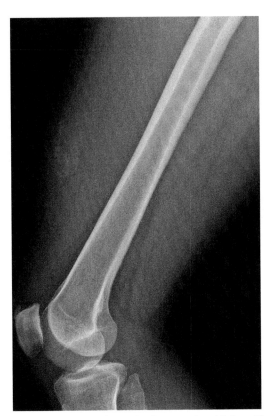

Fig. 8. Myositis ossificans in the anterior thigh, with peripheral mineralization.

unplanned excisions occurred in 37% of patients referred to a specialized cancer center.[30]

Following an unplanned excision, treatment generally depends on the histologic grade of the tumor and the surgical margin. For low-grade tumors with negative surgical margins, observation may be performed. For high-grade tumors, or tumors with positive margins, resection of the tumor bed is often performed along with radiation therapy. In either case, the patient must undergo proper staging studies, which include MR imaging with and without contrast of the tumor bed as well as a PET/CT and chest CT to evaluate for metastatic disease. Even following a wide resection of a contaminated tumor bed, patients will still be at a higher risk for developing local recurrence after an unplanned excision.[31,32]

COMMON POSTOPERATIVE COMPLICATIONS

Postoperative complications are common following soft tissue sarcoma resections. These complications often include wound dehiscence and postoperative infection. They are more prevalent in the lower extremities and following preoperative radiation, occurring in up to 30% to 40% of patients (**Fig. 10**).[33]

Several studies have attempted to reduce postoperative complications, using methods such as incisional wound vacuum therapy, hyperbaric oxygen, or aggressive use of soft tissue flap coverage. Unfortunately, these authors have reported no significant change in postoperative complications following these measures, with reported complication rates matching historic controls.[34–37]

Newer technology has emerged that has the potential to help reduce postoperative complications. Intraoperative use of indocyanine green fluorescence angiography has recently been shown to have a high positive predictive value in determining postoperative wound complications, especially in the lower extremity.[38] The use of this technology will allow surgeons to remove at-risk tissue during the procedure and may help decrease the rate of postoperative wound complications in patients who have received preoperative radiation therapy. This is an exciting new development for orthopedic oncology (**Fig. 11**).

POSTOPERATIVE SURVEILLANCE IMAGING

Routine surveillance imaging postoperatively is performed to identify early local recurrence or metastatic spread of disease. This imaging often consists of an MR imaging with and without contrast of the surgical site as well as a CT scan of the chest to evaluate for pulmonary nodules.

The cadence for obtaining postoperative surveillance imaging is variable, often dependent on institutional protocols rather than evidence based. Most institutions continue to follow patients with imaging for 5-years postoperatively as most recurrences occur during this period.[39]

Newer research has emerged that attempts to provide evidence-based guidelines for obtaining surveillance imaging. Based on the observed growth rates of local recurrences, the authors recommend performing an MR imaging of the extremity every 6 months.[40] Further research is necessary to determine the optimal timing of surveillance imaging to minimize unnecessary testing while still providing early detection of recurrent disease.

DEALING WITH RECURRENT DISEASE

Tumor recurrence can be devastating to patients and requires swift diagnosis and treatment. Recurrent disease can either present locally at the surgical site or due to the development of distant metastatic spread. Soft tissue sarcomas typically spread hematogenously, often seeding the lungs. Rarely, soft tissue sarcomas will spread to regional lymph nodes. Nodal spread is more common with

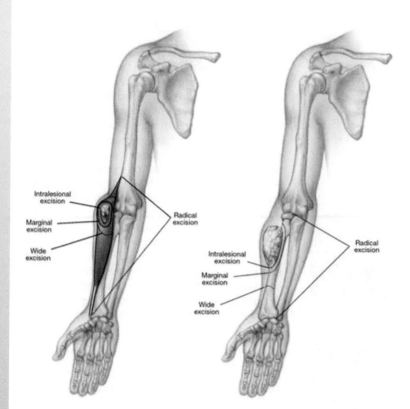

Fig. 9. An illustrative example of surgical margins as defined by Enneking.

certain histologic subtypes (synovial sarcoma, epithelioid sarcoma, clear cell sarcoma, and rhabdomyosarcoma).[41]

For suspicious masses in the tumor bed, often a repeat biopsy is necessary to confirm recurrence.

These biopsies are generally performed under image guidance. If tumor recurrence is confirmed, treatment is generally a wide resection of the area of recurrence. Additional radiation may be given, depending on the location relative to critical structures and cumulative dose. Locally recurrent tumors are generally of higher grade than the original lesion and portend a worse survival prognosis.[42]

For soft tissue sarcomas, metastatic disease is usually first diagnosed in the lungs on a chest CT. Pulmonary nodules >1 cm are concerning and are generally referred for a biopsy. Treatment

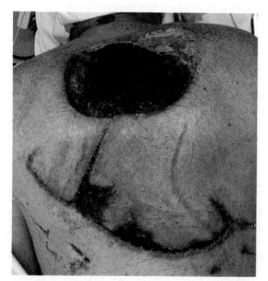

Fig. 10. A postoperative wound complication following a pedicled flap for wound closure. (*Courtesy of J. Post, DO, South Bend, Indiana.*)

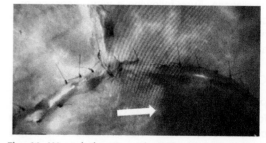

Fig. 11. Wound closure evaluated with ICG angiography. The dark area demonstrates an area of hypoperfusion (*arrow*). (*Courtesy of J. Post, DO, South Bend, Indiana.*)

of metastatic disease is variable, based on the tumor burden. For isolated pulmonary lesions, a wedge resection or radiation may be used, depending on accessibility. For multiple metastatic foci, chemotherapy is generally favored.[43]

SUMMARY

Soft tissue sarcomas are rare and often require a multidisciplinary approach at a specialized center to limit complications related to the diagnosis or management of these complex cases. It is imperative to work closely with the surgical team when planning the approach for a guided biopsy. The biopsy should be completed only after all advanced imaging of the mass is obtained and should be directed in line with the planned incision for tumor resection, taking care to avoid critical structures and intermuscular planes.

Preoperative imaging is important to help the surgical team plan the resection. It is important to note the tumor location relative to critical anatomic structures, and if a tissue plane is present. Encasement of structures such as nerves or blood vessels should be noted and requires resection of these structures at the time of surgery to avoid contamination of the wound.

Routine postoperative imaging is important to identify local recurrence or metastatic disease in a timely fashion. These recurrences are treated on an individual basis, often with repeat surgery for local recurrence, and resection, radiation, and/or chemotherapy for metastatic disease.

Above all, it is important to work in a multidisciplinary team and refer patients to a center specialized in sarcoma care in a timely fashion to optimize patient outcomes.

CLINICS CARE POINTS

- All masses larger than 5 cm that are superficial to the fascia, and all masses deep to the fascia should undergo advanced imaging and possible biopsy.
- Advanced imaging should be completed prior to obtaining a biopsy to avoid alteration of tissue planes and distortion of the imaging.
- Planned biopsy trajectories should be discussed with the surgeon planning to remove the mass to avoid errant biopsy placement.
- Routine surveillance imaging is necessary to detect local recurrence or metastatic spread.

DISCLOSURE

The authors have received research support from Summit Medical and the Desmoid Tumor Research Foundation.

REFERENCES

1. Tukiainen E, Bohling T, Huuhtanen R. Soft tissue sarcoma of the trunk and extremities. Scand J Surg 2003;92(4):257–63.
2. Siegel RL, Miller KD, Jemal A. Cancer statistics, 2020. CA Cancer J Clin 2020;70(1):7–30.
3. Mayerson JL, Scharschmidt TJ, Lewis VO, et al. Diagnosis and Management of Soft-tissue Masses. J Am Acad Orthop Surg 2014;22(11):742–50.
4. Bjerkehagen B, Smeland S, Walberg L, et al. Radiation-induced sarcoma: 25-year experience from the Norwegian Radium Hospital. Acta Oncol 2008; 47(8):1475–82.
5. Persson BM, Rydholm A. Soft-tissue masses of the locomotor system. A guide to the clinical diagnosis of malignancy. Acta Orthop Scand 1986;57(3): 216–9.
6. Lichtenstein L. Classification of primary tumors of bone. Cancer 1951;4(2):335–41.
7. Enneking WF, Spanier SS, Goodman MA. A system for the surgical staging of musculoskeletal sarcoma. Clin Orthop Relat Res 1980;(153):106–20.
8. Consensus Conference. Limb-sparing treatment of adult soft-tissue sarcomas and osteosarcomas. JAMA 1985;254(13):1791–4.
9. Sundaram M, McGuire MH, Herbold DR, et al. Magnetic resonance imaging in planning limb-salvage surgery for primary malignant tumors of bone. J Bone Joint Surg Am 1986;68(6):809–19.
10. Hudson TM, Schakel M 2nd, Springfield DS, et al. The comparative value of bone scintigraphy and computed tomography in determining bone involvement by soft-tissue sarcomas. J Bone Joint Surg Am 1984;66(9):1400–7.
11. Gustafson P. Soft tissue sarcoma. Epidemiology and prognosis in 508 patients. Acta Orthop Scand Suppl 1994;259:1–31.
12. Conrad EU 3rd, Morgan HD, Vernon C, et al. Fluorodeoxyglucose positron emission tomography scanning: basic principles and imaging of adult soft-tissue sarcomas. J Bone Joint Surg Am 2004;86-A(Suppl 2): 98–104.
13. Schuetze SM, Rubin BP, Vernon C, et al. Use of positron emission tomography in localized extremity soft tissue sarcoma treated with neoadjuvant chemotherapy. Cancer 2005;103(2):339–48.
14. Kubo T, Furuta T, Johan MP, et al. A meta-analysis supports core needle biopsy by radiologists for better histological diagnosis in soft tissue and bone sarcomas. Medicine (Baltimore) 2018;97(29):e11567.

15. Mankin HJ, Lange TA, Spanier SS. The hazards of biopsy in patients with malignant primary bone and soft-tissue tumors. J Bone Joint Surg Am 1982;64(8):1121–7.

16. Mankin HJ, Mankin CJ, Simon MA. The hazards of the biopsy, revisited. Members of the Musculoskeletal Tumor Society. J Bone Joint Surg Am 1996; 78(5):656–63.

17. Matsumoto K, Hukuda S, Ishizawa M, et al. MRI findings in intramuscular lipomas. Skeletal Radiol 1999; 28(3):145–52.

18. Hochman M, Adams DM, Reeves TD. Current knowledge and management of vascular anomalies: I. Hemangiomas. Arch Facial Plast Surg 2011;13(3): 145–51.

19. Rimon U, Garniek A, Galili Y, et al. Ethanol sclerotherapy of peripheral venous malformations. Eur J Radiol 2004;52(3):283–7.

20. Mavrogenis AF, Soucacos PN, Papagelopoulos PJ. Heterotopic ossification revisited. Orthopedics 2011;34(3):177.

21. Cable MG, Randall RL. Extremity soft tissue sarcoma: tailoring resection to histologic subtype. Surg Oncol Clin N Am 2016;25(4):677–95.

22. Gilbert NF, Cannon CP, Lin PP, et al. Soft-tissue sarcoma. J Am Acad Orthop Surg 2009;17(1):40–7.

23. Weitz J, Antonescu CR, Brennan MF. Localized extremity soft tissue sarcoma: improved knowledge with unchanged survival over time. J Clin Oncol 2003;21(14):2719–25.

24. Bakri A, Shinagare AB, Krajewski KM, et al. Synovial sarcoma: imaging features of common and uncommon primary sites, metastatic patterns, and treatment response. AJR Am J Roentgenol 2012; 199(2):W208–15.

25. Ferrari A, Gronchi A, Casanova M, et al. Synovial sarcoma: a retrospective analysis of 271 patients of all ages treated at a single institution. Cancer 2004;101(3):627–34.

26. Shieber W, Graham P. An experience with sarcomas of the soft tissues in adults. Surgery 1962;52:295–8.

27. Yang JC, Chang AE, Baker AR, et al. Randomized prospective study of the benefit of adjuvant radiation therapy in the treatment of soft tissue sarcomas of the extremity. J Clin Oncol 1998;16(1):197–203.

28. Nathenson MJ, Conley AP, Sausville E. Immunotherapy: A New (and Old) Approach to Treatment of Soft Tissue and Bone Sarcomas. Oncologist 2018;23(1):71–83.

29. Giuliano AE, Eilber FR. The rationale for planned reoperation after unplanned total excision of soft-tissue sarcomas. J Clin Oncol 1985;3(10):1344–8.

30. Lewis JJ, Leung D, Espat J, et al. Effect of reresection in extremity soft tissue sarcoma. Ann Surg 2000; 231(5):655–63.

31. Noria S, Davis A, Kandel R, et al. Residual disease following unplanned excision of soft-tissue sarcoma of an extremity. J Bone Joint Surg Am 1996;78(5): 650–5.

32. Davis AM, Kandel RA, Wunder JS, et al. The impact of residual disease on local recurrence in patients treated by initial unplanned resection for soft tissue sarcoma of the extremity. J Surg Oncol 1997;66(2): 81–7.

33. O'Sullivan B, Davis AM, Turcotte R, et al. Preoperative versus postoperative radiotherapy in soft-tissue sarcoma of the limbs: a randomised trial. Lancet 2002; 359(9325):2235–41.

34. Bedi M, King DM, DeVries J, et al. Does Vacuum-assisted Closure Reduce the Risk of Wound Complications in Patients With Lower Extremity Sarcomas Treated With Preoperative Radiation? Clin Orthop Relat Res 2019;477(4):768–74.

35. Peat BG, Bell RS, Davis A, et al. Wound-healing complications after soft-tissue sarcoma surgery. Plast Reconstr Surg 1994;93(5):980–7.

36. Siegel HJ. Management of open wounds: lessons from orthopedic oncology. Orthop Clin North Am 2014;45(1):99–107.

37. Cordeiro PG, Neves RI, Hidalgo DA. The role of free tissue transfer following oncologic resection in the lower extremity. Ann Plast Surg 1994;33(1):9–16.

38. Wilke BK, Schultz DS, Huayllani MT, et al. Intraoperative indocyanine green fluorescence angiography is sensitive for predicting postoperative wound complications in soft-tissue sarcoma surgery. J Am Acad Orthop Surg 2021;29(10):433–8.

39. Ezuddin NS, Pretell-Mazzini J, Yechieli RL, et al. Local recurrence of soft-tissue sarcoma: issues in imaging surveillance strategy. Skeletal Radiol 2018;47(12):1595–606.

40. King CS, Sebro R. Linear mixed-effects models for predicting sarcoma local recurrence growth rates: Implications for optimal surveillance imaging frequency. Eur J Radiol 2020;132:109308.

41. Gaakeer HA, Albus-Lutter CE, Gortzak E, et al. Regional lymph node metastases in patients with soft tissue sarcomas of the extremities, what are the therapeutic consequences? Eur J Surg Oncol 1988;14(2):151–6.

42. Pisters PW, Leung DH, Woodruff J, et al. Analysis of prognostic factors in 1,041 patients with localized soft tissue sarcomas of the extremities. J Clin Oncol 1996;14(5):1679–89.

43. Grimer R, Judson I, Peake D, et al. Guidelines for the management of soft tissue sarcomas. Sarcoma 2010;2010:506182.

MR Imaging of Benign Soft Tissue Tumors
Highlights for the Practicing Radiologist

Geoffrey M. Riley, MD[a],*, Steven Kwong, MD[a], Robert Steffner, MD[b],
Robert D. Boutin, MD[a]

KEYWORDS

• MR imaging • Soft tissue tumor • Benign neoplasm

KEY POINTS

- Benign soft tissue masses are commonly encountered and outnumber sarcomas by 100 to 1.
- Some benign lesions have unique MR imaging characteristics allowing for a specific diagnosis, but many lesions will generate a differential diagnosis.
- Among the most helpful MR imaging findings are the pattern of T1 and T2 signal intensity (SI) that reflect the presence of fatty, fibrous, myxomatous, mineralized, or hemorrhagic tissue.
- Differential diagnosis can be honed by other characteristics such as clinical history, size, anatomic location, and involved tissue (eg, muscle, nerve).
- The main value of contrast material is to differentiate lesions that are vascularized (solid) versus lesions that contain fluid or necrosis.

INTRODUCTION

Benign soft tissue neoplasms are more frequently encountered than their malignant counterparts with lipomas being the most common. When also including nonneoplastic lesions, such as ganglion cysts, the disproportionate number of benign to malignant lesions becomes even more noteworthy—and therefore it is of great practical importance. Only a small fraction of the many soft tissue masses can be covered here, and the focus is on those the general radiologist will likely encounter with MR imaging.

With all masses on MR imaging, it is essential to report the lesion size, location, and extent (local staging). Soft tissue masses with nonspecific MR imaging findings greater than 5 cm in size often proceed to tissue sampling with histologic diagnosis and thus, there is greater demand on radiologists to distinguish benign versus malignant soft tissue masses measuring less than 5 cm. In a recent large

MR imaging study of small soft tissue tumors (80% deep/20% superficial),[1] the frequency of malignancy significantly decreased with size (≤5 cm, 22%; ≤ 3 cm, 16%; ≤ 2 cm, 15%). The most common benign soft tissue mass is lipoma, comprising approximately 29% of superficial masses. While less likely, small masses are malignant in ~5% of patients, with undifferentiated pleomorphic sarcoma being the most common.[1]

The 2020 World Health Organization (WHO) classification for primary soft tissue masses categorizes tumors into several *families* (or *groups*) based on the cell type that they most closely resemble.[2] Within each family, such as lipomatous tumors, there are further divisions into *types* and *subtypes*.

Although soft tissue masses are frequently nonspecific, there are features characteristic of each type. (Of note, many soft tissue masses that occur in specific locations are not included in this review, such as Morton's neuroma,

[a] Department of Radiology, Stanford University School of Medicine, 453 Quarry Road, MC 5659, Palo Alto, CA 94304, USA; [b] Department of Orthopedic Musculoskeletal Tumor Surgery, Stanford University School of Medicine, 420 Broadway Street 1st Floor Pavilion D MC 6415, Palo Alto, CA 94063, USA
* Corresponding author.
E-mail address: GRILEY@STANFORD.EDU

Radiol Clin N Am 60 (2022) 263–281
https://doi.org/10.1016/j.rcl.2021.11.006

elastofibroma dorsi, and glomus tumor). Even with these hallmarks, MR imaging often cannot reliably distinguish between benign and malignant lesions. This article emphasizes the distinctive features of common benign tumors that facilitate a specific diagnosis or targeted differential diagnosis.

LIPOMATOUS (ADIPOCYTIC) LESIONS
Lipoma

The adipocytic family of tumors is a large group of which lipomas are the most common type. Lipomas occur in many locations, most commonly in superficial soft tissues. Composed almost entirely of mature adipocytes, as their imaging appearance reflects, lipomas and their variants can also contain foci of fibrous stroma, fat necrosis, and even calcification (Box 1.).

The uniform or near-uniform fat tissue signal intensity (SI) on all noncontrast sequences will usually allow a diagnosis without the need for contrast (Fig. 1). Superficial smaller lesions tend to be rounded, whereas lesions deep to subcutaneous fascia are more variable in shape and tend to be larger. At times, the only indication of a tumor may be a deformity of an adjacent structure, such as muscle or skin, and the presence of a thin capsule. Intramuscular lipomas can occasionally contain intermingled muscle fibers that mimic septations. This tissue, however, represents muscle fibers and is isointense with adjacent muscle on all sequences. A few strands of nonfatty tissue can be present in simple lipomas but should be thin (less than 2 mm). Strands of tissue within a true lipoma generally do not enhance avidly; such septal enhancement raises concern for a lesion other than a simple lipoma, such as an

atypical lipomatous tumor (ALT).[3] In addition to thick septae, nodularity, and enhancement, recent studies also have confirmed additional features significantly favoring ALT over lipoma: large lesion size, incomplete fat suppression, and increased architectural complexity.[4,5]

Nonfatty components may be identified in ~15% of lipomatous neoplasms, and when lesions are not uniformly fat SI, the differential diagnosis may include benign lipomatous lesions (eg, lipoma variants such as spindle cell lipoma, hibernoma, angiolipoma, or scar from trauma; see details later in discussion) and malignant neoplasms (statistically far less likely).[6] Liposarcomas characteristically have a heterogeneous appearance with nodularity or interrupted septa.[3] Further, they do not follow uniform fat signal on T1 and T2 fat-suppressed (T2FS) sequences and generally enhance. Other lesions containing both fatty and nonfatty tissue include fat necrosis, which has a markedly variable appearance (Fig. 2).[7] Fat necrosis can be included in the differential diagnosis of a fat-containing subcutaneous mass with heterogeneous SI and contrast enhancement.[8] When mass-like, fat necrosis can appear similar to an ALT.

Ultimately tissue sampling may be necessary to exclude lesions such as ALT or liposarcoma. When an indeterminant lipomatous lesion is biopsied, molecular testing generally includes fluorescence in situ hybridization (FISH) for MDM2 and CDK4 amplification to differentiate benign versus malignant lesions.

Spindle Cell Lipoma

SCLs are classically located in subcutaneous tissues of the posterior neck, upper back, and shoulders, and are at least twice as common in men than women.[2,9] SCLs are typically well-circumscribed with variable amounts of fat, spindle cells, and ropey collagen.[9]

On MR imaging, SCLs usually contain 50% to 90% fat and show variable contrast enhancement.[9] SCLs can pose a diagnostic challenge because of a wide spectrum of MR imaging appearances, including deep locations (up to one-third are intermuscular or intramuscular), hyperintense T2 SI (up to 88%, similar to a cystic or myxoid lesion), and sometimes little or no visible fat (<20%)[9–11] (Fig. 3). The MR imaging differential diagnosis of a soft tissue mass containing fat and other elements includes ALT, liposarcoma, and hibernoma.

Hibernoma

The name "hibernoma" was coined because these benign lesions contain brown fat similar to that

---

> **Box 1**
> **Fatty lesion highlights**
>
> - Lipomas are generally isointense with subcutaneous fat; thin (<2 mm) internal septations may be present
>
> - ATLs contain nonadipose tissues such as thickened (>2 mm) septations and small (<2 cm) nodules, increased T2 SI, and septal/nodular contrast enhancement
>
> - Fat necrosis has a variable appearance and can be included in the differential diagnosis of a fat-containing subcutaneous mass with heterogeneous SI and enhancement
>
> - Hibernomas generally contain tissue with lower T1 and higher T2 SI than subcutaneous fat, internal vessels, and variable contrast enhancement

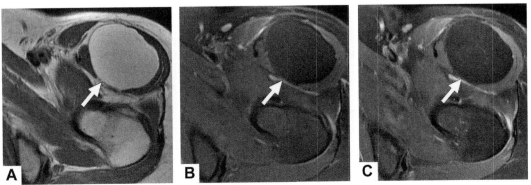

Fig. 1. Lipoma. A 59-year-old woman with intramuscular mass (*arrow*) in the tensor fascia lata muscle. The mass is homogenously isointense to fat on axial T1-weighted (*A*) and T2-weighted fat-suppressed (*B*) images. There is no enhancement on the postcontrast T1-weighted fat-suppressed image (*C*).

seen in hibernating animals. These rare lesions have a predilection for the trunk and proximal extremities, and often occur within muscle or subcutaneous fat.[12,13] On MR imaging, proposed criteria for diagnosing these lesions include hypointense T1 signal relative to subcutaneous fat, hyperintense T2 signal relative to subcutaneous fat, internal vascularity seen as flow voids on T1-weighted images, and variable contrast enhancement.[12–14] (**Fig. 4**). Hibernomas are conspicuous on PET scans owing to intense FDG tracer uptake.

PERIPHERAL NERVE SHEATH TUMORS

Peripheral nerve sheath tumors (PNSTs) are primarily made up of schwannomas and neurofibromas (NF). While some imaging features favor one over the other, it is often not possible to differentiate between them. Schwannomas, as opposed to solitary NFs, can frequently be removed while sparing the involved nerve, a distinction helpful for surgical planning and patient expectations of nerve function following surgery.[15] (**Box 2.**)

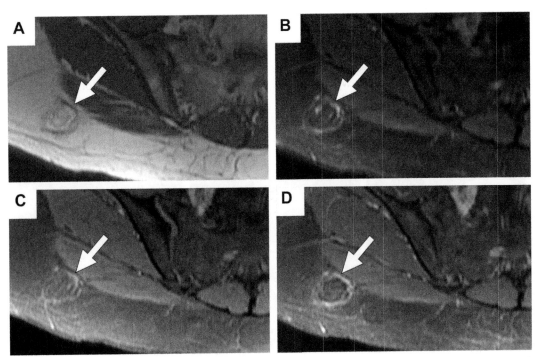

Fig. 2. Fat necrosis. A 49-year-old woman with a well-defined focal area (*arrow*) that is primarily isointense to fat on axial T1-weighted (*A*) and axial T2-weighted fat-suppressed (*B*) images with mild rim and central edema signal. Precontrast axial T1-weighted fat-suppressed image (*C*) shows a slight rim of increased T1 signal that enhances on the postcontrast image (*D*).

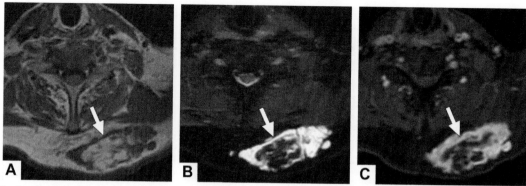

Fig. 3. Spindle cell lipoma. A 72-year-old man with a well-defined multilobulated complex mass (*arrow*) in the posterior neck subcutaneous layer. The mass contains a mix of nonenhancing adipose tissue and intensely enhancing nonadipose tissue on axial T1-weighted (*A*), axial T2-weighted fat-suppressed (*B*), and postcontrast axial T1-weighted fat-suppressed (*C*) images.

Neurofibroma

Ninety percent of NFs are of the localized type, often involving small cutaneous or subcutaneous nerves. Deeper lesions also occur whereby they may involve larger nerves. When associated with NF-1, NFs are often deeper, multiple, and involve larger nerves.[15] Plexiform NF is a subtype that is limited to, and pathognomonic of, NF-1. These consist of diffuse involvement along a long nerve segment and its branches.[16] Resection of plexiform NF results in the loss of nerve function.

Schwannoma (Neurilemoma)

Like NFs, schwannomas are most commonly solitary. A rare syndrome of schwannomatosis consists of multiple schwannomas without the hallmark vestibular nerve involvement typical of NF-2. This has been referred to as the "third form of neurofibromatosis."[17] Large schwannomas can undergo degenerative cystic change with necrosis and hemorrhage in which case they are referred to as ancient schwannomas, a WHO-recognized subtype. Although rare, they can transform into malignant PNST (MPNST).

Magnetic Resonance Imaging of Peripheral Nerve Sheath Tumors

On MR imaging, findings include an entering and exiting nerve, the target sign, the split-fat sign, the fascicular sign, and the thin hyperintense rim sign.[8] Of these, the target sign is most frequent, reportedly more common in NFs than schwannomas.[18] This sign consists of low-to-intermediate SI centrally due to fibrous tissue, with peripheral high T2 SI from myxoid tissue (**Fig. 5**). Postcontrast images may show reversal of the target with higher SI centrally (**Fig. 6**), but the enhancement pattern is variable and can be diffuse. The "split-fat sign" generally refers to the characteristic appearance of soft tissue tumors that arise in the

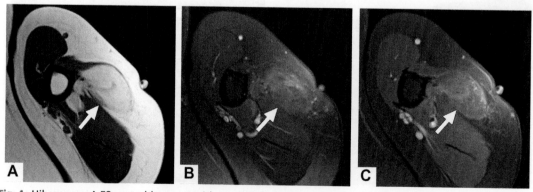

Fig. 4. Hibernoma. A 58-year-old woman with a multilobulated mass (*arrow*) in the anterolateral upper arm with signal intensity slightly less intense than subcutaneous fat on axial T1-weighted (*A*) and incomplete fat suppression on axial T2-weighted fat-suppressed (*B*) images. The postcontrast axial T1-weighted fat-suppressed image (*C*) shows faint heterogenous enhancement consistent with internal vascularity.

intermuscular fat plane and is seen most commonly with PNSTs. Less commonly, PNSTs also can occur within the muscle. *Intramuscular* masses with a "fatty rind" are most frequently due to PNSTs (especially schwannomas) and other benign lesions (eg, myxomas, venous malformations).[19,20]

Plexiform Neurofibroma

Plexiform NF are complex, histologically benign PNSTs that can grow to large sizes and cause significant morbidity (eg, neurologic deficits, refractory pain, deformity). It is the plexiform neurofibroma that results in the massive extremity enlargement known as elephantiasis.[15] The target sign can be present within the multiple lesions that follow a nerve distribution. Heterogeneous enhancement is typical and the pattern is more infiltrative (**Fig. 7**).

As with other soft tissue tumors, MR imaging is the imaging method of choice to document the location, extent, biological activity, and potential malignant transformation of plexiform NF. MR imaging techniques to evaluate these lesions include 3D volumetric measurements[21] combining multiple imaging features (eg, perilesional edema, intralesional necrosis, irregular margins), and assessment for diffusion restriction.[22] Biopsies to evaluate for malignant transformation may be omitted if there is a target sign and the lesion lacks perilesional edema or ill-defined margins.[23] MR imaging utilization is now also important with the advent of exciting new developments in drug treatments for plexiform NF.[24,25]

Malignant transformation of NFs can occur, mostly in the deep plexiform type in patients with NF-1.[26] Findings that suggest MPNST include rapid growth, an enhancing zone of perilesional edema-like SI, and cystic changes[27] (**Fig. 8**). Up to 50% of MPNST cases occur in patients with NF-1, and the 5-year survival rate is generally less than 50%.

VASCULAR ANOMALIES

Vascular tumors are classified in the literature according to 2 vastly different, discordant systems. In our practice, there has been a shift away from the traditional WHO guidelines for vascular tumors to the widely accepted International Society for the Study of Vascular Anomalies (ISSVA) classification system.[28,29] The ISSVA system divides vascular anomalies into 2 broad groups: tumors and malformations (VM). The vascular tumor group consists of true neoplasms of which benign hemangioma is the most common. The vast majority of hemangiomas in the ISSVA system occur in infancy and subsequently often involute.[30] (**Box 3**.)

VMs are generally divided into high-flow and low-flow lesions, which is an important distinction

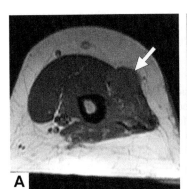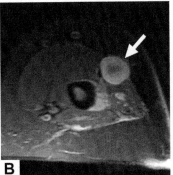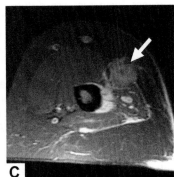

Fig. 5. Neurofibroma. A 26-year-old woman with neurofibromatosis type-1 and a well-circumscribed mass (*arrow*) along the course of the posterior cutaneous nerve. Signal intensity is nearly isointense to muscle on the axial T1-weighted (*A*) image, with hyperintense tissue peripherally, and a central area of low signal intensity (target sign), on the axial T2-weighted (*B*) image. The postcontrast axial T1-weighted fat-suppressed image (*C*) shows peripheral enhancement.

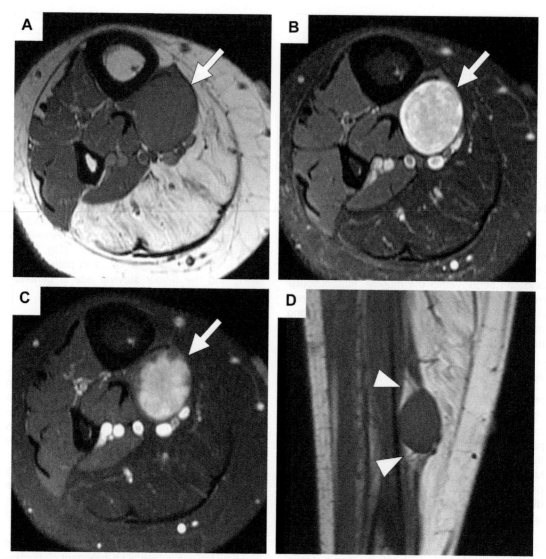

Fig. 6. Schwannoma. A 56-year-old woman with a well-circumscribed intermuscular mass (*arrow*) that is isointense to muscle on axial T1-weighted (*A*) and heterogeneously hyperintense on axial T2-weighted fat-suppressed (*B*) images. There is intense, diffuse central enhancement on the postcontrast axial T1-weighted fat-suppressed image (*C*). Axial T1-weighted image (*D*) shows a tapered rim of fat signal intensity (*arrowheads*) at the proximal and distal ends of the lesion (split fat sign). There is incidental severe fatty infiltration and atrophy of the soleus and gastrocnemius.

for treatment planning.[31] Lesions are considered high flow when any amount of arterial flow is present. These include arteriovenous malformations (AVM) and arteriovenous fistulas (AVF). With the exception of AVFs, which are secondary to trauma, VMs are congenital. The MR imaging hallmark of high-flow lesions is the presence of flow voids with dilated feeding arteries and draining veins (**Fig. 9**). When present, hemorrhage and thrombosis can lead to areas of high T1 SI. The lesions can appear infiltrative and cross tissue planes.

Low-flow lesions lack arterial flow and include venous (most common), lymphatic, capillary, and combined malformations.[28] The venous type is the most common type in the extremities,[32] while lymphatic malformations are most often in the neck. Capillary malformations are usually limited to the dermis.[32]

The MR imaging appearance of low-flow lesions reflects their composition of venous, lymphatic, and capillary components. These lesions often have a lobulated appearance with internal septa, usually without substantial mass effect on adjacent

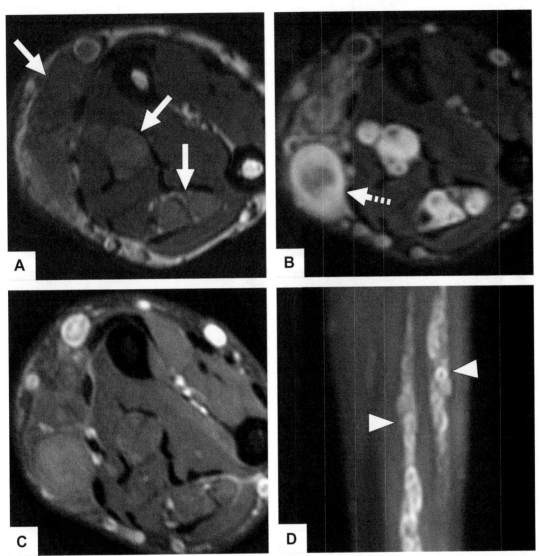

Fig. 7. Plexiform neurofibroma. A 19-year-old woman with extensive multilobulated lesions (*arrows*) along the major nerves in the forearm involving the subcutaneous soft tissues along the lateral forearm. Lesions are slightly hyperintense on axial T1-weighted imaging (*A*) with hyperintense rims (target signs) (dotted *arrow*) on the axial T2-weighted fat-suppressed image (*B*). An axial postcontrast T1-weighted fat-suppressed image (*C*) shows mild enhancement. The sagittal T2-weighted fat-suppressed image (*D*) shows the long segment nerve involvement in the forearm (*arrowheads*).

structures (**Fig. 10**).[33–35] With venous malformations, T1 SI is generally intermediate to hypointense, but foci of high T1 signal can result from areas of fat, acute thrombus, and recent hemorrhage. Low SI phleboliths can be mistaken for low SI flow voids (which would be the characteristic of a high-flow lesion), and therefore correlation with radiographs is helpful. Lymphatic malformations show high T2 SI with variably sized cystic areas. Fluid-fluid levels are characteristically seen in lymphatic malformations, but also can be present in other low-flow vascular malformations.[33,36]

The MR imaging differential diagnosis for VMs may sometimes include a varicose vein. However, varicose veins are more likely subcutaneous, extend over a long course, and involve the lower extremity of older patients. In atypical cases of vascular lesions, the differential diagnosis may include lesions such as a hypervascular sarcoma.[33]

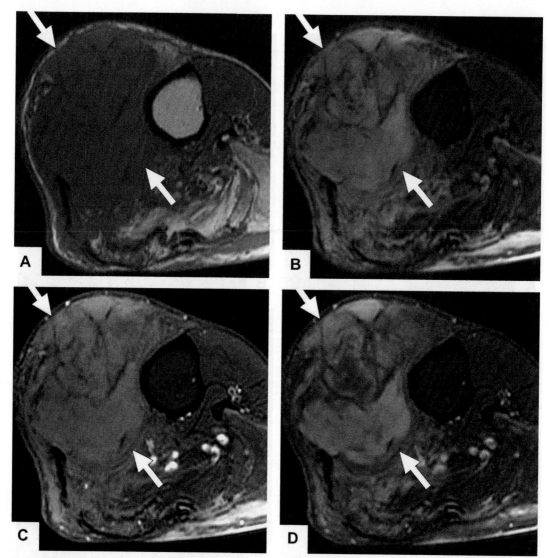

Fig. 8. Malignant transformation of plexiform neurofibroma. A 60-year-old man with a multilobulated lesion (*arrows*) in the medial calf showing signal intensity primarily isointense to muscle and areas of hypointense septations on the T1-weighted image (*A*). The axial T2-weighted fat-suppressed image (*B*) shows areas of low signal intensity septations, central nodularity, and peripheral edema. Precontrast T1-weighted fat-suppressed image (*C*) shows slight heterogeneity. Postcontrast T1-weighted fat-suppressed image (*D*) shows heterogenous enhancement.

Box 3
Vascular anomaly highlights

- Vascular malformations are generally divided into high-flow and low-flow lesions
- High-flow lesions have flow voids with dilated feeding arteries and draining veins
- Venous malformation is the most common low-flow vascular malformation
- Venous malformation should be considered when the MR imaging shows phleboliths or fat in the interstices of the lesion. Other findings may include feeding/draining vessels, fluid-fluid levels, and intralesional hemorrhage/thrombosis

MYXOMA

Myxomas are composed predominantly of myxoid tissue that has a gelatinous matrix with a very high water content, giving them their characteristic bright homogenous T2 SI. Although myxomas can be variable in size and location, in the extremities they are most often solitary intramuscular lesions (intermuscular and subcutaneous myxomas are rare).[37–39] Multiple intramuscular myxomas can be present in approximately 2% of patients with fibrous dysplasia, a condition termed Mazabraud syndrome.[40] The radiologist should also consider low-grade myxofibrosarcoma, which can have a similar appearance.

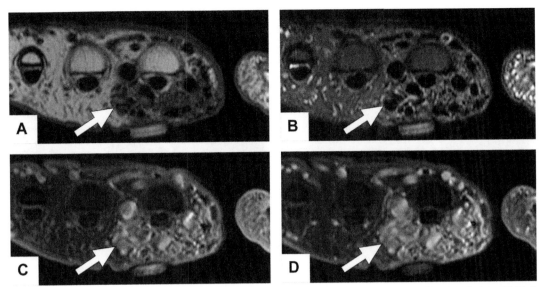

Fig. 9. High-flow vascular malformation. A 37-year-old man with multiple serpiginous flow voids (*arrow*) in the palmar aspect of the hand on axial T1-weighted fat-suppressed (*A*) and T2-weighted fat-suppressed (*B*) images. The presence of flow voids confirms an arterial component. Axial T1-weighted fat-suppressed precontrast (*C*) and postcontrast (*D*) images show the degree of contrast enhancement.

On MR imaging, myxomas generally appear well defined with diffuse fluid-like SI intensity, a rind of perilesional fat, and often some perilesional edema in the surrounding muscle (**Fig. 11**).[37,41] Given their fluid-like T2 SI, contrast-enhanced imaging may be necessary to confirm a solid lesion, typically with lacy internal enhancement.[38]

Benign lesions in the differential include cysts, PNSTs, and other myxoid lesions. Malignant tumors with bright T2 SI suggesting myxoid tissue include myxofibrosarcoma and myxoid liposarcoma. Unlike myxomas, myxoid liposarcoma will usually contain a small amount of fat. Low-grade myxofibrosarcomas will have a more pronounced enhancement than myxomas.

FIBROBLASTIC/MYOFIBROBLASTIC TUMORS

Within this large family of tumors, those discussed include nodular fasciitis, fibromatoses (superficial and deep), and fibroma of the tendon sheath.

Nodular Fasciitis

Nodular fasciitis usually presents as a small, rapidly growing lesion in young to middle-aged patients.[42,43] The most common location is the upper

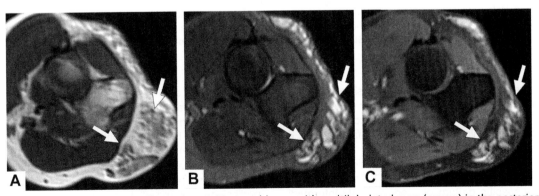

Fig. 10. Low-flow vascular malformation. A 35-year-old man with multilobulated mass (*arrows*) in the posterior elbow subcutaneous layer. The mass contains fat signal intensity within the lesion interstices and is predominantly hypointense on axial T1-weighted (*A*) and hyperintense on axial proton density fat-suppressed images (*B*). There are no flow-voids as are seen in the high-flow vascular malformation (see **Fig. 9**). The postcontrast axial T1-weighted fat-suppressed image (*C*) shows intense contrast enhancement.

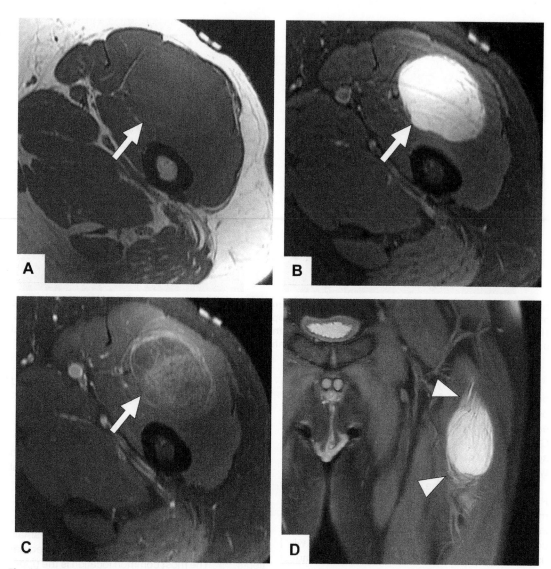

Fig. 11. Intramuscular myxoma. A 69-year-old man with a well-defined intramuscular mass (*arrow*) in the anterior thigh compartment showing T1-weighted signal intensity hypointense to muscle on the axial T1-weighted image (*A*) and fluid-like signal intensity on the axial T2-weighted fat-suppressed image (*B*). Postcontrast axial T1-weighted fat-suppressed image (*C*) shows peripheral rim and faint central heterogenous enhancement, which would not be present in a true cyst. Note the faint perilesional edema (*arrowheads*) on the coronal T2-weighted fat-suppressed image (*D*).

extremity (more than one-third of lesions), followed by the head/neck, trunk, and lower extremity.[44,45] They may be further classified according to the location within the subcutaneous fat, muscle, or tracking along fascia.

On MR imaging, nodular fasciitis is usually small (2–4 cm) (Fig. 12).[46] There is often a nonspecific pattern of predominantly intermediate T1 and increased T2 SI, but ancillary MR imaging signs also have been described. The "fascial tail sign" (linear extension of the lesion that resembles a tail) is reported in greater than

25% of cases and is significantly more frequent with nodular fasciitis than other soft tissue lesions.[45] The "inverted target sign" (nonenhancing central area of high T2 SI, with surrounding lower SI peripherally) has been described in greater than 10% of cases.[45] In less than 10% of cases the margins are ill-defined and associated with perilesional edema ("cloud sign"), which can appear similar to early myositis ossificans (Fig. 13). It is important to correlate with a clinical history of trauma, rapid growth, and subsequent size stability.

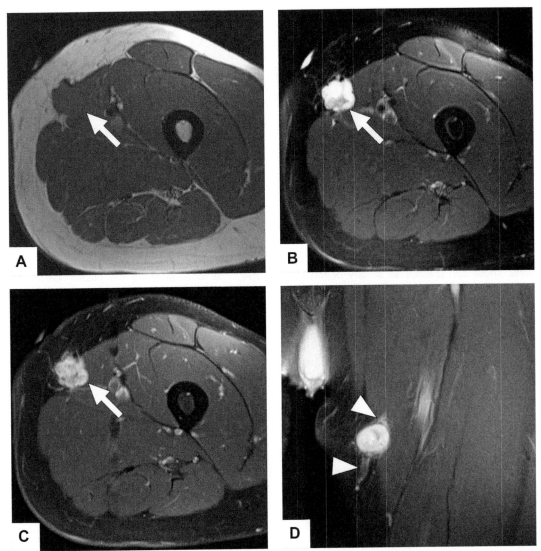

Fig. 12. Nodular fasciitis. A 55-year-old man with lobulated mass (*arrow*), likely arising from the fascia of the medial thigh. The lesion shows T1 signal intensity similar to muscle (*A*) and hyperintense signal on the axial T2-weighted fat-suppressed image (*B*). Postcontrast axial T1-weighted fat-suppressed image (*C*) displays intense, mildly heterogenous enhancement. Note the adjacent edema (*arrowheads*) on the coronal proton density-weighted fat-suppressed image (*D*).

Superficial Fibromatosis

Palmar fibromatosis

Palmar fibromatosis occurs in older patients and is usually diagnosed clinically.[47] Superficial palmar involvement occurs in hands and fingers and is often multifocal. Coalescence of aponeurotic nodules into fibrous cords involving flexor tendons results in a flexion contraction clinically known as Dupuytren's contracture. The clinical differential diagnosis may include stenosing flexor tendon tenosynovitis ("trigger finger").

Typical MR imaging findings consist of multiple nodular masses in the volar hand fascial structures. In the early stage, lesions show high T2 SI and contrast enhancement (owing to more cellularity and vascularity). In the later stage, lesions demonstrate low T1 and T2 SI, with diminished contrast enhancement (owing to dense collagen bundles) (**Fig. 14**). This distinction can be helpful for surgical planning as lesions in the initial proliferative stage more often recur after excision.[48]

Plantar fibromatosis

Foot lesions occur in a younger age group (usually 30–50 years of age) than their counterpart hand

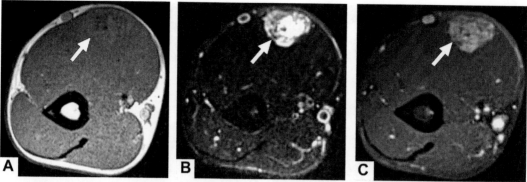

Fig. 13. Myositis ossificans. A 28-year-old man with an intramuscular upper arm mass with isointense signal intensity on axial T1-weighted (*A*) and hyperintense signal intensity on axial T2-weighted fat-suppressed images (*B*). There are punctate foci of low signal intensity on all sequences owing to small internal foci of mineralization. Postcontrast axial T1-weighted fat-suppressed image (*C*) shows lesion enhancement.

lesions. These can present as solitary or multiple nodules with a fascial tail, most commonly in the middle plantar fascia cord.[47] Imaging characteristics are similar to the palmar type with immature lesions showing higher T1 and T2 SI, while mature lesions appear as dark T1 and T2 intensity (**Fig. 15**).[43] The enhancement pattern is also similar to the palmar

type. The location along the plantar fascia and appearance suggests the correct diagnosis in most cases. Differential diagnostic considerations may include tenosynovial giant cell tumor (TGCT) and fibroma of the tendon sheath (FTS) (discussed later). Fibromatosis is less likely to show bony changes than TGCT or FTS.

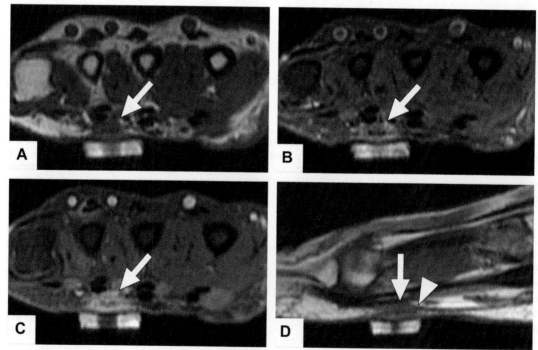

Fig. 14. Palmar fibromatosis. A 55-year-old woman with a small area of fusiform thickening at the palmar fascia (*arrow*) showing signal intensity isointense to muscle on axial T1-weighted image (*A*), intermediate signal intensity on axial T2-weighted fat-suppressed image (*B*), and enhancement on the postcontrast axial T1-weighted fat-suppressed image (*C*). Note the fascial tail that tapers along the palmar fascia (*arrowhead*) on the sagittal T1-weighted image (*D*) similar to the foot plantar fibromatosis on **Fig 15**.

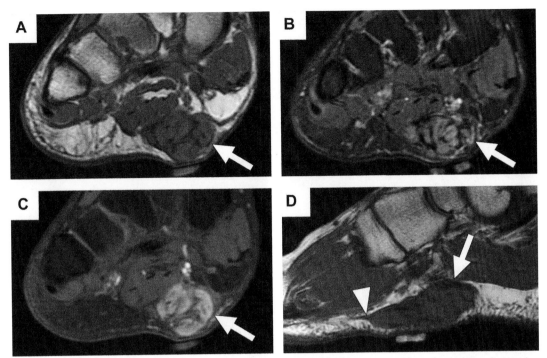

Fig. 15. Plantar fibromatosis. A 51-year-old man with fusiform thickening of the plantar fascia (*arrow*) that demonstrates signal intensity predominantly similar in signal intensity to muscle on axial T1-weighted image (*A*), intermediate signal intensity on axial T2-weighted fat-suppressed image (*B*), and contrast enhancement on the postcontrast T1-weighted fat-suppressed image (*C*). Note the fascial tail of tissue that tapers along the plantar fascia (*arrowhead*) on sagittal T1-weighted image (*D*).

Desmoid (Deep) Fibromatosis

The 2020 WHO classification uses the term *desmoid fibromatosis* (DF) to include both extraabdominal and abdominal subtypes of DF. Alternative terms for DF include *aggressive fibromatosis* and *desmoid tumor*. These neoplasms are classified as having intermediate biological aggressiveness.

The extraabdominal type of DF occurs in a variety of locations. The shoulder and upper arm regions are the most common locations, but other sites include the gluteal, lower extremity, and chest wall/back regions. DF is intimately associated with muscle and fascia,[49] and are occasionally multicentric.[47] The abdominal subtype arises from the musculoaponeurotic structures of the abdominal wall and tends to occur in young women (**Fig. 16**).

DFs may have either well-defined or ill-defined borders, and SI can be highly variable. As with the superficial fibromatoses, the T2 SI and amount of enhancement decrease as the lesion becomes less cellular, findings indicative of lesion maturation or effective treatment (**Fig. 17**). MR imaging signs associated with DF have been described; although not all are specific (**Box 4**).[50] Although the differential diagnosis of T2 hypointense soft

tissue masses is long,[51] the most common MR imaging differential considerations for DF include TGCT (which often occurs in different locations) and sarcoma (which often have heterogeneous, predominantly hyperintense T2 SI).

TENOSYNOVIAL GIANT CELL TUMOR

Within the *so-called fibrohistiocytic* group of lesions in the WHO 2020 classification, the most common is TGCT. TGCT has many manifestations that vary by the site (intraarticular vs extraarticular, bursa, or tendon), and extent (localized vs diffuse or multifocal). For the past decade, the term TGCT has been used as an overarching term to include lesions formerly referred to as *pigmented villonodular synovitis* (PVNS) and giant cell tumor of the tendon sheath.

When localized, the most common site affected in the hand and wrist, particularly targeting the tendon sheaths in the fingers. When diffuse, the knee is the most common site, within or around the joint. A helpful clinical clue to the diagnosis is recurrent, hemorrhagic joint effusions with hemorrhagic fluid on arthrocentesis.[52]

On MR imaging, the localized form of TGCT has well-defined margins with intermediate to low T1

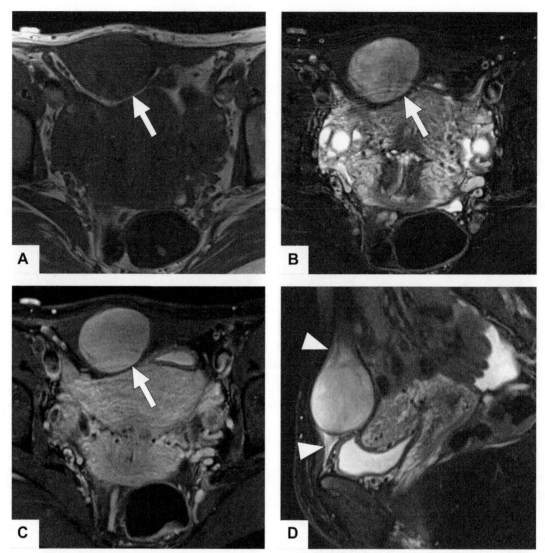

Fig. 16. Desmoid fibromatosis. A 32-year-old woman with a well-circumscribed mass (*arrow*) in the rectus abdominis muscle showing signal intensity isointense to muscle on axial T1-weighted image (*A*), increased signal intensity on axial T2-weighted fat-suppressed image (*B*), and enhancement on the postcontrast axial T1-weighted image (*C*). Note the fascial tail of edema-like signal (*arrowheads*) on the sagittal STIR image (*D*) is similar to that seen with nodular fasciitis (see **Fig. 12**).

SI. Lesions are characteristically hypointense on conventional T2 images, although increased T2 SI may be seen when fat-suppression changes the dynamic range of T2 images (**Fig. 18**). Diffuse lesions have irregular margins, and intraarticular lesions are associated with synovial thickening with nodularity. One of their hallmarks is low SI "blooming artifact" on gradient-echo images due to hemosiderin deposition (see **Fig. 18**). While this is a helpful finding when present, it is less common in localized TGCT. Pressure bone erosions, subcortical cysts, and bone marrow edema

are more common in smaller less capacious joints.[53] Contrast enhancement is usually present but variable in extent.[54]

Other neoplasms with dark T1 and T2 SI include DF and fibroma of the tendon sheath (described later). TGCT is favored over DF when blooming artifact is observed on gradient-echo images, and when lesions are located in joints and around tendons. When articular erosions are present, the differential diagnosis may include synovial chondromatosis, inflammatory/infectious arthritis, and hemophiliac arthropathy.

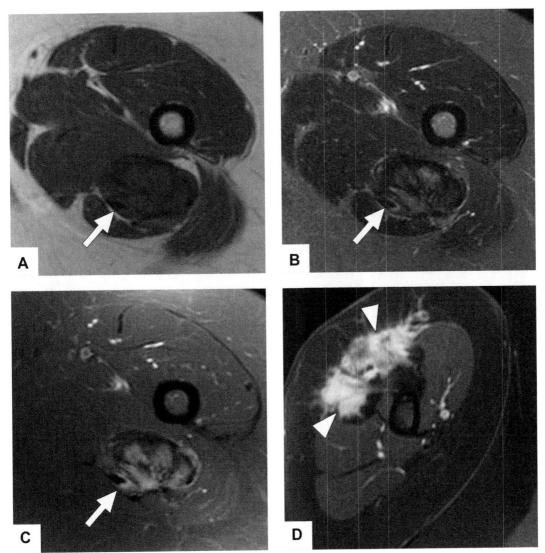

Fig. 17. Desmoid fibromatosis. A 52-year-old woman with a soft tissue mass (*arrow*) deep to the gluteus maximus muscle with bands of low signal intensity (band sign) on axial T1-weighted (*A*), axial T2-weighted fat-suppressed (*B*), and postcontrast axial T1-weighted fat-suppressed (*C*) images. In a different patient, a 48-year-old man, a postcontrast axial T1-weighted fat-suppressed image (*D*) shows internal enhancement with flame-shaped margins (flame sign) and a fascial tail anteriorly and a fascial tail anteriorly (*arrowheads*).

FIBROMA OF THE TENDON SHEATH

FTS, another lesion that can show foci of dark T1 and T2 SI, is most commonly found in the fingers and hand, whereby it involves the flexor surfaces. Other upper extremity locations are possible (Fig. 19).[55,56] Like several other tumors, the SI can vary depending on the amount of cellularity and myxoid tissue. Most, but not all, of these lesions lack overt contrast enhancement.[55] The main differential diagnosis for FTS is TGCT. FTS is considered rare in the lower extremity, and therefore TGCT would be favored in that location.

Box 4
Desmoid fibromatosis MR imaging signs

- Band sign - Linear areas of low T1 and T2 SI
- Flame sign - Feathery margins
- Fascial tail sign - Growth along fascial planes

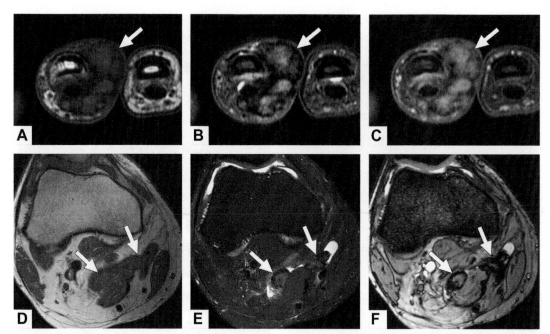

Fig. 18. Tenosynovial giant cell tumor. A 23-year-old woman with a lobulated lesion along the radial aspect of the fourth digit showing heterogenous low signal intensity on axial T1-weighted image (*A*) and heterogenous signal intensity on axial T2-weighted fat-suppressed image (*B*) with internal areas of increased signal intensity. The post-contrast axial T1-weighted fat-suppressed image (*C*) shows mild heterogenous enhancement. Images from a different patient, a 34-year-old man, show a lobulated lesion within a Baker's cyst with predominantly interme-diate signal intensity on the axial T1-weighted (*D*) and axial T2-weighted fat-suppressed image (*E*). Axial gradient-echo image (*F*) shows susceptibility artifact (*arrows*) (blooming), a hallmark of a tenosynovial giant cell tumor.

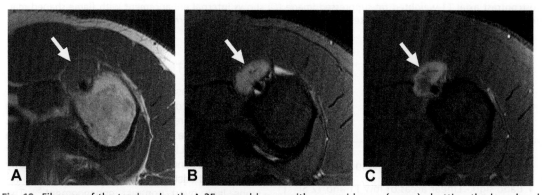

Fig. 19. Fibroma of the tendon sheath. A 35-year-old man with an ovoid mass (*arrow*) abutting the long head biceps tendon sheath with signal intensity isointense to muscle on axial T1-weighted (*A*) and hyperintense on axial T2-weighted fat-suppressed (*B*) images. Postcontrast axial T1-weighted fat-suppressed image (*C*) shows pe-ripheral enhancement.

Box 5
Some characteristic MR imaging features

- Lipoma - Purely or near purely fat SI
- Spindle cell lipoma - Partly fatty tumor in posterior neck
- Hibernoma – T1 SI that is similar but slightly lower than fat
- PNST – Target sign, split fat sign, nerves entering and exiting mass
- Nodular fasciitis - Can mimic other tumors, but are generally small and regresses
- Superficial fibromatosis - Dark T2 SI in hands and feet
- High-flow vascular malformations - Large vessels with flow voids
- Venous malformations – Vascular channels, intralesional fat, phleboliths
- Myxoma – Fluid-like T2 SI, occasionally with surrounding edema
- Desmoid - Flame sign, band sign
- Tenosynovial giant cell tumor - In or around joints, dark T2 SI
- Fibroma of the tendon sheath - Dark T2 lesion in upper extremity

---

SUMMARY

The overwhelming majority of soft tissue tumors are benign, and several have characteristic imaging features (**Box 5**.) While these features can be helpful in suggesting a diagnosis or specific differential diagnosis, many lesions require clinical correlation and imaging follow-up. When a benign diagnosis is in doubt, tissue sampling is appropriate to establish a definitive histopathologic diagnosis.

CLINICS CARE POINTS

- Most soft masses are benign.
- While often nonspecific there are some imaging features that help narrow the differential diagnosis.
- Clinical history, signal intensity, contrast enhancement, location, size and tissue involved are all factors that should be considered when providing a differential diagnosis.

DISCLOSURE

The authors have nothing to disclose.

REFERENCES

1. Gassert FG, Gassert FT, Specht K, et al. Soft tissue masses: distribution of entities and rate of malignancy in small lesions. BMC Cancer 2021;21(1):93.
2. Cancer WCoTEBStabtLFlAfRo. (WHO classification of tumours series te, 3). v. WHO Classification of Tumours Editorial Board. Soft tissue and bone tumours. 5th edition. Lyon (France): International Agency for Research on Cancer; 2020. p. 2020.
3. Gupta P, Potti TA, Wuertzer SD, et al. Spectrum of Fat-containing Soft-Tissue Masses at MR imaging: the common, the uncommon, the characteristic, and the sometimes confusing. Radiographics 2016;36(3):753–66.
4. Nardo L, Abdelhafez YG, Acquafredda F, et al. Qualitative evaluation of MRI features of lipoma and atypical lipomatous tumor: results from a multicenter study. Skeletal Radiol 2020;49(6):1005–14.
5. Knebel C, Neumann J, Schwaiger BJ, et al. Differentiating atypical lipomatous tumors from lipomas with magnetic resonance imaging: a comparison with MDM2 gene amplification status. BMC Cancer 2019;19(1):309.
6. Berkeley R, Okereke O, Malhotra K, et al. The incidence and relevance of non-fatty components in trunk and extremity lipomatous soft tissue masses. Br J Radiol 2021;94(1122):20201403.
7. Burkholz KJ, Roberts CC, Lidner TK. Posttraumatic Pseudolipoma (Fat Necrosis) Mimicking Atypical Lipoma or Liposarcoma on MRI. Radiol Case Rep 2007;2(2):56–60.
8. Lee SA, Chung HW, Cho KJ, et al. Encapsulated fat necrosis mimicking subcutaneous liposarcoma: radiologic findings on MR, PET-CT, and US imaging. Skeletal Radiol 2013;42(10):1465–70.
9. Jelinek JS, Wu A, Wallace M, et al. Imaging of spindle cell lipoma. Clin Radiol 2020;75(5):396.e15-21.
10. Kirwadi A, Abdul-Halim R, Fernando M, et al. MR imaging features of spindle cell lipoma. Skeletal Radiol 2014;43(2):191–6.
11. Bancroft LW, Kransdorf MJ, Peterson JJ, et al. Imaging characteristics of spindle cell lipoma. AJR Am J Roentgenol 2003;181(5):1251–4.
12. Liu W, Bui MM, Cheong D, et al. Hibernoma: comparing imaging appearance with more commonly encountered

benign or low-grade lipomatous neoplasms. Skeletal Radiol 2013;42(8):1073–8.

13. Ritchie DA, Aniq H, Davies AM, et al. Hibernoma–correlation of histopathology and magnetic-resonance-imaging features in 10 cases. Skeletal Radiol 2006;35(8):579–89.

14. Lee JC, Gupta A, Saifuddin A, et al. Hibernoma: MRI features in eight consecutive cases. Clin Radiol 2006;61(12):1029–34.

15. Murphey MD, Smith WS, Smith SE, et al. From the archives of the AFIP. Imaging of musculoskeletal neurogenic tumors: radiologic-pathologic correlation. Radiographics 1999;19(5):1253–80.

16. Yilmaz S, Ozolek JA, Zammerilla LL, et al. Neurofibromas with imaging characteristics resembling vascular anomalies. AJR Am J Roentgenol 2014; 203(6):W697–705.

17. Koontz NA, Wiens AL, Agarwal A, et al. Schwannomatosis: the overlooked neurofibromatosis? AJR Am J Roentgenol 2013;200(6):W646–53.

18. Jee WH, Oh SN, McCauley T, et al. Extraaxial neurofibromas versus neurilemmomas: discrimination with MRI. AJR Am J Roentgenol 2004;183(3):629–33.

19. Sung J, Kim JY. Fatty rind of intramuscular soft-tissue tumors of the extremity: is it different from the split fat sign? Skeletal Radiol 2017;46(5):665–73.

20. Lee SK, Kim JY, Lee YS, et al. Intramuscular peripheral nerve sheath tumors: schwannoma, ancient schwannoma, and neurofibroma. Skeletal Radiol 2020;49(6):967–75.

21. Cai W, Steinberg SM, Bredella MA, et al. Volumetric MRI Analysis of Plexiform Neurofibromas in Neurofibromatosis Type 1: Comparison of Two Methods. Acad Radiol 2018;25(2):144–52.

22. Wilson MP, Katlariwala P, Low G, et al. Diagnostic Accuracy of MRI for the Detection of Malignant Peripheral Nerve Tumors: A Systematic Review and Meta-Analysis. AJR Am J Roentgenol 2021;28:1–9.

23. Martin E, Geitenbeek RTJ, Coert JH, et al. A Bayesian approach for diagnostic accuracy of malignant peripheral nerve sheath tumors: a systematic review and meta-analysis. Neuro Oncol 2020; 23(4):557–71.

24. Ronsley R, Hounjet CD, Cheng S, et al. Trametinib therapy for children with neurofibromatosis type 1 and life-threatening plexiform neurofibroma or treatment-refractory low-grade glioma. Cancer Med 2021. https://doi.org/10.1002/cam4.3910.

25. Fisher MJ, Shih CS, Rhodes SD, et al. Cabozantinib for neurofibromatosis type 1-related plexiform neurofibromas: a phase 2 trial. Nat Med 2021;27(1): 165–73.

26. Tucker T, Wolkenstein P, Revuz J, et al. Association between benign and malignant peripheral nerve sheath tumors in NF1. Neurology 2005;65(2):205–11.

27. Wasa J, Nishida Y, Tsukushi S, et al. MRI features in the differentiation of malignant peripheral nerve

sheath tumors and neurofibromas. AJR Am J Roentgenol 2010;194(6):1568–74.

28. ISSVA Classification of Vascular Anomalies ! 2018 International Society for the Study of Vascular Anomalies. Available at: issva.org/classification. Accessed October 16, 2018.

29. Kuhn KJ, Cloutier JM, Boutin RD, et al. Soft tissue pathology for the radiologist: a tumor board primer with 2020 WHO classification update. Skeletal Radiol 2021;50(1):29–42.

30. Ahlawat S, Fayad LM, Durand DJ, et al. International Society for the Study of Vascular Anomalies Classification of Soft Tissue Vascular Anomalies: Survey-Based Assessment of Musculoskeletal Radiologists' Use in Clinical Practice. Curr Probl Diagn Radiol 2019;48(1):10–6.

31. McCafferty IJ, Jones RG. Imaging and management of vascular malformations. Clin Radiol 2011;66(12): 1208–18.

32. Fayad LM, Hazirolan T, Bluemke D, et al. Vascular malformations in the extremities: emphasis on MR imaging features that guide treatment options. Skeletal Radiol 2006;35(3):127–37.

33. Moukaddam H, Pollak J, Haims AH. MRI characteristics and classification of peripheral vascular malformations and tumors. Skeletal Radiol 2009;38(6): 535–47.

34. Donnelly LF, Adams DM, Bisset GS 3rd. Vascular malformations and hemangiomas: a practical approach in a multidisciplinary clinic. AJR Am J Roentgenol 2000;174(3):597–608.

35. Flors L, Leiva-Salinas C, Maged IM, et al. MR imaging of soft-tissue vascular malformations: diagnosis, classification, and therapy follow-up. Radiographics 2011;31(5):1321–40 [discussion: 1340–1].

36. Hussein A, Malguria N. Imaging of Vascular Malformations. Radiol Clin North Am 2020;58(4): 815–30.

37. Petscavage-Thomas JM, Walker EA, Logie CI, et al. Soft-tissue myxomatous lesions: review of salient imaging features with pathologic comparison. Radiographics 2014;34(4):964–80.

38. Baheti AD, Tirumani SH, Rosenthal MH, et al. Myxoid soft-tissue neoplasms: comprehensive update of the taxonomy and MRI features. AJR Am J Roentgenol 2015;204(2):374–85.

39. Baltu Y, Arikan ŞM, Dölen UC, et al. Intramuscular myxoma: clinical and surgical observation notes on eleven cases. Int Orthop 2017;41(4):837–43.

40. Majoor BCJ, van de Sande MAJ, Appelman-Dijkstra NM, et al. Prevalence and Clinical Features of Mazabraud Syndrome: A Multicenter European Study. J Bone Joint Surg Am 2019;101(2):160–8.

41. Bancroft LW, Kransdorf MJ, Menke DM, et al. Intramuscular myxoma: characteristic MR imaging features. AJR Am J Roentgenol 2002;178(5): 1255–9.

42. Coyle J, White LM, Dickson B, et al. MRI character-istics of nodular fasciitis of the musculoskeletal sys-tem. Skeletal Radiol 2013;42(7):975–82.

43. Walker EA, Petscavage JM, Brian PL, et al. Imaging features of superficial and deep fibromatoses in the adult population. Sarcoma 2012;2012:215810.

44. Lu L, Lao IW, Liu X, et al. Nodular fasciitis: a retro-spective study of 272 cases from China with clinico-pathologic and radiologic correlation. Ann Diagn Pathol 2015;19(3):180–5.

45. Wu SY, Zhao J, Chen HY, et al. MR imaging features and a redefinition of the classification system for nodular fas-ciitis. Medicine (Baltimore) 2020;99(45):e22906.

46. Dinauer PA, Brixey CJ, Moncur JT, et al. Pathologic and MR imaging features of benign fibrous soft-tissue tu-mors in adults. Radiographics 2007;27(1):173–87.

47. Murphey MD, Ruble CM, Tyszko SM, et al. From the archives of the AFIP: musculoskeletal fibromatoses: radiologic-pathologic correlation. Radiographics 2009;29(7):2143–73.

48. Yacoe ME, Bergman AG, Ladd AL, et al. Dupuytren's contracture: MR imaging findings and correlation between MR signal intensity and cellularity of le-sions. AJR Am J Roentgenol 1993;160(4):813–7.

49. Shinagare AB, Ramaiya NH, Jagannathan JP, et al. A to Z of desmoid tumors. AJR Am J Roentgenol 2011;197(6):W1008–14.

50. Braschi-Amirfarzan M, Keraliya AR, Krajewski KM, et al. Role of imaging in management of desmoid-type fibromatosis: a primer for radiologists. Radio-graphics 2016;36(3):767–82.

51. Finkelstein D, Foremny G, Singer A, et al. Differential diagnosis of T2 hypointense masses in musculoskel-etal MRI. Skeletal Radiol 2021. https://doi.org/10.1007/s00256-021-03711-0.

52. Garner HW, Ortiguera CJ, Nakhleh RE. Pigmented villonodular synovitis. Radiographics 2008;28(5):1519–23.

53. Walker EA, Fenton ME, Salesky JS, et al. Magnetic resonance imaging of benign soft tissue neoplasms in adults. Radiol Clin North Am 2011;49(6):1197–217, vi.

54. Murphey MD, Rhee JH, Lewis RB, et al. Pigmented villonodular synovitis: radiologic-pathologic correla-tion. Radiographics 2008;28(5):1493–518.

55. Fox MG, Kransdorf MJ, Bancroft LW, et al. MR imag-ing of fibroma of the tendon sheath. AJR Am J Roentgenol 2003;180(5):1449–53.

56. Emori M, Takashima H, Iba K, et al. Differential diag-nosis of fibroma of tendon sheath and giant cell tu-mor of tendon sheath in the finger using signal intensity on T2 magnetic resonance imaging. Acta Radiol 2020. https://doi.org/10.1177/0284185-120976915. 284185120976915.

Soft Tissue Tumors
Imaging Features of Primary Soft Tissue Malignancies

Felipe Souza, MD[a], Fabiano Nassar Cardoso, MD[a], Chase Cortes[a],
Andrew Rosenberg, MD[b], Ty K. Subhawong, MD[a],*

KEYWORDS

• Soft tissue sarcoma • MR imaging • Tumor • Musculoskeletal oncology • Radiology

KEY POINTS

- STS comprise a heterogeneous group of malignancies that are categorized by the normal mesenchymal tissue that they morphologically resemble
- Key imaging findings that aid in ensuring radiologic-pathologic concordance include macroscopic fat for adipocytic tumors; areas of spontaneous tumor necrosis that denote higher histologic grade, and peritumoral edema associated with locally infiltrative growth.
- Awareness of particular patterns of disease spread is important for appropriate staging of some subtypes:
    o myxoid liposarcoma →bone and soft tissue (early)
    o rhabdomyosarcoma, epithelioid sarcoma, clear cell sarcoma, and angiosarcoma →regional lymph nodes

INTRODUCTION

Soft tissue sarcomas (STS) comprise a heterogeneous group of neoplasms, with more than 50 recognized histologic subtypes.[1] Although STS putatively derive from a population of mesenchymal stem cells, they are conventionally classified according to the type of adult tissue they histologically resemble. STS may arise in almost any location, but are most common in the extremities, the lower and upper extremities accounting for 28% and 12% of cases, respectively. Visceral sites of disease account for 22% of STS, most frequently gastrointestinal stromal tumors (GISTs) and uterine leiomyosarcomas (LMS).[2] In this review, we discuss the multimodality imaging features—with an emphasis on MR imaging —of nonvisceral STS, highlighting representative tumors from the various WHO subtypes. We focus on STS with metastatic potential and on imaging features which may aid the radiologist in categorizing tumor subtype and grade to optimize local staging.

PREDICTING TUMOR GRADE AND STAGING

Histologic grading of STS generally follows a three-tiered system whereby points are assigned based on the degree of differentiation, mitotic count, and tumor necrosis; such systems have been devised by the French Federation of Cancer Centers Sarcoma Group and the National Cancer Institute. Numerous studies have shown histologic grade correlates with more aggressive biologic behavior, and that it is singularly most predictive of metastatic potential and overall survival.[3]

The main goal of this staging system was to garner the most important prognostic factors into

[a] Department of Radiology, Sylvester Comprehensive Cancer Center, University of Miami Miller School of Medicine/Jackson Memorial Hospital, 1611 NorthWest 12th Avenue, JMH WW 279, Miami, FL 33136, USA;
[b] Department of Pathology, Sylvester Comprehensive Cancer Center, University of Miami Miller School of Medicine, 1120 NorthWest 14th St #1407, Miami, FL 33136, USA
* Corresponding author.
E-mail address: tsubhawong@miami.edu

Radiol Clin N Am 60 (2022) 283–299
https://doi.org/10.1016/j.rcl.2021.11.007

one single classification system to evaluate the risk of recurrence and regional or distant metastasis, provide implications for surgical management, and outline guidelines for the use of adjunct therapies (Table 1).[4,5] The Musculoskeletal Tumor Society promptly adopted the Enneking system as the basis for multicenter studies. Although its content has remained unchanged as its inception, the Enneking MSTS staging system is still used by orthopedic surgeons.[4]

On the other hand, the American Joint Committee on Cancer TNM staging system has undergone several revisions since its first publication in 1977 and is currently on its 8th edition (Tables 2 and 3). This staging system is determined by tumor size, histologic grade, and disease spread.[6] The most current edition has dispensed with tumor depth as a factor in the T component of the TNM staging system, and instead relies solely on tumor maximum diameter. Of note, several STS subtypes have a propensity for metastatic spread to lymph nodes, including rhabdomyosarcoma (RMS), clear cell sarcoma, and epithelioid sarcoma (Table 4), such that sentinel node biopsy may be justified for initial staging.[7,8]

Because biopsy may suffer from sampling error, establishing radiologic-pathologic concordance is important to avoid undergrading of STS. MR imaging findings of peritumoral edema and central necrosis have also been found to correlate with higher histologic grade.[9,10] Therefore, tumors with these features should be thoroughly sampled, ideally with image guidance. However, it should be stressed that some high-grade STS do not exhibit peritumoral edema, and that the lack of reactive changes in the surrounding soft tissues should not be taken as evidence of biologic indolence. Standard staging systems do not yet account for more advanced or functional imaging features, despite emerging evidence that such information can be prognostic. Nomograms have also been developed to allow for a personalized computation of various outcome probabilities, such as local recurrence and disease-specific survival, based on patient-specific and tumor-specific characteristics.[11]

TUMOR SUBTYPES

STS subtypes are organized according to the adult tissue types they morphologically resemble; tumors with no obvious normal mesenchymal counterpart are placed under the category of uncertain differentiation. Although the imaging appearance of STS is often indeterminate even with advanced imaging, familiarity with these entities is important for the radiologist in formulating a relevant differential diagnosis, especially when certain characteristic features may be present. Knowledge of tumor subtypes is also important in planning biopsy to target the highest grade or least differentiated tumor component, while also avoiding purely necrotic tissue.[1] Ultimately, close collaboration between radiologists and pathologists, surgeons, and medical and radiation oncologists in a multidisciplinary setting is crucial in ensuring diagnostic congruence between radiologic and pathologic findings, and in synthesizing optimal treatment plans. While not exhaustive, the following discussion provides an overview of the major WHO STS subtypes with representative imaging and histologic findings.

Adipocytic

Lipomatous tumors represent the most common type of STS, comprising approximately 20% to 25% of all STS.[2] These tumors may be recognized as adipocytic in origin by demonstrating macroscopic fat, which may be evident both radiographically and on MR imaging. The recognized liposarcoma subtypes include well-differentiated/dedifferentiated, myxoid/round cell, and pleomorphic liposarcomas.[12]

Atypical lipomatous tumor/well-differentiated/dedifferentiated liposarcoma

While atypical lipomatous tumor and well-differentiated liposarcoma are histologically identical, the term "well-differentiated liposarcoma" (WDL) is reserved for those tumors found within the abdomen, retroperitoneum, spermatic cord, or mediastinum. "Atypical lipomatous tumor" (ALT) is used for tumors in the extremities. Increasing age, larger tumor size, the presence of thick (>2 mm) septations, areas of hyperintensity on fluid-sensitive

Table 1
Enneking/MSTS staging system for soft tissue sarcomas

Stage	Grade	Site	Metastases
IA	Low	Intracompartmental	—
IB	Low	Extracompartmental	—
IIA	High	Intracompartmental	—
IIB	High	Extracompartmental	—
III	Any	Any	Present (regional or distant)

Malignant lesions are classified using roman numerals and letters, and benign lesions using Arabic numerals 1, 2, and 3 to designate latent, active, and aggressive lesions, respectively.

Table 2
Local tumor T definitions for anatomic sites

Primary Tumor Site	Trunk and Extremity	Retroperitoneum	Head and Neck	Visceral Site
TX	Primary tumor cannot be assessed	Primary tumor cannot be assessed	Primary tumor cannot be assessed	Primary tumor cannot be assessed
T0	No primary tumor evidence	No primary tumor evidence	N/A	N/A
T1	Tumor ≤ 5 cm dimension	Tumor ≤ 5 cm dimension	Tumor ≤ 2 cm	Organ confined
T2	Tumor > 5 cm to ≤ 10 cm dimension	Tumor > 5 cm to ≤ 10 cm dimension	>2 cm to ≤ 4 cm	Tumor invasion of tissue beyond organ
T3	Tumor > 10 cm to ≤ 15 cm dimension	Tumor > 10 cm to ≤ 15 cm dimension	>4 cm	Tumor invasion of another organ
T4	Tumor >15 cm dimension	Tumor >15 cm dimension	Tumor invasion to adjoining structures	Multifocal tumor involvement
T4a	N/A	N/A	Tumor with orbital, central compartment viscera, facial skeleton invasion	Multifocal tumor involvement (2 sites)
T4b	N/A	N/A	Tumor with brain parenchymal, prevertebral muscle, central system invasion	Multifocal tumor involvement (3–5 sites)
T4c	N/A	N/A	N/A	Multifocal tumor involvement (>5 sites)

Adapted from Part IX Soft Tissue Sarcoma. Amin MB, Edge S, Greene F, et al. AJCC Cancer Staging Manual. 8th edition. Springer International Publishing; 2017. 214-239. Used with permission of the American College of Surgeons, Chicago, Illinois. The original source for this information is the AJCC Cancer Staging System (2020).

sequences, and nodular areas of nonfatty soft tissue density/signal raise the likelihood of WDL/ALT over lipoma.[13] However, significant imaging overlap with benign fatty tumors exists due to possible involutional changes within lipomas as well as several lipoma variants (such as spindle cell lipoma) that can mimic WDL/ALT or dedifferentiated liposarcoma.[14,15] Moreover, the sclerosing variant of WDL may exhibit little macroscopic fat with variable enhancing nonlipomatous elements and an increased propensity for dedifferentiation.[16] As with WDL from which they arise, 90% of dedifferentiated liposarcomas (DDLS) show amplification and overexpression of the MDM2, HMGA2, and CDK4 oncogenes. The dedifferentiated component may be comprised of undifferentiated pleomorphic sarcoma (UPS), RMS, LMS, osteosarcoma, or chondrosarcoma.[14] Radiologically, it may manifest as a small soft tissue nodule within a larger well-differentiated tumor, or overtake and replace the low-grade component as the dominant morphologic component (**Fig. 1**).[12] It is the dedifferentiated component which metastasizes, most frequently to lung, with median survival rates of DDLS reported to be approximately 43% in the retroperitoneum and 67% in the extremities.[17]

Myxoid/ round cell liposarcoma
Approximately 30% to 40% of extremity liposarcomas are of the myxoid/round-cell subtype, with higher round cell components associated with poorer prognosis.[18] They often occur in the intermuscular fascial planes and more frequently occur in the medial thigh and popliteal regions and show varying amounts of macroscopic fat (**Fig. 2**).[18,19] These tumors may simulate cysts on fluid sensitive sequences due to the high water content of the myxomatous tumor elements. Avid contrast-

Table 3
American joint committee on cancer staging system for soft tissue sarcomas

Stage	Tumor	Nodes	Metastases	Grade	Brief Summary of the Stage
IA	T1	N0	M0	G1, Gx	Low-grade tumors < 5 cm
IB	T2, T3, or T4	N0	M0	G1, Gx	Low-grade tumors > 5 cm
II	T1	N0	M0	G2, G3	High-grade tumors < 5 cm
IIIA	T2	N0	M0	G2, G3	High-grade tumors 5–10 cm
IIIB	T3 or T4	N0	M0	G2, G3	High-grade tumors > 10 cm
IVA	Any	N1	M0	Any G	Any tumor involving the lymph node
IVB	Any	Any N	M1	Any G	Any tumor with distant metastases

Gx = grade cannot be assessed, G1 = French Federation of Cancer Centers Sarcoma (Fédération Nationale des Center de Lutte Contre le Cancer [(FNCLCC)] grade 1, total differentiated, mitotic count, and necrosis score of 2 or 3, G2 = FNCLCC grade 2, total differentiated, mitotic count, and necrosis score of 4 or 5, G3 = FNCLCC grade 3, total differentiated, mitotic count, and necrosis score of 2 or 3, M0 = no distant metastasis, M1 = distant metastasis, N0 = no regional lymph node metastasis (or status unknown), N1 = regional lymph node metastasis, Tx = primary tumor cannot be assessed, T0 = no evidence of primary tumor, T1 = tumor ≤ 5 cm in greatest dimension, T2 = tumor greater than 5 cm and ≤ 10 cm in greatest dimension, T3 = tumor greater than 10 cm and ≤ 15 cm in greatest dimension, T4 = tumor greater than 15 cm in greatest dimension.

enhancement has been correlated with worse prognosis,[20] as have select radiomics features that quantify tumor heterogeneity.[21] Importantly for staging and surveillance, the commonest sites of early metastatic disease are extrapulmonary and include the soft tissues and bone, with pulmonary metastases usually occurring later.[22,23] Of note, bone lesions in this disease may be occult on CT[24]; therefore, spine or whole-body MR imaging is justified for initial staging and during surveillance.

Pleomorphic liposarcoma

Pleomorphic liposarcoma is a rare but aggressive liposarcoma variant that frequently demonstrates

Table 4
STS with nodal metastases

Soft Tissue Sarcoma Subtype	Incidence
Rhabdomyosarcoma	20%–55% (alveolar highest)
Clear cell sarcoma	19%–23%
Epithelioid sarcoma	15%–20%
Myxoid/Round Cell liposarcoma	19%
Ewing sarcoma	14%
Angiosarcoma	8%–12%
Synovial sarcoma	3%–4%
Overall	5%

Incidence of regional nodal metastases by sarcoma subtype. Despite prior suggestions of heightened risk of nodal metastases with synovial sarcoma, recent data from the SEER registry suggest this risk is in line with the overall rate of STS nodal metastases of approximately 5%.

internal hemorrhage but little to no macroscopic fat on imaging (**Fig. 3**). The presence of lipoblasts constitutes the defining histologic feature of this subtype, and areas of necrosis and an infiltrative growth pattern are frequent.[25] Lung metastases are frequent and prognosis is poor compared with other liposarcoma subtypes, with 5-year survival rates reported to be around 60%.[26]

Fibroblastic/Myofibroblastic

Fibroblastic/myofibroblastic tumors are a heterogeneous group of neoplasms composed of neoplastic spindle-shaped fibroblasts admixed with plumper myofibroblasts that contain more cytoplasm and conspicuous nucleoli. The cell populations of these tumors often show different staining patterns.[27] We discuss 3 of the more commonly encountered subtypes.

Myxofibrosarcoma

Myxofibrosarcoma (MFS) is one of the most common STS in the elderly. It is characterized by a high rate of local recurrence, with 5-year local recurrence rate estimated at 18%, and 5-year overall survival of 77%.[28] These tumors produce a myxoid matrix—a gelatinous, watery substance composed of sulfated (chondroitin sulfate, keratan sulfate) and nonsulfated (hyaluronic acid) glycosaminoglycans.[29] Whereas most STS grow as discrete round or oval masses, MFS often has an infiltrative border (macroscopically and microscopically) that extends into surrounding tissues for substantial distances along normal anatomic planes, particularly fascial planes, resulting in distant microscopic tumor deposits that predispose to local recurrence after resection.[30] At MR imaging, this infiltrative spread may manifest

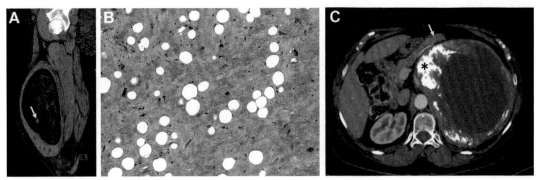

Fig. 1. Well-differentiated liposarcoma with focal intratumoral dedifferentiation. (A) Sagittal CT shows a small 1 cm nonlipomatous soft tissue nodule (arrow) that was proven histologically to be dedifferentiated liposarcoma, completely surrounded by well-differentiated tumor which shows numerous thickened septations superiorly. In such cases, marginal resection of the well-differentiated component is generally considered adequate, as it achieves wide negative margins for the dedifferentiated component. (B) H&E stain of well-differentiated liposarcoma shows the tumor cells mimic adipocytes and are present amidst a background of pink collagenous stroma (C) Axial CT in a different patient demonstrates a large retroperitoneal (note anterior displacement of the pancreas, arrow) dedifferentiated liposarcoma with extensive coarse calcifications (*) but no macroscopically visible fat.

as curvilinear projections, or "tails", that extend from the primary mass of the MFS (Fig. 4).[31] Radiologists should stress enhancing tails as indicative of fascial spread to facilitate complete tumor resection. Moreover, an infiltrative pattern may be seen as the first manifestation of local recurrence, and because it can simulate posttreatment changes and granulation tissue, may lead to delay in diagnosis during surveillance imaging.[32]

Low-grade fibromyxoid sarcoma

Low-grade fibromyxoid sarcoma (LGFMS) is a rare sarcoma subtype predominantly affecting younger adults, with equal predilection for males and females, and estimated to comprise fewer than 5% of STS.[33] Histologically, LGFMS is composed of contrasting fibrous and myxoid areas, and moderate to low cellularity. The spindle cells are bland with minimal nuclear pleomorphism and rare mitotic figures, and display a swirling, whorled growth pattern.[33,34] Despite their deceptive low-grade histology, up to 45% of patients may develop metastatic disease, usually to the chest. Of note, metastases can appear several years after definitive surgery.[34] LGFMS is usually solitary and well-circumscribed, although it may present as an infiltrating mass (Fig. 5).[35] On MR imaging, LGFMS is inhomogeneous, owing to its 2 distinct internal zones: myxoid and fibrous. Generally, the low T1/T2 signal and slight enhancement correspond to fibrous components, while low T1/high T2 signal and variable enhancements correspond to the myxoid components.[35,36] A gyriform pattern of alternating hypointense and hyperintense signal

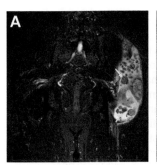
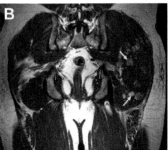
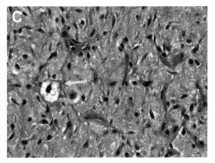

Fig. 2. Myxoid liposarcoma. (A) Coronal fat-suppressed T2 and (B) T1-weighted MR imaging shows a large tumor in the left gluteal soft tissues with numerous globules of macroscopic fat (arrows) encompassed in a T2 hyperintense myxoid matrix in this myxoid liposarcoma. The amount of macroscopic fat identifiable radiologically in myxoid liposarcomas varies considerably and may be absent entirely. (C) H&E stain shows that myxoid liposarcoma contains spindle and stellate cells enmeshed in a myxoid stroma with a plexiform vascular tree and scattered lipoblasts (arrow).

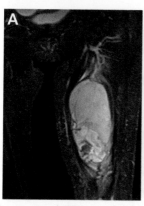 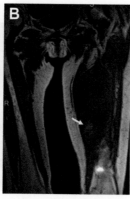 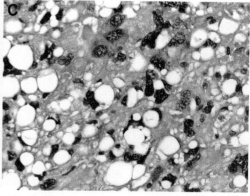

Fig. 3. Pleomorphic liposarcoma. (*A*) Coronal fat-suppressed T2 and (*B*) T1-weighted MR imaging show a large tumor in the left thigh, with only a small component of macroscopic fat identifiable in the inferior aspect (*arrow*) in this pleomorphic liposarcoma. (*C*) H&E stain shows the characteristic pleomorphic lipoblasts of pleomorphic liposarcoma, cells with enlarged pleomorphic nuclei, and fat vacuoles.

or internal nodularity is identified in a majority of cases.[35]

Undifferentiated

UPS is an STS that lacks histologic or molecular markers for any specific line of differentiation and is therefore considered a diagnosis of exclusion.[37] In the same way that many phenotypically defined sarcomas have well-recognized pleomorphic variants, we feel that many tumors that fall into the wastebasket designation of UPS are better characterized as high-grade pleomorphic fibroblastic/myofibroblastic sarcomas.[38] Conceptually, this is also a natural extension in recognizing a high-grade variant of low-grade myofibroblastic sarcoma, but we retain UPS here for purposes of familiarity. CT or MR imaging generally reveals a nonspecific rounded or oval mass that heterogeneously enhances and may contain areas of necrosis and internal hemorrhage (Fig. 6). Most are in the lower extremities (thigh > leg > > upper extremity > retroperitoneum > trunk). The tumor may erode or invade adjacent bone and intratumoral calcification is seen in approximately 15% of cases.[39] High-grade UPS may demonstrate aggressive regional infiltration at presentation, with tumor spreading from the dominant mass in a "tail-like" fashion, similar to that of MFS. Furthermore, MFS with less than 10% myxoid component displays a similar recurrence risk to high-grade UPS.[40] Attempts to uncover actionable driver mutations through next-generation sequencing in this tumor have been disappointing—only one of the 18 patients with UPS had a clinically relevant mutation.[41]

Smooth Muscle

LMS is one of the more common STS, comprising approximately 10% to 20% of malignant mesenchymal neoplasms.[42] LMS metastasizes with high frequency to the lungs, and patients with LMS have 5-year overall survival rates of approximately 70%; increasing size, grade, and tumor depth adversely affect prognosis.[43] LMS may arise in various anatomic sites but can be broadly divided into uterine and extrauterine tumors. Extrauterine tumors may arise within or in close association with the vascular wall, resulting in obliteration of the vessel lumen (Fig. 7). Absent this vascular origin, the imaging findings at CT or MR imaging are nonspecific, showing heterogeneous enhancement.[44,45] This is especially problematic in the uterus, whereby benign leiomyomas may be difficult to distinguish from LMS.[46] Unfortunately, their imaging similarities may lead to unplanned excisions or morcellation of uterine LMS that significantly worsens outcome due to peritoneal seeding.[47] Investigators using histogram analysis have found that LMS is marked by higher signal intensity voxels on T2-weighted images, specifically the mean of the bottom 10th percentile on histogram analysis.[48] Recent work has suggested that optimizing radiomics models may permit more accurate detection of LMS than radiologists.[49]

Skeletal Muscle

The term RMS designates a mesenchymal tumor differentiating like striated muscle. However, RMS typically arises in sites lacking striated muscle.[50] RMS is the most common STS in children, representing more than 50% of all childhood sarcomas, with approximately 80% occurring in individuals younger than 10 years.[51] Histologically, they can be classified into 4 major subtypes: embryonal, the most common type, accounting for about 60% of cases and predominantly seen in children; alveolar, responsible for 30% of cases and also mostly seen in children; pleomorphic, occurring exclusively in the adult population; and spindle cell/sclerosing RMS, which affects both children and adults.[51,52] In pediatrics, unfavorable prognostic factors include alveolar histology,

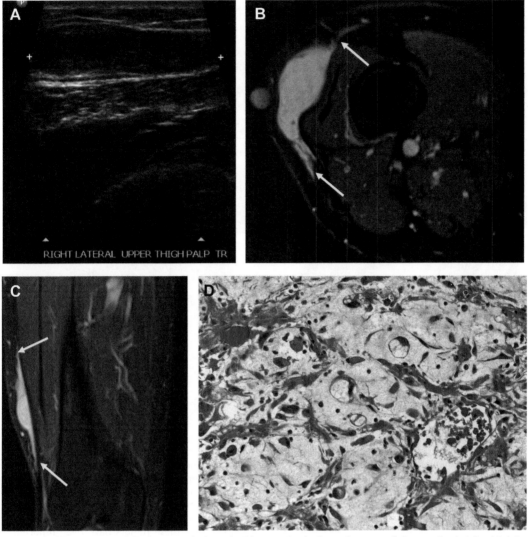

Fig. 4. Myxofibrosarcoma. (*A*) Ultrasound of a palpable mass in the lateral aspect of the proximal right thigh in a 46-year-old woman shows an elongated mass isoechoic to the adjacent subcutaneous fat, simulating a subcutaneous lipoma. (*B*) Axial and (*C*) coronal fat-suppressed PD-weighted images demonstrated a hyperintense tumor growing along the fascia of the vastus lateralis, with tails extending both transversely and craniocaudally (*arrows*). Myxofibrosarcoma was confirmed at biopsy. Careful inspection for these tails is mandatory when planning surgical resection, and generous cuffs of tissue remote from the main soft tissue mass should be anticipated so that wide negative margins can be achieved. In such cases, delaying definitive wound closure pending final histologic margin status may be warranted. (*D*) Histologically the tumor is composed of large polyhedral cells in a myxoid stroma that contains branching blood vessels.

tumor location, lymph node involvement, tumor size greater than 5 cm, and patient age $\geq$10 years.[53] Fusion status has also emerged as a strong independent predictor.[54] An important consideration for staging is that RMS has a high propensity for nodal metastases, with locoregional nodal involvement seen in up to 55% of cases. In transit nodal disease is particularly common in alveolar subtypes.[55,56]

MR imaging characteristics of RMS are nonspecific, usually demonstrating intermediate T1 signal and intermediate to hyperintense T2 signal, with heterogeneous enhancement[57] (**Fig. 8**).

The head and neck are the most common site of involvement of the embryonal subtype, accounting for 50% of all RMS. The most common variant of embryonal RMS is the botryoid variant, its name deriving from its macroscopic resemblance to a bunch of grapes (botryoid in Greek). This variant

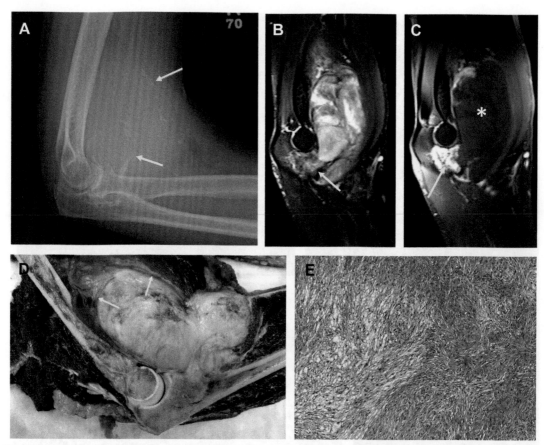

Fig. 5. Low-grade fibromyxoid sarcoma. 32-year-old man with mass in the right elbow. (A) Lateral radiograph demonstrates a large peripherally mineralized soft tissue mass arising from the antecubital fossa. (B) Sagittal fat-suppressed PD-weighted MR imaging demonstrates the heterogeneously hyperintense mass with erosion into the coronoid base and proximal ulna (arrow). (C) Sagittal fat-suppressed contrast-enhanced MR imaging shows enhancement in this invasive intraosseous component (arrow), but otherwise the majority of the tumor shows central nonenhancement (*). (D) Gross specimen after amputation through the upper arm shows the pale tan/white tumor invading the ulna and a surrounding fibrous pseudocapsule (arrows) in this low-grade fibromyxoid sarcoma. Despite their relatively bland cellular morphology, these tumors have been reported to metastasize in up to 45% of cases. (E) H&E stain shows a moderately cellular proliferation of spindle cells with limited atypia in a variable myxocollagenous stroma.

arises in the genitourinary system, which is the second most common site of embryonal RMS after the head and neck.[52] Although not always seen, this type of RMS may sometimes present as a multicystic mass with areas of high signal on T2 corresponding to the areas of the myxoid component, aiding in the diagnosis.[58]

Nerve Sheath

Malignant soft tissue neurogenic tumors are called malignant peripheral nerve sheath tumors (MPNSTs), and account for 3% to 10% of all malignant soft tissue neoplasms.[59,60] About 25% to 50% of cases of MPNSTs are associated with neurofibromatosis type-1, which is the single most important risk factor for developing an MPNST. Patients with deep-seated plexiform

neurofibromas are at particularly high risk because they have a greater potential for malignant transformation.[61] Frequently, they can be identified arising from or in association with a peripheral nerve (Fig. 9). Several studies have described MR imaging characteristics more commonly seen with MPNSTs, which might help differentiate them from benign PNSTs (Table 5).[59,60,62] In addition, DWI might be of help in distinguishing these 2 entities, with values lower than 1.0×10^{-3} mm^2/s^2 and 1.15×10^{-3} mm^2/s^2 for the minimum and mean apparent diffusion (ADC) values, respectively, suggestive of MPNSTs.[60,63,64]

Vascular

Angiosarcoma is a rare STS subtype, representing less than 1% of all STS. It carries a poor prognosis

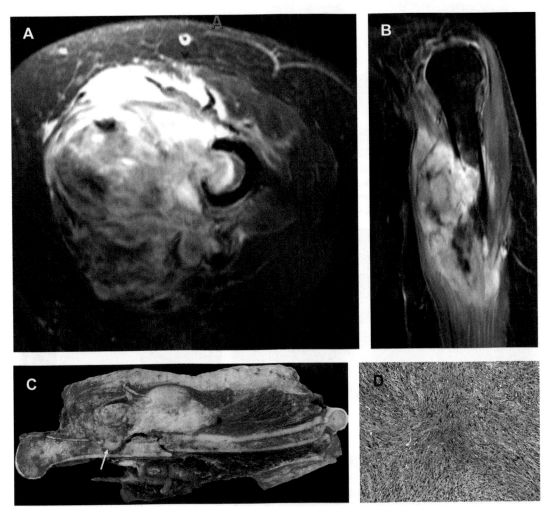

Fig. 6. Leiomyosarcoma. (*A*) Axial fat-suppressed T2-weighted MR imaging demonstrates a large mass in the anterior upper arm, invading the humerus, and peritumoral edema extending into the posterior compartment. (*B*) Coronal fat-suppressed contrast-enhanced T1-weighted MR imaging shows the solidly-enhancing tumor invading bone and infiltrating adjacent musculature. (*C*) Gross specimen after disarticulation shows the tan/white mass along the length of the humerus with osseous invasion (*arrow*); note pathologic fracture through the mid-diaphysis. (*D*) H&E stain highlights the pleomorphic nature of tumor with storiform arrangement of spindle cells with enlarged nuclei in this grade 3 fibroblastic/myofibroblastic sarcoma.

with overall survival ranging from 6 to 16 months.[65,66] Morphologically, angiosarcomas can form poorly organized vessels and solid masses or nodules. Almost half of angiosarcomas arise in the scalp, while only 10% arise in the deep soft tissues.[65] Risk factors include chronic lymphedema (Stewart–Treves syndrome) or prior radiation, with most cases of postradiation angiosarcoma in the breast reported within 5 to 10 years of treatment.[67] Imaging features of deep soft tissue angiosarcomas are generally nonspecific, with CT showing irregular enhancement in a solid mass, and MR imaging depicting infiltration into the surrounding soft tissues[65] (**Fig. 10**). Internal hemorrhage or necrosis may be present. In cutaneous angiosarcomas of

the scalp or radiated breast, skin thi-ckening may be the only salient radiologic finding. This can be difficult to differentiate from radiation-induced induration.[68] Metastases are often to lung and bone, and regional nodal metastases have been reported to occur in approximately 10% of cases.[7]

Tumors of Uncertain Differentiation

There are more than 20 different types of tumors classified under this designation according to the World Health Organization,[69] and a thorough review of each is beyond the scope of this article. Only a few representative malignant entities will be discussed here.

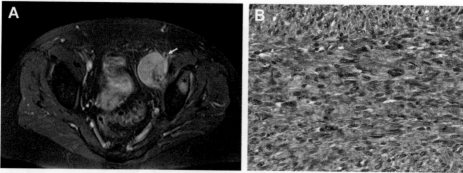

Fig. 7. Leiomyosarcoma. (*A*) Axial contrast-enhanced fat-suppressed T1-weighted MR imaging shows a left pelvic mass obliterating the left iliac vein, proven to be a grade 2 leiomyosarcoma. Note the pulsation artifact of the adjacent iliac artery (*arrow*) and synchronous metastasis to the left iliac bone (*). (*B*) H&E stain exhibiting spindle cells arranged in fascicles intersecting one another at right angles, a feature of leiomyosarcoma.

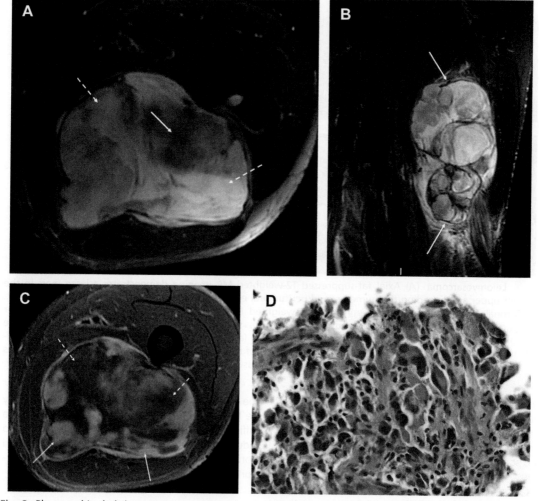

Fig. 8. Pleomorphic rhabdomyosarcoma. 58-year-old male with history of an enlarging mass in the posterior aspect of the left thigh for 6 months. (*A*) Axial fat-suppressed T2-weighted MR imaging portrays a large heterogeneous intramuscular mass within the adductor magnus muscle with solid (*solid arrow*) and cystic/necrotic components (dashed *arrows*). Final diagnosis was consistent with a pleomorphic rhabdomyosarcoma. (*B*) Coronal fat-suppressed T2-weighted MR imaging demonstrates the full extension of the mass craniocaudally (*arrows*) in the posterior aspect of the thigh. Peritumoral soft tissue edema is associated with higher histologic grade tumors. (*C*) Axial contrast-enhanced fat-suppressedT1-weighted MR imaging illustrates heterogenous enhancement of the mass, with strongly enhancing regions that correlate with the more cellular regions of tumor. Also note multiple regions without enhancement, corresponding to tumor necrosis (dashed *arrows*) that is, a marker of high histologic grade. (*D*) Pleomorphic rhabdomyosarcoma is composed of large atypical cells with abundant densely eosinophilic cytoplasm.

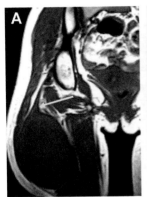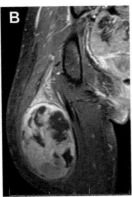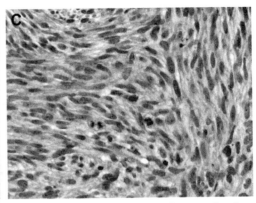

Fig. 9. MPNST. (*A*) Coronal T1 weighted MR imaging in 20-year-old woman with right thigh mass, showing a large tumor arising from the right sciatic nerve (*arrow*). (*B*) Coronal contrast-enhanced fat-suppressed T1-weighted MR imaging shows heterogeneous enhancement; nonenhancing centrally necrotic components denote high grade. (*C*) H&E stain shows that MPNST is hypercellular and composed of fascicles of atypical spindle cells.

Synovial sarcoma

Synovial sarcoma (SS) is the fourth most common STS, accounting for about 2.5% to 10% of all STS worldwide. It frequently involves the extremities (80%–95% of cases), particularly the thigh, and is commonly seen in young adults (15–40 years of age).[70] Because they may behave indolently, the average time to diagnosis can range from 2 to 4 years.[71] SS infrequently involves a joint (5%–10%), and more often due to secondary invasion from a juxta-articular tumor rather than from true intraarticular origin.[70] The designation "synovial" in its name refers to its histologic *resemblance* to

synovium, and not its *histogenesis.* The positive prognostic significance of prominent calcification remains to be confirmed in larger studies.[72] Radiographs can be normal in up to 50% of cases, particularly with small lesions, while calcifications can be seen in up to one-third of plain films, whereby they are eccentric or peripheral within the mass.[70]

On MR imaging, SS are most often well-defined and multilobulated with internal septa, with more than 40% showing high signal on both T1 and T2, consistent with hemorrhage. Fluid-fluid levels are present in approximately 20%, and more

---

Table 5
Conventional MR imaging characteristics of MPNST versus BPNST

MR Characteristic	MPNST	BPNST
T1-W Images[a]	Isointense to muscles; homogenous or heterogeneous	Isointense to muscles; homogenous
T2-W Images	Heterogeneous SI	Heterogeneous SI
Size	Large (>5 cm)	Small (<5 cm)
Margins	Ill-defined/infiltrative	Well-defined
Necrosis/Cystic Change	Common	Uncommon
Perilesional Edema	Present	Absent
Split Fat Sign[b]	Absent	Present
Fascicular Sign[c]	Absent	Present
Target Sign[d]	Absent	Present

Abbreviations: BPNST, benign peripheral nerve sheath tumor; MPNST, malignant peripheral nerve sheath tumor; SI, signal intensity.

[a] If heterogenous on T2-WI and heterogenous on T1-WI with hyperintense areas indicative of hemorrhage, strongly suggestive of MPNST diagnosis.

[b] split-fat sign: suggests a tumor origin in the intermuscular space about the neurovascular bundle.

[c] fascicular sign: multiple ring-like prominent hypointense structures seen on T2-W sequences, possibly reflecting the enlarged fascicular bundles seen on histology.

[d] target sign: related to a central low or intermediate SI surrounded by a rim of higher SI on T2-W sequences, representing the centrally located cellular area, peripherally surrounded by a myxoid region.

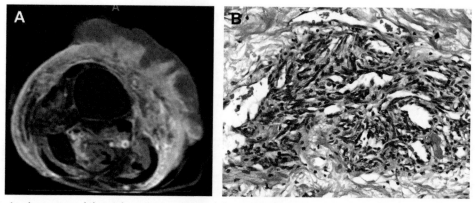

Fig. 10. Angiosarcoma. (*A*) Axial contrast-enhanced fat-suppressed T1 weighted MR imaging in an 80-year-old man demonstrates a large fungating mass at the anteromedial aspect of the right lower leg, with ill-defined nearly circumferential infiltration of the subcutaneous soft tissues. (*B*) H&E stain shows that angiosarcoma is composed of malignant spindle cells delineating irregular vascular structures.

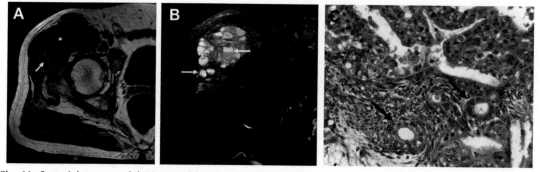

Fig. 11. Synovial sarcoma. (*A*) 56-year-old male complaining of a slow growing painless mass in his right hip for about 1 year. Axial T1-weighted MR imaging shows a soft tissue mass (***) growing between the sartorius and rectus femoris muscles. There are scattered areas of mild hyperintensity (*arrows*), consistent with hemorrhage, not fat. (*B*) Axial fat-suppressed T2-weighted MR imaging highlights internal heterogeneity with multiple fluid levels (*arrows*) secondary to spontaneous intratumoral hemorrhage with hematocrit effect. Signal heterogeneity, with low-, intermediate-, and high-signal areas on fluid-sensitive sequences has been described as the "triple-sign" feature of synovial sarcomas, albeit one that is, nonspecific and can be seen in other STS. (*C*) H&E stain reveals cuboidal cells forming glands (*arrows*) surrounded by fascicles of uniform spindle cells in this biphasic synovial sarcoma.

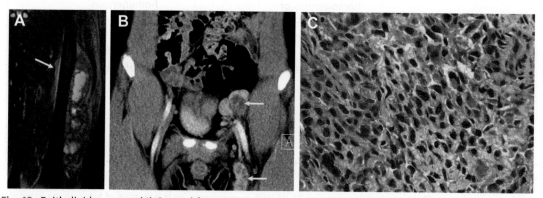

Fig. 12. Epithelioid sarcoma. (*A*) Coronal fat-suppressed T2-weighted MR imaging of the left thigh shows a large heterogeneous hyperintense mass centered in the lateral mid-thigh, with peritumoral edema extending posteromedially around the femoral shaft (*arrow*). Peritumor edema is suggestive of higher grade STS and an infiltrative growth pattern. (*B*) Coronal contrast-enhanced CT of the pelvis demonstrates left inguinal and iliac chain lymphadenopathy (*arrows*); epithelioid sarcoma has a propensity for regional nodal metastases, and patients should be staged appropriately. (*C*) H&E stain reveals aggregates of cytologically malignant epithelioid cells.

than one-third demonstrate the "triple-sign" (Fig. 11), whereby areas of iso-, hyper-, and hypo-intensity can be seen concomitantly within the tumor, due to a combination of solid and cystic components, associated with hemorrhage, necrosis, and fibrous tissue.[73,74] When using advanced MR techniques, SS demonstrates significantly restricted diffusion and avid early enhancement on dynamic sequences.[71]

Epithelioid sarcoma

Epithelioid sarcoma is an STS that usually presents in the subcutaneous or dermis in the distal aspect of the extremities of adolescents and young adults between 10 and 35 years of age.[75] The most common location is the distal aspect of the upper extremity, specifically the hands and forearms, seen in 58% of cases, followed by the distal and proximal lower extremity in 15% and 12% of cases, respectively. Histologically, it often presents as a multinodular proliferation of epithelioid and spindle-shaped cells with cytologic atypia.[76]

Subcutaneous tumors normally present as firm solitary or irregular multinodular masses which elevate the skin surface, becoming ulcerated within weeks or months. When deep-seated, they are typically larger, firmly attached to tendons and fascia, and notoriously known for high recurrence potential.[75] On MR imaging, epithelioid sarcomas display heterogenous T1 and T2 signal, depending on the amount of hemorrhage, necrosis, and cystic degeneration. They are also associated with frequent peritumoral edema denoting fascial spread and a high rate of regional nodal involvement (Fig. 12).[77]

Alveolar soft part sarcoma

Alveolar soft part sarcoma (ASPS) is rare, comprising approximately 0.5% to 1% of all STS.

ASPS is a slow-growing tumor, and symptoms are commonly overlooked by patients, leading to late diagnosis.[78] Consequently, approximately 65% of adults and 30% of children present with metastases at diagnosis, mainly to the lungs, brain, bone, or lymph nodes, with poor prognosis.[79] It occurs most commonly in young adults, from 15 to 35 years of age, involving the deep muscles of the extremities (60%), primarily in the thighs, or trunk (20%).[80] ASPS consistently presents as a highly vascularized intramuscular mass, with high signal on T1, absence of central necrosis, and large intra- and peritumoral vessels that manifest as hypointense "flow-voids" (Fig. 13).[79–81] Given its highly vascular nature, a treatment regimen blocking tumor angiogenesis with a VEGF receptor tyrosine-kinase inhibitor coupled with an anti-PD-1 immune checkpoint inhibitor recently showed promising results, achieving 3-month progression-free survival of 73%.[82]

FUTURE DIRECTIONS AND CONCLUSIONS

The nosologic evolution of STS is certain to continue using new diagnostic schema as additional genetic and signaling pathway abnormalities are uncovered.[83] Ultimately, tumor classification may be organized by molecular biomarkers or immune microenvironments in a paradigm shift that would emphasize actionable treatment targets.[84] For example, designations of histologic differentiation may matter less than information that reveals susceptibility to MEK- or immune checkpoint inhibitors. The ability to identify circulating blood-based tumor components (including tumor cells, cell-free nucleic acids, tumor-derived exosomes, and certain metabolites) may also revolutionize strategies in assessing treatment response and conducting tumor surveillance.[85]

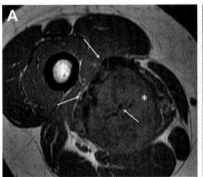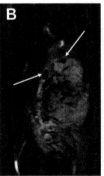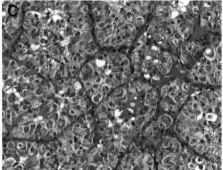

Fig. 13. Alveolar soft part sarcoma. (*A*) 34-year-old woman with history of a painful and enlarging soft tissue mass in the posteromedial aspect of her right thigh. Axial T1-weighted MR imaging demonstrates a predominantly iso-intense intramuscular mass (*) within the adductor magnus muscle, and multiple peritumoral and intratumoral "flow-voids" (*arrows*) corresponding to high-flow vessels. (*B*) Coronal fat-suppressed T2-weighted MR imaging also demonstrates these characteristic large peritumoral and intratumoral vessels throughout the soft tissue mass (*arrows*), a common feature of ASPS. (*C*) H&E stain of ASPS shows large polyhedral cells with abundant eosinophilic cytoplasm arranged in alveolar-like aggregates or rounded nests.

Despite the frequently nonspecific radiologic appearance of STS, several imaging clues may be suggestive of certain histologic subtypes or point toward higher grade neoplasms. Appreciation of these findings aids in establishing radiologic-pathologic concordance. Familiarity with STS that have a propensity for local infiltrative growth (eg, myxofibrosarcoma) or characteristic patterns of metastasis (eg, myxoid liposarcoma) also informs surgical planning, initial disease staging, and posttreatment surveillance.

CLINICS CARE POINTS

- STS comprise a heterogeneous group of mesenchymal neoplasms organized according to the type of tissue they resemble morphologically
- STS are staged according to tumor size, histologic grade, and extent of disease spread to regional lymph nodes or distant metastases (6)
- Identification of internal fat suggests an adipocytic origin, which is particularly important in establishing radiologic-pathologic congruence when histology suggests dedifferentiated liposarcoma
- Infiltrative growth, as often seen in myxofibrosarcoma, manifests as peritumoral edema and tails of enhancement that should be included in planning for complete tumor excision
- Staging studies should account for characteristic patterns of spread in some STS subtypes, which includes metastases to bone and soft tissues in myxoid liposarcoma, as well as regional nodal involvement in RMS, clear cell sarcoma, extraskeletal Ewing sarcoma, epithelioid sarcoma, and angiosarcoma

CONFLICT OF INTERESTS

The authors declare no conflicts of interest.

FUNDING/DISCLOSURES

T.K. Subhawong has received grant support from the Toshiba America Medical Systems/RSNA Research Seed Grant (#RSD1635), and grant support from the Desmoid Tumor Research Foundation; honoraria from iiCME for speaking activities unrelated to the preparation of this article; he has served as a consultant for Agios Pharmaceuticals and Arog Pharmaceuticals but has received no funding related to the preparation of this article.

REFERENCES

1. Kuhn KJ, Cloutier JM, Boutin RD, et al. Soft tissue pathology for the radiologist: a tumor board primer with 2020 WHO classification update. Skeletal Radiol 2021;50(1):29–42.
2. Hui JYC. Epidemiology and etiology of sarcomas. Surg Clin North Am 2016;96(5):901–14.
3. Coindre J-M. Grading of soft tissue sarcomas: review and update. Arch Pathol Lab Med 2006; 130(10):1448–53.
4. Steffner RJ, Jang ES. Staging of bone and soft-tissue sarcomas. J Am Acad Orthop Surg 2018; 26(13):e269–78.
5. Jawad MU, Scully SP. In brief: classifications in brief: mirels' classification: metastatic disease in long bones and impending pathologic fracture. Clin Orthop 2010;468(10):2825–7.
6. Amin MB, Edge SB, Greene FL, et al, editors. AJCC Cancer staging manual. 8th edition. New York: Springer; 2017.
7. Gusho CA, Fice MP, O'Donoghue CM, et al. A population-based analysis of lymph node metastasis in extremity soft tissue sarcoma: an update. J Surg Res 2021;262:121–9.
8. Jacobs AJ, Morris CD, Levin AS. Synovial sarcoma is not associated with a higher risk of lymph node metastasis compared with other soft tissue sarcomas. Clin Orthop 2018;476(3):589–98.
9. Zhao F, Ahlawat S, Farahani SJ, et al. Can MR imaging be used to predict tumor grade in soft-tissue sarcoma? Radiology 2014;272(1):192–201.
10. Fernebro J, Wiklund M, Jonsson K, et al. Focus on the tumour periphery in MRI evaluation of soft tissue sarcoma: infiltrative growth signifies poor prognosis. Sarcoma 2006;2006:21251.
11. Callegaro D, Miceli R, Mariani L, et al. Soft tissue sarcoma nomograms and their incorporation into practice. Cancer 2017;123(15):2802–20.
12. Rizer M, Singer AD, Edgar M, et al. The histological variants of liposarcoma: predictive MRI findings with prognostic implications, management, follow-up, and differential diagnosis. Skeletal Radiol 2016; 45(9):1193–204.
13. Kransdorf MJ, Bancroft LW, Peterson JJ, et al. Imaging of fatty tumors: distinction of lipoma and well-differentiated liposarcoma1. Radiology 2002;224(1): 99–104.
14. Gupta P, Potti TA, Wuertzer SD, et al. Spectrum of fat-containing soft-tissue masses at MR imaging: the common, the uncommon, the characteristic, and the sometimes confusing. Radiogr Rev Publ Radiol Soc N Am Inc 2016;36(3):753–66.
15. Berkeley R, Okereke O, Malhotra K, et al. The incidence and relevance of non-fatty components in trunk and extremity lipomatous soft tissue masses. Br J Radiol 2021;94(1122):20201403.

16. Bestic JM, Kransdorf MJ, White LM, et al. Sclerosing variant of well-differentiated liposarcoma: relative prevalence and spectrum of CT and MRI features. AJR Am J Roentgenol 2013;201(1):154–61.

17. Gootee J, Aurit S, Curtin C, et al. Primary anatomical site, adjuvant therapy, and other prognostic variables for dedifferentiated liposarcoma. J Cancer Res Clin Oncol 2019;145(1):181–92.

18. Saifuddin A, Whelan J, Pringle JA, et al. Malignant round cell tumours of bone: atypical clinical and imaging features. Skeletal Radiol 2000;29(11):646–51.

19. Murphey MD, Arcara LK, Fanburg-Smith J. From the archives of the AFIP: imaging of musculoskeletal liposarcoma with radiologic-pathologic correlation. Radiogr Rev Publ Radiol Soc N Am Inc 2005;25(5):1371–95.

20. Tateishi U, Hasegawa T, Beppu Y, et al. Prognostic significance of MRI findings in patients with myxoid-round cell liposarcoma. AJR Am J Roentgenol 2004;182(3):725–31.

21. Crombé A, Le Loarer F, Sitbon M, et al. Can radiomics improve the prediction of metastatic relapse of myxoid/round cell liposarcomas? Eur Radiol 2020;30(5):2413–24.

22. Fuglø HM, Maretty-Nielsen K, Hovgaard D, et al. Metastatic pattern, local relapse, and survival of patients with myxoid liposarcoma: a retrospective study of 45 patients. Sarcoma 2013;2013:548628.

23. Muratori F, Bettini L, Frenos F, et al. Myxoid liposarcoma: prognostic factors and metastatic pattern in a series of 148 patients treated at a single institution. Int J Surg Oncol 2018;2018:8928706.

24. Visgauss JD, Wilson DA, Perrin DL, et al. Staging and surveillance of myxoid liposarcoma: follow-up assessment and the metastatic pattern of 169 patients suggests inadequacy of current practice standards. Ann Surg Oncol 2021;28(12):7903–11.

25. Anderson WJ, Jo VY. Pleomorphic liposarcoma: updates and current differential diagnosis. Semin Diagn Pathol 2019;36(2):122–8.

26. Gebhard S, Coindre J-M, Michels J-J, et al. Pleomorphic liposarcoma: clinicopathologic, immunohistochemical, and follow-up analysis of 63 cases: a study from the French Federation of Cancer Centers Sarcoma Group. Am J Surg Pathol 2002;26(5):601–16.

27. Slack JC, Bründler M-A, Nohr E, et al. Molecular alterations in pediatric fibroblastic/myofibroblastic tumors: an appraisal of a next generation sequencing assay in a retrospective single centre study. Pediatr Dev Pathol 2021;24(5):405–21, 10935266211015558.

28. Sanfilippo R, Miceli R, Grosso F, et al. Myxofibrosarcoma: prognostic factors and survival in a series of patients treated at a single institution. Ann Surg Oncol 2011;18(3):720–5.

29. Lefkowitz RA, Landa J, Hwang S, et al. Myxofibrosarcoma: prevalence and diagnostic value of the "tail sign" on magnetic resonance imaging. Skeletal Radiol 2013 Jun;42(6):809–18.

30. Iwata S, Araki A, Funatsu H, et al. Optimal surgical margin for infiltrative soft tissue sarcomas: Assessing the efficacy of excising beyond the infiltration. J Surg Oncol 2018;118(3):525–31.

31. Spinnato P, Sambri A, Fujiwara T, et al. Myxofibrosarcoma: clinical and prognostic value of MRI features. Curr Med Imaging 2021;17(2):217–24.

32. Daniels C, Wang W, Madewell JE, et al. Pattern of recurrence of myxofibrosarcoma is not associated with pattern at presentation or rate of delayed diagnosis. Iran J Radiol 2017;14(1):e13469. https://doi.org/10.5812/iranjradiol.32548.

33. Chamberlain F, Engelmann B, Al-Muderis O, et al. Low-grade fibromyxoid sarcoma: treatment outcomes and efficacy of chemotherapy. Vivo Athens Greece 2020;34(1):239–45.

34. Evans HL. Low-grade fibromyxoid sarcoma: a clinicopathologic study of 33 cases with long-term follow-up. Am J Surg Pathol 2011;35(10):1450–62.

35. Hwang S, Kelliher E, Hameed M. Imaging features of low-grade fibromyxoid sarcoma (Evans tumor). Skeletal Radiol 2012;41(10):1263–72.

36. Miyake M, Tateishi U, Maeda T, et al. CT and MRI features of low-grade fibromyxoid sarcoma in the shoulder of a pediatric patient. Radiat Med 2006;24(7):511–4.

37. Widemann BC, Italiano A. Biology and management of undifferentiated pleomorphic sarcoma, myxofibrosarcoma, and malignant peripheral nerve sheath tumors: state of the art and perspectives. J Clin Oncol Off J Am Soc Clin Oncol 2018;36(2):160–7.

38. Rosenberg AE. WHO classification of soft tissue and bone, fourth edition: summary and commentary. Curr Opin Oncol 2013;25(5):571–3.

39. Levy AD, Manning MA, Al-Refaie WB, et al. Soft-tissue sarcomas of the abdomen and pelvis: radiologic-pathologic features, Part 1-Common sarcomas: from the radiologic pathology archives. Radiogr Rev Publ Radiol Soc N Am Inc 2017;37(2):462–83.

40. Yoshimoto M, Yamada Y, Ishihara S, et al. Comparative study of myxofibrosarcoma with undifferentiated pleomorphic sarcoma: histopathologic and clinicopathologic review. Am J Surg Pathol 2020;44(1):87–97.

41. Lewin J, Garg S, Lau BY, et al. Identifying actionable variants using next generation sequencing in patients with a historical diagnosis of undifferentiated pleomorphic sarcoma. Int J Cancer 2018;142(1):57–65.

42. George S, Serrano C, Hensley ML, et al. Soft tissue and uterine leiomyosarcoma. J Clin Oncol 2018;36(2):144–50.

43. Harati K, Daigeler A, Lange K, et al. Somatic leiomyosarcoma of the soft tissues: a single-institutional analysis of factors predictive of survival in 164 patients. World J Surg 2017;41(6):1534–41.

44. Bathan AJ, Constantinidou A, Pollack SM, et al. Diagnosis, prognosis, and management of

leiomyosarcoma: recognition of anatomic variants. Curr Opin Oncol 2013;25(4):384–9.

45. O'Sullivan PJ, Harris AC, Munk PL. Radiological imaging features of non-uterine leiomyosarcoma. Br J Radiol 2008;81(961):73–81.

46. DeMulder D, Ascher SM. Uterine leiomyosarcoma: Can MRI differentiate leiomyosarcoma from benign leiomyoma before treatment? Am J Roentgenol 2018;211(6):1405–15.

47. Bogani G, Cliby WA, Aletti GD. Impact of morcellation on survival outcomes of patients with unexpected uterine leiomyosarcoma: a systematic review and meta-analysis. Gynecol Oncol 2015; 137(1):167–72.

48. Gerges L, Popiolek D, Rosenkrantz AB. Explorative Investigation of whole-lesion histogram MRI Metrics for differentiating uterine leiomyomas and leiomyosarcomas. Am J Roentgenol 2018;210(5): 1172–7.

49. Xie H, Hu J, Zhang X, et al. Preliminary utilization of radiomics in differentiating uterine sarcoma from atypical leiomyoma: Comparison on diagnostic efficacy of MRI features and radiomic features. Eur J Radiol 2019;115:39–45.

50. McHugh K, Boothroyd AE. The role of radiology in childhood rhabdomyosarcoma. Clin Radiol 1999; 54(1):2–10.

51. Saboo SS, Krajewski KM, Zukotynski K, et al. Imaging features of primary and secondary adult rhabdomyosarcoma. AJR Am J Roentgenol 2012;199(6): W694–703.

52. Inarejos Clemente EJ, Navallas M, Barber Martínez de la Torre I, et al. MRI of Rhabdomyosarcoma and Other Soft-Tissue Sarcomas in Children. Radiogr Rev Publ Radiol Soc N Am Inc 2020;40(3):791–814.

53. Arndt CAS, Bisogno G, Koscielniak E. Fifty years of rhabdomyosarcoma studies on both sides of the pond and lessons learned. Cancer Treat Rev 2018; 68:94–101.

54. Gallego S, Zanetti I, Orbach D, et al. Fusion status in patients with lymph node-positive (N1) alveolar rhabdomyosarcoma is a powerful predictor of prognosis: Experience of the European Paediatric Soft Tissue Sarcoma Study Group (EpSSG). Cancer 2018;124(15):3201–9.

55. Carli M, Colombatti R, Oberlin O, et al. European intergroup studies (MMT4-89 and MMT4-91) on childhood metastatic rhabdomyosarcoma: final results and analysis of prognostic factors. J Clin Oncol Off J Am Soc Clin Oncol 2004;22(23):4787–94.

56. Nishida Y, Tsukushi S, Urakawa H, et al. High incidence of regional and in-transit lymph node metastasis in patients with alveolar rhabdomyosarcoma. Int J Clin Oncol 2014;19(3):536–43.

57. Vilanova JC, Woertler K, Narváez JA, et al. Soft-tissue tumors update: MR imaging features according to the WHO classification. Eur Radiol 2007;17(1):125–38.

58. Kobi M, Khatri G, Edelman M, et al. Sarcoma botryoides: MRI findings in two patients. J Magn Reson Imaging JMRI 2009;29(3):708–12.

59. Li C-S, Huang G-S, Wu H-D, et al. Differentiation of soft tissue benign and malignant peripheral nerve sheath tumors with magnetic resonance imaging. Clin Imaging 2008;32(2):121–7.

60. Yun JS, Lee MH, Lee SM, et al. Peripheral nerve sheath tumor: differentiation of malignant from benign tumors with conventional and diffusion-weighted MRI. Eur Radiol 2021;31(3):1548–57.

61. Wasa J, Nishida Y, Tsukushi S, et al. MRI features in the differentiation of malignant peripheral nerve sheath tumors and neurofibromas. AJR Am J Roentgenol 2010;194(6):1568–74.

62. Soldatos T, Fisher S, Karri S, et al. Advanced MR imaging of peripheral nerve sheath tumors including diffusion imaging. Semin Musculoskelet Radiol 2015;19(2):179–90.

63. Demehri S, Belzberg A, Blakeley J, et al. Conventional and functional MR imaging of peripheral nerve sheath tumors: initial experience. AJNR Am J Neuroradiol 2014;35(8):1615–20.

64. Ahlawat S, Blakeley JO, Rodriguez FJ, et al. Imaging biomarkers for malignant peripheral nerve sheath tumors in neurofibromatosis type 1. Neurology 2019; 93(11):e1076–84.

65. Gaballah AH, Jensen CT, Palmquist S, et al. Angiosarcoma: clinical and imaging features from head to toe. Br J Radiol 2017;90(1075):20170039.

66. Young RJ, Brown NJ, Reed MW, et al. Angiosarcoma Lancet Oncol 2010;11(10):983–91.

67. Virtanen A, Pukkala E, Auvinen A. Angiosarcoma after radiotherapy: a cohort study of 332,163 Finnish cancer patients. Br J Cancer 2007;97(1): 115–7.

68. Chesebro AL, Chikarmane SA, Gombos EC, et al. Radiation-associated angiosarcoma of the breast: what the radiologist needs to know. AJR Am J Roentgenol 2016;207(1):217–25.

69. WHO Classification of Tumours Editorial Board. Soft tissue and bone tumours. Lyon (France): International Agency for Research on Cancer; 2020.

70. Murphey MD, Gibson MS, Jennings BT, et al. From the archives of the AFIP: Imaging of synovial sarcoma with radiologic-pathologic correlation. Radiogr Rev Publ Radiol Soc N Am Inc 2006;26(5): 1543–65.

71. Ashikyan O, Bradshaw SB, Dettori NJ, et al. Conventional and advanced MR imaging insights of synovial sarcoma. Clin Imaging 2021;76:149–55.

72. Mariño-Enríquez A, Hornick JL. 3 - Spindle cell tumors of adults. In: Hornick JL, editor. Practical soft tissue pathology: a diagnostic approach. Second Edition. Philadelphia: Elsevier; 2019. Available at: https://www.sciencedirect.com/science/article/pii/B9780323897714500003X.

73. O'Sullivan PJ, Harris AC, Munk PL. Radiological features of synovial cell sarcoma. Br J Radiol 2008; 81(964):346–56.

74. Jones B, Sundaram M, Kransdorf M. Synovial sarcoma: MR imaging findings in 34 patients. Am J Roentgenol 1993;161(4):827–30.

75. Hanna SL, Kaste S, Jenkins JJ, et al. Epithelioid sarcoma: clinical, MR imaging and pathologic findings. Skeletal Radiol 2002;31(7):400–12.

76. Tateishi U, Hasegawa T, Kusumoto M, et al. Radiologic manifestations of proximal-type epithelioid sarcoma of the soft tissues. AJR Am J Roentgenol 2002;179(4):973–7.

77. McCarville MB, Kao SC, Dao TV, et al. Magnetic resonance and computed tomography imaging features of epithelioid sarcoma in children and young adults with pathological and clinical correlation: a report from Children's Oncology Group study ARST0332. Pediatr Radiol 2019;49(7):922–32.

78. Suh JS, Cho J, Lee SH, et al. Alveolar soft part sarcoma: MR and angiographic findings. Skeletal Radiol 2000;29(12):680–9.

79. McCarville MB, Muzzafar S, Kao SC, et al. Imaging features of alveolar soft-part sarcoma: a report from Children's Oncology Group Study ARST0332. AJR Am J Roentgenol 2014;203(6):1345–52.

80. Crombé A, Brisse HJ, Ledoux P, et al. Alveolar soft-part sarcoma: can MRI help discriminating from other soft-tissue tumors? A study of the French sarcoma group. Eur Radiol 2019;29(6):3170–82.

81. Viry F, Orbach D, Klijanienko J, et al. Alveolar soft part sarcoma-radiologic patterns in children and adolescents. Pediatr Radiol 2013;43(9):1174–81.

82. Wilky BA, Trucco MM, Subhawong TK, et al. Axitinib plus pembrolizumab in patients with advanced sarcomas including alveolar soft-part sarcoma: a single-centre, single-arm, phase 2 trial. Lancet Oncol 2019;20(6):837–48.

83. Kallen ME, Hornick JL. The 2020 WHO Classification: what's new in soft tissue tumor pathology? Am J Surg Pathol 2021;45(1):e1–23.

84. Petitprez F, de Reyniès A, Keung EZ, et al. B cells are associated with survival and immunotherapy response in sarcoma. Nature 2020;577(7791): 556–60.

85. Li X, Seebacher NA, Hornicek FJ, et al. Application of liquid biopsy in bone and soft tissue sarcomas: Present and future. Cancer Lett 2018;439:66–77.

Common Soft Tissue Mass-like Lesions that Mimic Malignancy

Sina Habibollahi, MD[a], Santiago Lozano-Calderon, MD, PhD[b,c],
Connie Y. Chang, MD[a,c],*

KEYWORDS

- MR imaging • Soft tissue tumor • Myositis • Calcinosis • Geyser • Myonecrosis • Gout

KEY POINTS

- In myositis ossificans, "rim of ossification" is the characteristic imaging finding, but it may not be visible in the early stages, even on cross-sectional imaging. Ossification rate in myositis ossificans is similar to fracture healing and is faster in younger individuals.
- Acute traumatic hematomas are typically associated with a history of trauma or anticoagulation and have greater perilesional edema on fluid-sensitive MR imaging compared with hemorrhagic malignant tumors.
- Tumoral calcinosis and hemorrhagic sarcoma can both demonstrate "fluid-fluid" levels, but the fluid-fluid levels are denser in tumoral calcinosis.
- Gouty tophus can be mass-like and enhance on MR imaging, mimicking a soft tissue malignancy. If a differential consideration, dual-energy CT can confirm the diagnosis.
- Myonecrosis can present as a soft tissue mass and appear heterogeneous on MR imaging, mimicking malignancy. Patient history is key in diagnosis.

INTRODUCTION

Every week our radiology group has a combined conference with Orthopedic Oncology, Pathology, and Radiology to review the imaging and management of patients with musculoskeletal (MSK)-related conditions of neoplastic and nonneoplastic origin. The collection of benign soft tissue mass-like lesions discussed in this review was all presented at our conference and is considered common mimickers of soft tissue malignancies. In fact, all of these cases were called "malignancies" and were referred to our institution for further evaluation and care. As with most findings on imaging, the finding alone may be deceiving, but the knowledge of the history and demographics can often prevent false-positive diagnosis of a malignancy.

"Post-Traumatic" Mimics

There are several soft tissue mass-like lesions considered "traumatic" in etiology that can be confused for malignancy. "Trauma" is placed in quotations because the damage results from small and repetitive events rather than a single traumatic event or the trauma was mild such that the patient does not recall a specific inciting event.

a Division of Musculoskeletal Imaging and Intervention, Department of Radiology, Massachusetts General Hospital, 55 Fruit Street Yawkey 6E, Boston, MA 02114, USA; b Division of Orthopedics, Massachusetts General Hospital, 55 Fruit Street Yawkey 3B, Boston, MA 02114, USA; c Harvard Medical School, 25 Shattuck St, Cambridge, MA, 02115, USA
* Corresponding author. Division of Musculoskeletal Imaging and Intervention, Department of Radiology, Massachusetts General Hospital, 55 Fruit Street Yawkey 6E, Boston, MA 02114, USA.
E-mail address: cychang@mgh.harvard.edu

Radiol Clin N Am 60 (2022) 301–310
https://doi.org/10.1016/j.rcl.2021.11.008

Myositis ossificans (MO) is the quintessential soft tissue tumor mimic. It tends to occur in the extremities of young people (25 ± 10 years).[1–4] The etiology is unknown, but trauma is thought to play a role in at least some of the cases.[5] MO often seems ominous on MR imaging—it typically involves a very long segment of muscle and has pronounced and intense surrounding edema and enhancement (Fig. 1).[6] Contrast the appearance of the MO in Fig. 1 with the osteosarcoma recurrence with acute hemorrhage in Fig. 2, whereby there is very little surrounding soft tissue edema.[7] The lack of edema should not be used to exclude a malignant diagnosis entirely, but if a worrisome-looking mass is encountered in association with edema, it is important to consider other benign diagnoses such as MO.

The hallmark of MO is the developing rim of ossification.[8] In the early stages, the rim of ossification may not be detected, even on cross-sectional imaging.[9] When it does develop, it begins in the periphery of the lesion and slowly progresses to the center (see Fig. 1).[10] However, if the diagnosis is at all suspected, holding off a biopsy for a few weeks and following up with a radiograph is prudent, as a soft tissue mass with osteoid can be mistaken for an osteosarcoma

histologically.[11] The rate of ossification can also be variable and can be thought of as similar to the expected rate of fracture healing. In a young person, at least some ossification is expected within 2 to 3 weeks.[12,13] Simon and colleagues detected ossification in MO lesions by ultrasonography in 26% at the initial visit, in 59% by the third week after trauma, and in 70% by the fourth week after trauma.[3] As with fracture healing, ossification of MO can be delayed in older individuals. In a study by Yaghmai and colleagues, subjects under age 30 had ossification by 10 weeks, but for the only patient who was over 50, ossification occurred at 14 weeks.[14] However, as MO is unusual in this demographic, and cancer is more common, earlier decision to proceed with biopsy would be prudent.

Acute traumatic hematoma can also be confused with a malignancy.[15] In Fig. 3, there seems to be a central, enhancing mass-like region. However, comparison with the T1 noncontrast image reveals that it is intrinsically T1 hyperintense. In combination with the more central region, which is hypointense on all sequences, this "mass" is consistent with a clot, containing different stages of blood degradation.[16] The more peripheral, fluid-signal intensity region is T1 hyperintense to

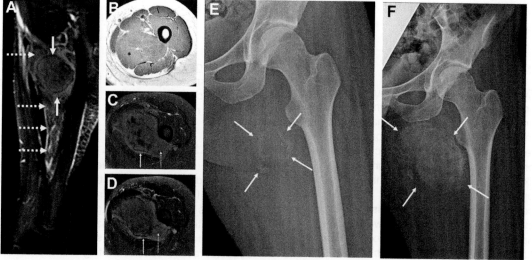

Fig. 1. 30-year-old with rapidly enlarging, painful soft tissue mass in the thigh. The patient did not recall any trauma. (A) Sagittal T2 fat-suppressed image of the thigh demonstrates a hyperintense mass with a low signal intensity rim (solid arrows). There is extensive surrounding edema (dashed arrows). (B) Axial T1 image of the thigh demonstrates the mass is slightly T1 hyperintense to the surrounding muscle (*). (C) Axial T1 postcontrast fat-suppressed and (D) axial T2 fat-suppressed image demonstrates low signal intensity rim around the mass (solid arrows), with extensive surrounding soft tissue edema and enhancement (dashed arrows). (E) AP image of the left thigh at the time of the MR imaging demonstrates faint rim of peripheral ossification in the medial thigh soft tissues. (F) AP image of the left thigh 20 days later demonstrates increased, mature-appearing ossification in the medial thigh soft tissues. These findings are compatible with myositis ossificans. Nine months later, the patient had persistent discomfort in the seated position, and an orthopedic oncologist resected the mass. Anatomic pathology confirmed the diagnosis of myositis ossificans.

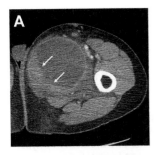

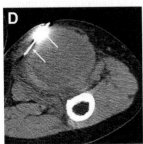

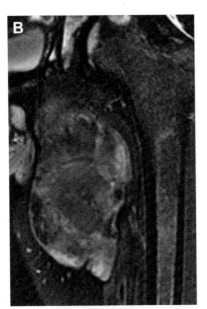

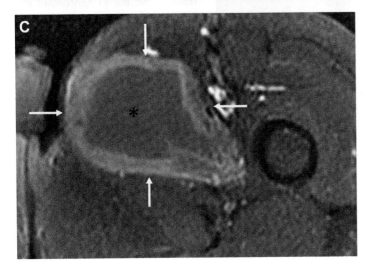

Fig. 2. 15-year-old with history of osteosarcoma of the pubis treated with radiation and resection, presents with acute medial thigh mass after "air kick." (A) Contrast-enhanced axial CT image of the mid-thigh at initial presentation demonstrates a predominantly low-density mass (*). There is a "rind" of soft tissue density along the right posterior aspect of the mass (arrows). Note that the area is not in the dependent region of the mass and is therefore not a "meniscus" or "fluid-fluid level." Given the questionable history of trauma and the possibility that this could be hematoma, our multi-disciplinary team agreed to bring the patient back after 1 month for repeat imaging, (B) Coronal T2 fat-suppressed and (C) axial T1 post-contrast fat-suppressed images at 1-month follow-up demonstrate the same mass, which has slightly decreased in size. However, there remains a thick rim of enhancement (arrows). There is a central area of nonenhancement, which is intermediate signal intensity on T2 (not fluid signal intensity) (*). While it still could be hematoma, the mass did not decrease in size a sufficient amount to be reassuring, and the central nonenhancing area was more complex than expected for an organizing hematoma. Therefore, the patient was brought back for biopsy. (D) Axial noncontrast CT image obtained during from biopsy demonstrates the needle in the "rind" (arrows). Anatomic pathology confirmed this mass to be osteosarcoma recurrence. The central nonenhancing area was a combination of hemorrhage and necrosis.

the surrounding muscle, consistent with acute blood products. The thin linear peripheral enhancement is a common finding and is likely due to gadolinium leakage from torn blood vessels.[16] The primary question to consider is whether this is a tumor with acute hemorrhage. Key information to glean from the patient medical record is the history of trauma or anticoagulation, which was the case in Fig. 3. The substantial surrounding muscle edema seen on the sagittal T2 fat-suppressed image is also helpful to decrease suspicion. However, these features do not rule out malignancy as the cause for the hematoma.[17–19] Clinical follow-up is prudent, and short-term imaging follow-up (6–8 weeks is typically used at our institution) or biopsy may be warranted.[17–19]

When the clinical picture is unclear, repeat MR imaging can help distinguish a lesion with an evolving rim of blood products that is slowly getting smaller from a growing mass with rehemorrhage. Typically, hematomas are not treated.[20] In this case, the hematoma was large, and the combination of patient discomfort and orthopedist concern for developing compartment syndrome prompted an ultrasound-guided aspiration, which yielded 70 mL of blood. The patient felt immediate symptomatic improvement. As the aspiration was performed, the sample was sent for cytology, and no malignant cells were found. The patient's symptoms also did not recur.

Geyser lesion is a name that arises from the era whereby arthrography was the primary modality

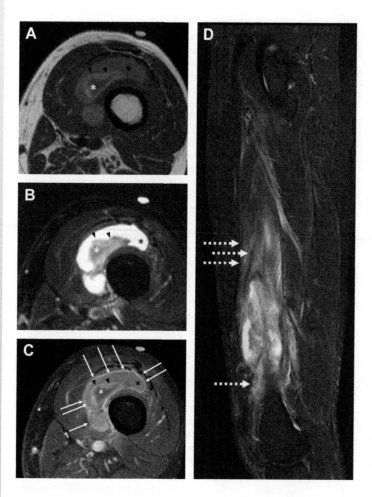

Fig. 3. 60-year-old on Plavix for cardiac stent who developed immediate swelling of the thigh after being tackled while playing family backyard football. (*A*) Axial T1 noncontrast MR imaging, (*B*) axial T2 fat-suppressed, and (*C*) axial T1 fat-suppressed postcontrast images through the mid-thigh demonstrates a mass in the vastus intermedius. There are 3 zones. The most peripheral zone is T1 hyperintense and T2 hyperintense to muscle (black *). This is the liquid blood and plasma. This zone has thin linear enhancement on the postcontrast images (*white arrows*), and is due to leaky blood vessels, some of which probably tore and resulted in this hematoma. The middle zone is more mass-like, and on the postcontrast image seems to have nodular, peripheral enhancement (*black arrowheads*). However, on the T1 noncontrast image, this area is intrinsically T1 hyperintense, consistent with clot (*black arrowheads*). The central zone is hypointense on all sequences and is the oldest, most mature clot, likely containing some hemosiderin (white *). (*D*) Sagittal T2 fat-suppressed image of the thigh shows the long segment of surrounding muscle edema (*dashed white arrow*). This mass was aspirated, and cytology confirmed hemorrhage and no malignant cells.

for diagnosing rotator cuff tears. In the setting of a chronic, full-thickness rotator cuff tear *and* severe acromioclavicular joint degenerative change, contrast injected into the glenohumeral joint could extend through the rotator cuff defect and acromioclavicular joint capsule into the subcutaneous soft tissues superior to the joint, creating the appearance of a geyser, particularly if the contrast was injected forcefully.[21] Clinically, the patient presents with a slowly growing mass in their shoulder, and thus the concern for malignancy. The mass is essentially an acromioclavicular joint synovial cyst.[21,22] The MR imaging geyser sign is the MR imaging equivalent of the arthrographic finding. As seen in **Fig. 4**, there is a fluid signal intensity lesion with no peripheral enhancement centered above the severely degenerated acromioclavicular joint. The superior and inferior acromioclavicular ligaments are torn, as is the rotator cuff. This particular example is relatively straightforward, as there is no synovitis or other complex feature of the cyst. If there

are any suspicious features, then the case should be carefully reevaluated. In the case seen in **Fig. 5**, there is a chronic full-thickness rotator cuff tear and severe acromioclavicular degenerative change, just like the case in **Fig. 4**. Because of these findings and a suspected connection via a small channel extending to the acromioclavicular joint, the possibility of a geyser lesion was raised. However, there are a few features that make this suggestion very unlikely. First, the T2 hyperintense portion of the lesion is complex, with multiple internal septations. While this finding alone is not sufficient to raise suspicion, it is summative with the other atypical features of this lesion. Second, the T2 hyperintense portion of the lesion is not centered on the acromioclavicular joint; it is offset medially. Third, the T2 hyperintense portion of this lesion is intrinsically T1 hyperintense, suggesting hemorrhage, which would be atypical for a geyser lesion. Lastly, postcontrast imaging of the entire clavicle demonstrates a solid, enhancing portion of the

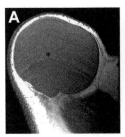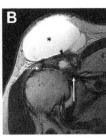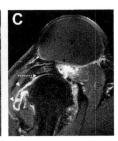

Fig. 4. 62-year-old with slowly enlarging shoulder mass. (A) Axial T1, (B) Coronal T2, and (C) Sagittal T1 fat-suppressed postcontrast images of the right shoulder demonstrate a T1 isointense and T2 hyperintense to muscle, nonenhancing mass (*) centered on the acromioclavicular joint (black arrowheads); there is severe degeneration of the acromioclavicular joint, and the superior and inferior acromioclavicular ligaments are torn. There is a chronic, retracted full-thickness rotator cuff tear (arrow), with superior subluxation of the humeral head with respect to the glenoid and acetabularization of the acromion (dashed arrow). The synovium is enhancing, consistent with synovitis (white arrowheads). The mass is consistent with a geyser lesion.

lesion more medially. This portion was poorly visualized on the original shoulder MR imaging. If a lesion has any concerning features, care should be taken to ensure that the entire lesion is adequately imaged on the MR imaging. The lesion in Fig. 5 was biopsied and anatomic pathology demonstrated angiosarcoma.

Nontraumatic Mimics

Tumoral calcinosis (TC) is a condition that can have a dramatic clinical and imaging presentation. The etiology can be either congenital or idiopathic in nature.[23] The congenital type manifests as a metabolic disorder with 2 subtypes, one associated with hyperphosphatemia (hFTC) and the other with normophosphatemia (nFTC). Three genes that regulate phosphate metabolism, namely fibroblast growth factor (FGF)-23, GALNT3, and α-Klotho, have been linked to the hFTC subtype. In the hFTC subtype, mutations of these genes cause increased renal phosphate reabsorption and hFTC. The SAM9 gene has been linked to the nFTC subtype. Although bone mineral metabolism is intact in this subtype the SAM9 gene encodes a protein believed to cause an abnormal response to skin trauma. Both subtypes are associated with ectopic calcification due to calcium phosphate deposition, which is most common in periarticular tissues. In the nFTC subtype, hyperpigmented skin lesions and gingivitis can also be found.[24,25] The idiopathic type is most commonly seen in the setting of

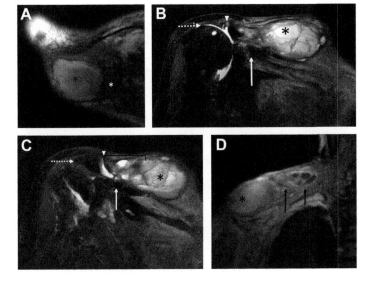

Fig. 5. 86-year-old with slowly enlarging shoulder mass. (A) Axial T1, (B) and (C) Coronal T2 fat-suppressed, and (D) Coronal T1 fat-suppressed postcontrast images of the right shoulder demonstrate a predominantly intrinsically T1 hyperintense (black *) and T2 hyperintense mass to muscle. Intrinsic T1 hyperintensity is consistent with hemorrhage. There are multiple internal septations. Like the lesion in Fig. 6, there is a chronic, full thickness, retracted rotator cuff tear (white arrow), superior subluxation of the humeral with acetabularization of the acromion (white dashed arrow), and severe degeneration of the acromioclavicular joint with torn the superior and inferior acromioclavicular ligaments (white arrowheads). In (C), there is a suggestion of a tract connecting to the acromioclavicular joint (black bracket). Additional larger field of images of the chest wall obtained at a later date seen in (D) showed an enhancing component more medially (black arrows). This component was partially visible as a T1 isotense to mass muscle on the original shoulder MR imaging (white *). The enhancing component was biopsied, and anatomic pathology showed angiosarcoma.

chronic renal disease. Of note, the use of the term "tumoral calcinosis" in this setting is controversial.[23,26]

The idiopathic form, one-third of which is familial with autosomal dominant transmission of abnormal FGF-23, is demonstrated in **Fig. 6**. Calcium hydroxyapatite is deposited around large joints, most commonly the hip, shoulder, elbow, foot, and wrist. On radiographs, TC seems as an amorphous, multilobulated, mineralized lesion in the periarticular tissues or bursae.[6] Serum calcium is normal, but there can be elevated serum phosphate levels. **Fig. 7** demonstrates secondary TC, which occurs in about 1% of chronic renal failure patients.[26] It is often but not always associated with hyperparathyroidism.[27] As these masses are large, it can be difficult to determine on radiograph if there is an osseous component, and cross-sectional imaging may be needed to confirm the extraosseous location of the mass.[6] As acute TC is largely a liquid suspension, fluid-fluid levels can be seen on cross-sectional imaging.[6] Hemorrhage within a sarcoma can also seem as fluid-fluid levels, but hemorrhage is not as dense as calcium on CT.[28] On T1-weighted MR imaging, TC is a homogeneous lesion with low signal intensity. On T2-weighted MR imaging, generally, 2 patterns can be detected: (1) diffuse low signal intensity or (2) alternating high and low signal with a nodular pattern.[6]

Gout is another disease that can manifest as a periarticular mass with mineralization and can mimic soft tissue sarcoma. Gout can be classified into acute, intermediate, and chronic forms. In chronic gout, a soft tissue mass-like tophus can form which contains deposits of urate, protein matrix, inflammatory cells, and foreign body giant cells. Gouty tophus can develop in the intraarticular space, synovial recesses, bursae, peri-articular subcutaneous tissues, tendons, ligaments, cartilage, and bone.[29] Radiographic findings in chronic gout include juxta-articular erosions with overhanging margins, eccentric soft tissue swelling, and preservation of joint space until the late stage of the disease.[29] On both T1 and T2 images, tophi seem as homogenous or heterogeneous low to intermediate signal intensity masses (**Fig. 8**). Tophi may also enhance on postgadolinium images, which can be confused for enhancement within a soft tissue malignancy, especially when the enhancing tophus is located outside the joint proper. When intraarticular, the differential diagnosis for a mineralized mass includes chronic rheumatoid arthritis, intraarticular tenosynovial giant cell tumor, chronic mycobacterial arthritis, chronic hemarthrosis, amyloidosis, and calcium pyrophosphate dihydrate deposition (CPPD)

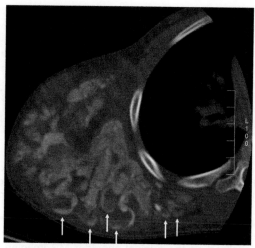

Fig. 6. 8-year-old with painless enlarging mass around the right shoulder extending along the right chest wall. Axial noncontrast CT image demonstrates a large soft tissue mass with fluid-fluid levels (*arrows*). Anatomic pathology of the mass confirmed calcium hydroxyapatite deposition, consistent with tumoral calcinosis.

arthropathy.[30] Intraarticular soft tissue malignancies are extremely rare. Dual-energy CT can be helpful for distinguishing these masses, as it is specific for monosodium crystal deposition. DECT can also help to determine the acuity of the gout attack and assess for response to gout treatment.[29,31] If the amount of monosodium urate detected is out of proportion to the degree of joint inflammation, a parallel disease process may also need to be considered.[32]

The sarcomas most often associated with intratumoral calcification include synovial sarcoma,

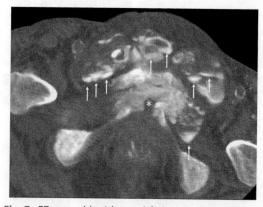

Fig. 7. 57-year-old with renal failure and parathyroid hormone level of 1313. Axial noncontrast CT image demonstrates a large soft tissue with fluid-fluid levels (*arrows*) around the pubic symphysis (*). This mass was presumed to be tumoral calcinosis based on the patients' history and the imaging appearance.

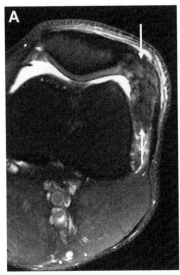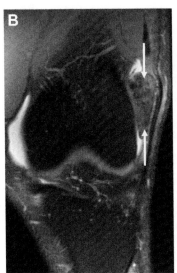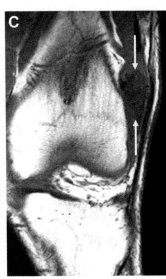

Fig. 8. 44-year-old with chronic pain in the left knee. (*A*) Axial T2 fat-suppressed, (*B*) Coronal T2 fat-suppressed, and (*C*) Coronal T1 MR imaging images of the knee show an intraarticular mass in the lateral aspect of the knee, with multiple foci of low signal intensity on all sequences, consistent with mineralization (*arrows*). There is no erosion or marrow edema of the adjacent patella and femur. Percutaneous and excisional biopsy both confirmed the diagnosis of tophaceous gout.

undifferentiated pleomorphic sarcoma (UPS), well-differentiated liposarcoma, and the rarer extraskeletal osteosarcoma and extraskeletal myxoid chondrosarcoma. Calcifications can be found in up to 41% of synovial sarcomas and typically appear as nonspecific eccentric or peripheral intratumoral calcifications on radiographs or CT.[33] UPS can manifest with calcifications on radiographs in 5%-20% of cases whereby they appear peripheral curvilinear or punctate.[34] Well-differentiated liposarcomas can be calcified in 10% to 32% of cases and calcifications can be single or multiple and tend to be rounded.[35–37] Calcifications occur in about 50% of extraosseous osteosarcomas and are best seen on CT whereby they appear as mineralized osteoid located eccentric within the lesion, rather than unmineralized osteoid in the center of the lesion.[38,39] As both extraosseous osteosarcoma and MO have dense calcifications, it can also be challenging to distinguish these lesions from each other; however, the ossification in MO is peripheral and matures over weeks, whereas in extraskeletal osteosarcoma it remains immature.[38]

Myonecrosis is a confusing entity that can be mistaken for a malignancy because it looks "ugly" and can present as a soft tissue mass. There are multiple etiologies that can lead to disrupted muscular blood flow and the development of muscle infarction or myonecrosis, including compartment syndrome, diabetes, trauma, exercise, heatstroke, radiation, infection, metabolic disorders, seizures, envenomation, toxins, medicinal or illicit drug use, vasculitis, and infection.[40,41] On ultrasound, linear muscle fibers can be seen traversing the lesion.[41] On MR imaging, myonecrosis is typically isointense or slightly hyperintense to adjacent muscle on T1 imaging due to the hemorrhage and/or protein within the liquefied infarcted muscle. On T2 imaging, the lesion is typically heterogeneous with areas that can be as hyperintense as fluid. On postcontrast images, there is often a "serpentine" appearance.[40,42] This "buzz-word" is typically used for osteonecrosis, and is also appropriate here, as it is a similar process, but in a different tissue. The "stipple" sign, which is due to residual viable or inflammatory muscle tissue, can also be observed.[40] Soft tissue malignancy may also have necrosis, but there is usually a more solid, nodular enhancing component. **Fig. 9** illustrates the typical findings of myonecrosis in a 37-year-old with type II diabetes who presented with a new left hip mass and 85-pound weight loss after a prolonged hospitalization for diabetic gastroparesis. Without the knowledge of the patient history, a soft tissue malignancy could be the top differential consideration. Fortunately, the history was provided in the examination indication and myonecrosis was provided as the favored diagnosis. Regarding the exact etiology of myonecrosis, diabetes or prolonged pressure during hospitalization was the most likely. Given the location immediately adjacent to the greater trochanter and the involvement

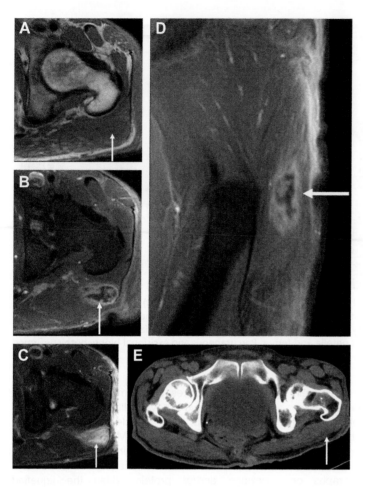

Fig. 9. 37-year-old with type II diabetes who presented with new left hip mass and 85-pound weight loss after a prolonged hospitalization. (A) Axial T1, (B) Axial T1 fat-suppressed postcontrast, and (C) Axial T2 fat-suppressed MR imaging images of the left hip demonstrate a geographic, serpentine, rim-enhancing, T2-hyperintense mass in the gluteus maximus. (D) Sagittal T1 fat-suppressed postcontrast image of the left hip again shows irregular peripheral enhancement. (E) Axial non-contrast CT image 2 months later demonstrates complete resolution of the mass, without any specific treatment. Due to the patient history, this mass was favored to represent myonecrosis.

of only one muscle rather than multiple muscles as is common in diabetic-induced myonecrosis, the prolonged pressure etiology was preferred. The patient did not have any specific treatment of this finding, and 2 months later, it spontaneously resolved, confirming the presumed diagnosis.

SUMMARY

Distinguishing benign and malignant soft tissue tumors solely on imaging can be challenging. However, there are distinctive imaging features that can direct the radiologist to the correct diagnosis when observed in conjunction with demographical and historical information. MO is most often encountered in young individuals in their third and fourth decade of life and can be distinguished from more ominous lesions by their rim of ossification. Acute traumatic hematomas are commonly found in patients with a history of trauma or anticoagulation and on imaging they usually demonstrate thin linear peripheral enhancement which is indicative of gadolinium leakage from torn blood vessels. The geyser lesion is seen in the setting of chronic full-thickness rotator cuff tear and severe acromioclavicular degenerative change and is typically cyst-like with no nodular enhancement. TC is usually periarticular and often demonstrates fluid-fluid levels that are denser than tumor-associated hemorrhage. Gouty tophus forms in patients with chronic gout. When gout is in the differential, dual-energy CT can confirm the diagnosis. Myonecrosis results from the disruption of muscular blood flow and the imaging findings can mimic a soft tissue malignancy. Patient history is very important for making this diagnosis. Knowledge of the typical imaging and clinical patterns of these common mass-like soft tissue tumor mimics can help avoid unnecessary workup and patient anxiety.

CLINICS CARE POINTS

- If the patient is not in a typical demographic for cancer, consider MO as a diagnosis.
- Non-contrast T1 images are helpful for making the diagnosis of hematoma.

- Geyser lesions are very common and should be considered in the setting of a fluid-filled lesion centered on the acromioclavicular joint, in a patient with a full-thickness rotator cuff tear.

- Tumoral calcinosis is most commonly associated with chronic renal insufficiency.

- Dual-energy CT can be helpful for making the diagnosis of gout.

- Myonecrosis can appear mass-like. Query the patient for potential history of localized or diffuse muscular blood flow disruption.

REFERENCES

1. Tyler P, Saifuddin A. The imaging of myositis ossificans. Semin Musculoskelet Radiol 2010;14(2):201–16.

2. Wang H, Nie P, Li Y, et al. MRI findings of early myositis ossificans without calcification or ossification. Biomed Res Int 2018;2018.

3. Simon T, Guillodo Y, Madouas G, et al. Myositis ossificans traumatica (circumscripta) and return to sport: A retrospective series of 19 cases. Joint Bone Spine 2016;83(4):416–20.

4. Colman MW, Lozano-Calderon S, Raskin KA, et al. Non-neoplastic soft tissue masses that mimic sarcoma. Orthop Clin North Am 2014;45(2):245–55.

5. King JB. Post-traumatic ectopic calcification in the muscles of athletes: a review. Br J Sports Med 1998;32(4):287–90.

6. May DA, Disler DG, Jones EA, et al. Abnormal signal intensity in skeletal muscle at MR Imaging: patterns, pearls, and pitfalls. RadioGraphics 2000;20(suppl_1):S295–315.

7. Yarmish G, Klein MJ, Landa J, et al. Imaging characteristics of primary osteosarcoma: nonconventional subtypes. RadioGraphics 2010;30(6):1653–72.

8. Kransdorf MJ, Meis JM. From the archives of the AFIP. Extraskeletal osseous and cartilaginous tumors of the extremities. Radiogr Rev Publ Radiol Soc N Am Inc 1993;13(4):853–84.

9. Kransdorf MJ, Meis JM, Jelinek JS. Myositis ossificans: MR appearance with radiologic-pathologic correlation. AJR Am J Roentgenol 1991;157(6):1243–8.

10. Nuovo MA, Norman A, Chumas J, et al. Myositis ossificans with atypical clinical, radiographic, or pathologic findings: a review of 23 cases. Skeletal Radiol 1992;21(2):87–101.

11. Murphey D. The Many Faces of Osteosarcom. Radiographics 1997;17(5):27.

12. Isaacson BM, Potter BK, Bloebaum RD, et al. Determining the mineral apposition rate of heterotopie ossification in military healthcare system patients after total joint replacement: a case series. Bone Tissue Regen Insights 2016;7:S38041. BTRI.

13. Marsell R, Einhorn TA. The biology of fracture healing. Injury 2011;42(6):551–5.

14. Yaghmai I. Myositis ossificans: diagnostic value of arteriography. Am J Roentgenol 1977;128(5):811–6.

15. Gomez P, Morcuende J. High-grade sarcomas mimicking traumatic intramuscular hematomas. Iowa Orthop J 2004;24:106–10.

16. De Smet AA. Magnetic resonance findings in skeletal muscle tears. Skeletal Radiol 1993;22(7):479–84.

17. Stacy GS, Dixon LB. Pitfalls in MR image interpretation prompting referrals to an orthopedic oncology clinic. Radiogr Rev Publ Radiol Soc N Am Inc 2007;27(3):805–26.

18. Kontogeorgakos VA, Martinez S, Dodd L, et al. Extremity soft tissue sarcomas presented as hematomas. Arch Orthop Trauma Surg 2010;130(10):1209–14.

19. Jahed K, Khazai B, Umpierrez M, et al. Pitfalls in soft tissue sarcoma imaging: chronic expanding hematomas. Skeletal Radiol 2018;47(1):119–24.

20. Popov M, Sotiriadis C, Gay F, et al. Spontaneous intramuscular hematomas of the abdomen and pelvis: a new multilevel algorithm to direct transarterial embolization and patient management. Cardiovasc Intervent Radiol 2017;40(4):537–45.

21. Cooper HJ, Milillo R, Klein DA, et al. The MRI geyser sign: acromioclavicular joint cysts in the setting of a chronic rotator cuff tear. Am J Orthop Belle Mead NJ 2011;40(6):E118–21.

22. Hiller AD, Miller JD, Zeller JL. Acromioclavicular joint cyst formation. Clin Anat N Y N 2010;23(2):145–52.

23. Steinbach LS, Johnston JO, Tepper EF, et al. Tumoral calcinosis: radiologic-pathologic correlation. Skeletal Radiol 1995;24(8):573–8.

24. Farrow EG, Imel EA, White KE. hyperphosphatemic familial tumoral calcinosis (FGF23, GALNT3, αKlotho). Best Pract Res Clin Rheumatol 2011;25(5):735–47.

25. Folsom LJ, Imel EA. Hyperphosphatemic familial tumoral calcinosis: genetic models of deficient FGF23 action. Curr Osteoporos Rep 2015;13(2):78–87.

26. Olsen KM, Chew FS. Tumoral calcinosis: pearls, polemics, and alternative possibilities. Radiogr Rev Publ Radiol Soc N Am Inc 2006;26(3):871–85.

27. Eisenberg B, Tzamaloukas AH, Hartshorne MF, et al. Periarticular tumoral calcinosis and hypercalcemia in a hemodialysis patient without hyperparathyroidism: a case report. J Nucl Med 1990;31(6):1099–103.

28. Tsai JC, Dalinka MK, Fallon MD, et al. Fluid-fluid level: a nonspecific finding in tumors of bone and soft tissue. Radiology 1990;175(3):779–82.

29. Dhanda S, Quek ST, Bathla G, et al. Intra-articular and peri-articular tumours and tumour mimics-what a clinician and onco-imaging radiologist

should know. Malays J Med Sci MJMS 2014;21(2): 4–19.

30. Chen CK, Yeh LR, Pan HB, et al. Intra-articular gouty tophi of the knee: CT and MR imaging in 12 patients. Skeletal Radiol 1999;28(2):75–80.

31. Karcaaltincaba M, Aktas A. Dual-Energy Ct revisited with multidetector ct: review of principles and clinical applications. Available at: http://www.openaccess. hacettepe.edu.tr:8080/xmlui/handle/11655/15891. Accessed September 13, 2021.

32. Desai MA, Peterson JJ, Garner HW, et al. Clinical utility of dual-energy ct for evaluation of tophaceous gout. RadioGraphics 2011;31(5):1365–75.

33. Murphey MD, Gibson MS, Jennings BT, et al. From the archives of the AFIP: Imaging of synovial sarcoma with radiologic-pathologic correlation. Radiogr Rev Publ Radiol Soc N Am Inc 2006;26(5):1543–65.

34. Murphey MD, Gross TM, Rosenthal HG. From the archives of the AFIP. Musculoskeletal malignant fibrous histiocytoma: radiologic-pathologic correlation. RadioGraphics 1994;14(4):807–26.

35. Murphey MD, Arcara LK, Fanburg-Smith J. Imaging of musculoskeletal liposarcoma with radiologic-pathologic correlation. RadioGraphics 2005;25(5):1371–95.

36. Kransdorf MJ, Meis JM, Jelinek JS. Dedifferentiated liposarcoma of the extremities: imaging findings in four patients. AJR Am J Roentgenol 1993;161(1):127–30.

37. Tuoheti Y, Okada K, Miyakoshi N, et al. Unusual variant of liposarcoma with multiple punctate calcifications. Skeletal Radiol 2002;31(11):666–70.

38. Mc Auley G, Jagannathan J, O'Regan K, et al. Extra-skeletal osteosarcoma: spectrum of imaging findings. Am J Roentgenol 2012;198(1):W31–7.

39. Roller LA, Chebib I, Bredella MA, et al. Clinical, radiological, and pathological features of extraskeletal osteosarcoma. Skeletal Radiol 2018;47(9): 1213–20.

40. Smitaman E, Flores DV, Mejía Gómez C, et al. MR imaging of atraumatic muscle disorders. RadioGraphics 2018;38(2):500–22.

41. Stacy GS, Kapur A. Mimics of bone and soft tissue neoplasms. Radiol Clin North Am 2011;49(6): 1261–86.

42. Jelinek JS, Murphey MD, Aboulafia AJ, et al. Muscle infarction in patients with diabetes mellitus: MR imaging findings. Radiology 1999;211(1):241–7.

Bone and Soft Tissue Tumors
Interventional Techniques for Diagnosis and Treatment

Rupert O. Stanborough, MD[a],*, Jeremiah R. Long, MD[b], Hillary W. Garner, MD[a]

KEYWORDS

- Bone tumor • Soft tissue tumor • Biopsy • Ablation • Cementoplasty

KEY POINTS

- Patient history and imaging should be reviewed before all bone and soft tissue tumor biopsies.
- Radiology-pathology correlation of biopsied bone and soft tissue tumors is an essential component of patient care.
- Local tumor control and pain palliation are 2 indications for radiologists to treat bone metastases.
- Cementoplasty should be considered in weightbearing bones at risk for pathologic fracture.

INTRODUCTION

Radiologists play an integral role in the multi-disciplinary management of benign and malignant musculoskeletal (MSK) tumors and tumor-like conditions. In the review, we discuss common interventional techniques performed by radiologists to diagnose and treat these diseases.

DIAGNOSTIC BIOPSY
Indications

Percutaneous MSK biopsy tissue sampling is most often performed for the histologic differentiation of a benign process from a malignant process when a definitive diagnosis of a benign lesion cannot be made by imaging features alone. Other common indications for percutaneous MSK biopsy include the confirmation of metastatic disease when multiple bone lesions are present and/or a primary malignancy is known or highly suspected; marrow sampling (biopsy and aspiration) for a known or suspected hematologic malignancy; sampling of a suspected infectious process to confirm diagnosis and for culture and antibiotic sensitivity testing; muscle sampling in the setting of myositis; and obtaining additional material from a known malignancy to assess treatment response or for advanced testing (eg, special stains, genetic sequencing).[1-6] In general, a percutaneous biopsy is indicated when the results of the biopsy could alter patient management.[1]

Contraindications

Contraindications to biopsy are infrequent, but include lack of a safe needle path, inadequate needle length, acute or ongoing non-MSK infection, soft tissue infection overlying the target, uncorrected bleeding diathesis, or an uncooperative patient.[1-6] The majority of percutaneous MSK biopsy sites are superficial and readily compressible whereby bleeding can usually be detected and controlled. Therefore, the Society of Interventional Radiology (SIR) considers bone and soft tissue biopsy is low risk in most anatomic locations. However, biopsies of the spine and deep soft tissues (eg, intraabdominal, retroperitoneal, and pelvic

a Department of Radiology, Mayo Clinic Florida, 4500 San Pablo Road, Jacksonville, FL 32224, USA;
b Department of Radiology, Mayo Clinic Arizona, 5777 E. Mayo Boulevard, Phoenix, AZ 85054, USA
* Corresponding author.
E-mail address: stanborough.rupert@mayo.edu

Radiol Clin N Am 60 (2022) 311–326
https://doi.org/10.1016/j.rcl.2021.11.009
0033-8389/22/© 2021 Elsevier Inc. All rights reserved.

compartments) are considered high risk.[7] Given a low overall complication rate (generally <5%),[2,8–14] some investigators suggest foregoing routine pre-procedural coagulation testing (platelet count, prothrombin time, international normalized ratio).[15,16] Furthermore, the SIR's 2019 Consensus Guidelines do not recommend testing for patients with minimal bleeding risk who are undergoing low-risk procedures.[7]

Target Selection

Preprocedural planning is an essential step for the safe and successful performance of a percutaneous MSK biopsy. Proper planning begins with a thorough review of relevant prior imaging. If appropriate imaging has not been obtained, this should be requested before proceeding with biopsy. Occasionally, biopsy can be avoided if a definitive diagnosis of benignity can be achieved with imaging alone, such as in cases of hemangioma or lipoma. If a lesion remains indeterminate or suspicious after imaging review, the radiologist can assess the likelihood of a primary malignancy versus a metastasis. In cases with multiple available targets, the target that is the safest and easiest access should be selected. For example, a lesion within the posterior ilium would generally be chosen over a lesion in the vertebral body.

The goal of biopsy is to obtain a representative sample of the lesion to maximize accuracy in pathologic diagnosis. The most aggressive-appearing component of the lesion corresponds to the most metabolically active tumor cells and should be included within the needle path. In general, targeting regions of new growth, bone destruction, avid MRI or CT enhancement, or greatest PET/CT hypermetabolism will increase the likelihood of capturing diagnostic tissue [Fig. 1].

Needle Path Selection

When considering a needle path, the shortest distance to the target may not be the optimal choice. When a primary tumor is suspected, the radiologist should assume that limb-sparing surgery will be an option for local disease control. Therefore, the biopsy path should be along the same plane as what would be used for tumor resection as most surgeons will resect the tumor and biopsy tract en bloc to remove possible tumor seeding along the needle tract.[17] Biopsy path considerations before limb-sparing surgery are discussed further in Goulding and colleagues' article, "Skeletal Sarcomas: Diagnosis, Treatment, and Follow-up from the Orthopedic Oncologist Perspective," in this issue and Wilke and colleagues' article, "Soft Tissue Tumors: Diagnosis,

Treatment, and Follow-up from the Orthopedic Oncologist Perspective," in this issue and in the literature.[18,19] However, it is important to reiterate that in cases whereby lesion origin, whether primary or metastatic, cannot be clearly discerned, the selected approach should reflect the assumption that the target is a primary tumor.[4] An inappropriate biopsy path could adversely affect patient outcome, including increasing the risk of local recurrence and limb amputation.[20] Although tumor seeding along a percutaneous biopsy tract has been reported[21–23] [Fig. 2], the concept remains controversial in the literature.[21–28] Overall, it is prudent to work in conjunction with the oncologic surgeon to ensure the needle path aligns with potential operative approach.

Individualized Patient Considerations

Knowledge of the patient's allergy profile, particularly regarding local anesthesia and moderate sedation medications, as well as contrast, is mandatory. Furthermore, sensitivities to skin cleansers, latex, and adhesives should be addressed.

Patient informed consent is a mandatory component of any procedure and should include a face-to-face discussion of procedural risks, anticipated benefits, and reasonable alternatives along with the opportunity to ask questions about the procedure.[29] The institutional preprocedural protocol for confirming the patient's identity, the procedure, and the specific location should be followed (eg, "time-out" protocol).

Percutaneous biopsy of a soft tissue tumor and of the soft tissue component of a bone tumor can usually be performed with local anesthesia alone. In our experience, bone biopsy is also typically well tolerated with local anesthesia alone when thorough periosteal numbing is accomplished. However, moderate sedation may be beneficial, especially if there is high patient anxiety or if the target lesion is densely sclerotic. General anesthesia is another option but is typically reserved for patients who cannot readily cooperate with positioning (eg, pediatric patients), patients at high risk for moderate sedation, and patients with high narcotic tolerance.

Image Guidance

The primary modalities available to most radiologists for biopsy image guidance are CT, ultrasound (US), and fluoroscopy. Although MRI can also be used, it is not as common. The modality chosen is primarily based on lesion location and conspicuity on prior imaging. The decision is also influenced by operator preference/familiarity as

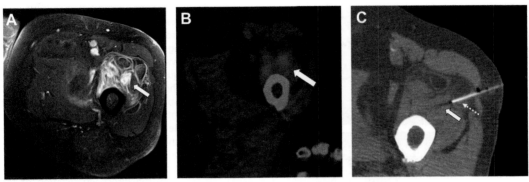

Fig. 1. 84-year-old man with a known long-standing left thigh mass presenting with recent growth of the mass. Axial post-contrast fat-suppressed T1-weighted MRI image (*A*) and an axial PET/CT image (*B*) show a fat-containing mass with an enhancing and FDG-avid nonadipose nodule within the anterior left thigh (*arrows*). Subsequent axial noncontrast CT image (*C*) shows placement of a biopsy introducer needle (*dotted arrow*) at the lateral margin of the nodule (*arrow*) immediately before coaxial placement of the biopsy needle into the nodule (not shown). Pathology showed dedifferentiated liposarcoma.

well as local equipment capabilities and availability.

CT guidance is best for deep lesions, intraosseous lesions, and cases whereby direct visualization of nearby neurovascular bundles and vital organs is essential [**Fig. 3**]. Benefits of CT guidance include availability and user familiarity. Even when CT-occult, lesions can be localized anatomically based on preprocedure PET or MRI[30][**Fig. 4**]. CT guidance also allows for immediate postprocedural imaging to evaluate for complications such as pneumothorax or hematoma [see **Fig. 3**]. Disadvantages of CT guidance include ionizing radiation, dependence on straight axial needle orientation, and the potential space constraints for clearing the CT gantry when using longer needles. Strategies to reduce patient dose can be used, including limiting the field of view on localization imaging, decreasing tube current and voltage, and increasing pitch.[31] As with all

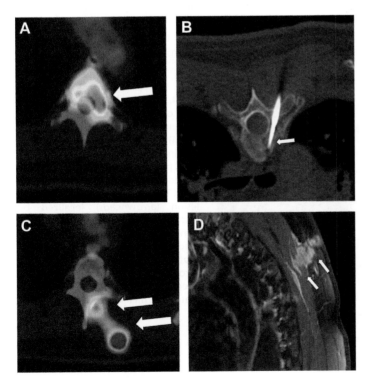

Fig. 2. 35-year-old woman with breast cancer presenting with pack pain. An axial image from the initial PET/CT (*A*) shows a focal FDG-avid lesion within the T4 vertebral body and left pedicle (*arrow*). Subsequent axial prone noncontrast CT image (*B*) shows placement of a biopsy needle in the corresponding T4 lytic lesion during CT-guided biopsy (*arrow*) with pathology showing metastatic breast cancer. Follow-up axial PET/CT image (*C*) and sagittal postcontrast fat-suppressed T1-weighted MR image (*D*) 9 months after biopsy show new FDG-avid and enhancing tumor nodules (*arrows*) seeding the biopsy tract.

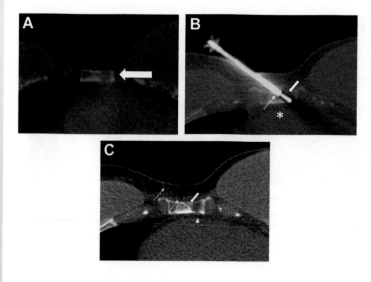

Fig. 3. 31-year-old woman with a history of breast cancer. An axial image from the initial staging PET/CT image(A) shows a focal FDG-avid lesion within the sternum (*arrow*). A subsequent axial noncontrast CT image (*B*) shows placement of a coaxial bone biopsy needle with the larger gauge introducer needle positioned just deep to the cortex (*dotted arrow*) and the smaller gauge inner biopsy needle (*arrow*) positioned within the corresponding lytic lesion (*arrow*). Note the direct visualization of the pericardium and heart (*asterisk*) deep to the tip of the biopsy needle. Immediate postprocedural axial noncontrast CT image (*C*) shows expected foci of air along the needle path (*dotted arrows*), the biopsy tract within the sternum (*arrow*), and the normal appearance of the subjacent pericardium and heart (*arrowhead*). Pathology confirmed metastatic breast cancer.

imaging modalities that use ionizing radiation, the as low as reasonably achievable (ALARA) principle should be applied when using CT guidance. Regarding the technical challenges inherent to needle placement, multiplanar reconstructions can be performed to maintain the orientation of the needle tip to the target[32,33][Fig. 5].

US is a widely available and versatile modality for percutaneous biopsy guidance. It is well suited for the biopsy of soft tissue masses and soft tissue components of bone tumors. Advantages of US include direct real-time needle visualization,

flexibility in the selection of the plane for needle approach, ability to identify vascularity with Doppler imaging or contrast material, and lack of ionizing radiation [Fig. 6]. US guidance can be technically challenging for deep biopsy targets and in patients with a large body habitus.

Fluoroscopy is another widely available modality for biopsy guidance and is best suited for bone lesions that are either visible radiographically or can be safely localized using surrounding osseous landmarks. Similar to US, fluoroscopy systems can produce real-time images for accurate needle

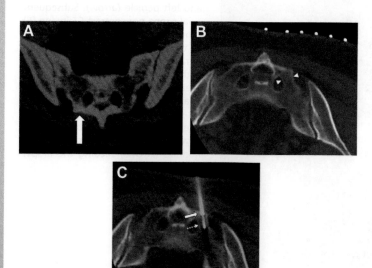

Fig. 4. 65-year-old woman with a history of melanoma of the heel. An axial image from a surveillance PET/CT (*A*) shows a focal FDG-avid lesion within posterior right sacrum (*arrow*). Axial prone noncontrast CT image obtained during the biopsy (*B*) shows the CT occult area of the FDG-avid lesion (*arrowheads*) localized by osseous landmarks. Subsequent axial noncontrast CT image (*C*) shows the placement of the biopsy needle (*dotted arrow*) with coaxial technique through the larger gauge introducing needle (*arrow*). Pathology confirmed metastatic melanoma.

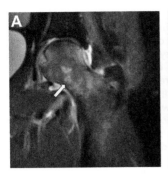
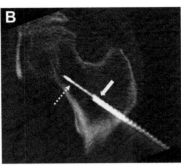

Fig. 5. 55-year-old woman with lung cancer presenting with left hip pain. Initial coronal postcontrast fat-suppressed T1-weighted MR image (A) shows an enhancing marrow-replacing lesion centered within the left femoral neck (arrow). Subsequent noncontrast CT imaging was reformatted into the coronal plane during the procedure. The reformatted coronal CT image (B) shows the placement of a soft tissue biopsy needle (dotted arrow) with coaxial technique through the larger gauge introducing bone needle positioned just lateral to the lytic lesion (arrow). Pathology confirmed metastatic lung cancer.

visualization. With a C-arm configuration, fluoroscopy can be oriented to facilitate the selection of the optimal plane for the needle approach. One specific advantage of fluoroscopy over CT lies in its ability to image around metal implants without beam hardening artifact. This can be particularly helpful when targeting lesions around spinal fixation or fracture fixation constructs [Fig. 7]. Fluoroscopy imparts ionizing radiation to both the patient and operator and is generally not an appropriate choice for soft tissue lesions.

MRI guidance can be valuable for lesions that are occult on other imaging modalities.[34,35] This modality has also been promoted due to its lack of ionizing radiation, which makes it a particularly attractive option for pediatric and pregnant patients[36] [Fig. 8]. Limitations include the need for MR compatible instruments and increased procedural time when compared with CT and US[35] as well as its lower availability and higher cost.

As percutaneous MSK biopsy has grown in popularity and imaging equipment has improved, many operators choose to combine guidance modalities to leverage the unique advantages of different modalities and improve diagnostic outcomes and patient safety. Given its portability and excellent soft tissue contrast, US is often chosen as an adjunct modality for needle guidance. In cases whereby important superficial structures are not well visualized, we have used US during initial

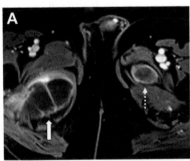
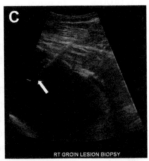
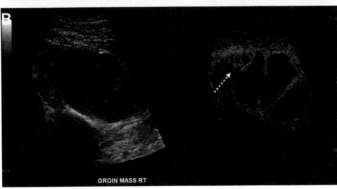

Fig. 6. 59-year-old man status postrenal transplant with leg pain, disseminated nocardia infection presenting with clinical suspicion for posttransplant lymphoproliferative disorder. Initial axial postcontrast fat-suppressed T1-weighted MR image (A) shows a rim enhancing mass in the medial aspect of the left thigh (dotted arrow) and a rim and septal enhancing mass in the medial aspect of the right thigh (arrow). Subsequent ultrasound images of the right thigh mass (B) obtained immediately before (left) and following ultrasound microbubble contrast (right) shows multiple internal enhancing septa (dotted arrow). Ultrasound image (C) during percutaneous biopsy shows the needle (arrow) sampling the internal enhancing septa. Pathology showed acute inflammation and necrosis with reactive stromal changes and culture was positive for nocardia farcinica.

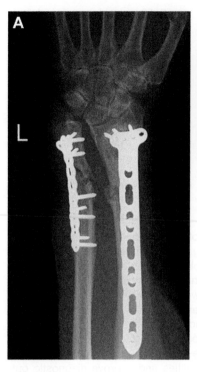
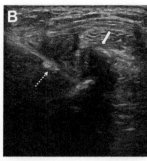
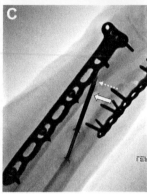

Fig. 7. 78-year-old woman with open fractures of the distal radius and ulna, both of which went on to nonunion. Biopsy was requested for histology and culture to exclude infection before planned revision with bone grafting. Initial PA radiograph of the left wrist (A) shows plate and screw fixation constructs across both fracture sites. Ultrasound images obtained immediately before and during needle placement (not shown) confirmed that the needle path avoided major vascular structures. Subsequent ultrasound image (B) shows the needle (dotted arow) into the radius fracture defect with the radial cortical margin identified (arrow). Intraprocedural fluoroscopic image (C) shows the coaxial bone biopsy needle set with the introducer needle (arrow) placed at the radius bone edge and the biopsy needle (dotted arrow) within the radius. Pathology showed devitalized bone and testing for infection was negative.

needle advancement to confidently avoid these structures [see **Fig. 7**]. Technologic advances in imaging equipment have also aided in combining modalities. For example, the addition of cone-beam CT to fluoroscopy units allows seamless integration during bone biopsies to ensure proper lesion targeting [**Fig. 9**]. In the setting of bone biopsies, simplified planning and decreased procedure times have been cited as advantages of this combination.[37]

Biopsy Devices

Familiarity with the different biopsy needle systems is key. There are several core needle biopsy sets of various design, length, and gauge currently on the market. In general, percutaneous MSK biopsy can be performed without or with coaxial needle technique. Of note, coaxial needle technique has several advantages, including improved efficiency when multiple biopsy samples are needed and reduced need for additional imaging guidance between biopsy needle passes. For this reason, coaxial technique is particularly valuable for deeper lesions and lesions within bone, whereby cortical penetration only needs to be performed once during the initial needle placement.

Soft tissue lesions can be biopsied with side cutting or end-cutting soft tissue core needles. These generally include a spring-loaded component that facilitates tissue cutting and capture. Different needle lengths and calibers are available

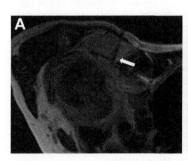
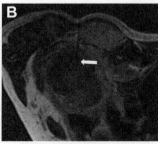

Fig. 8. 28-year-old pregnant woman with a history of NF1 and a known brachial plexus mass presenting with recent onset left scapular and chest pain radiating to the forearm as well as left-hand weakness. Axial T2-weighted MR images obtained during MRI-guided biopsy with the patient in the prone position of a mass in the subcutaneous tissues of the left upper back at the T1 level (A) and of a mass in the apex of the left lung (B) show titanium alloy biopsy needles (arrows) within each mass. Pathology showed neurofibroma at each site.

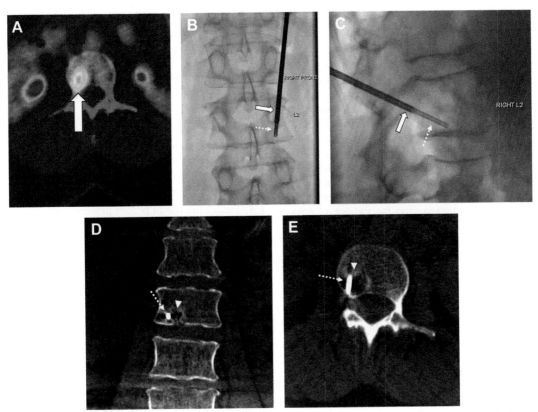

Fig. 9. 65-year-old woman with breast cancer. An axial image obtained during surveillance PET/CT (*A*) shows a focal FDG-avid lesion within L2 vertebral body (*arrow*). Subsequent frontal (*B*) and lateral (*C*) fluoroscopic images show a coaxial bone biopsy needle set with the introducing needle crossing through the right pedicle into the vertebral body (*arrows*) and the biopsy needle passing into the L2 vertebral body (*dotted arrows*). Cone beam CT images in the coronal (*D*) and axial (*E*) planes obtained at the same time confirmed the biopsy needle (*dotted arrows*) is positioned within the lateral margin of the targeted lytic lesion. Pathology confirmed metastatic breast cancer.

and can be selected depending on target depth and size. With side cutting needles the most distal 2 to 3 mm of the needle tip are part of the cutting component of the needle and do not capture tissue. When visualizing the distal tip of the biopsy needle within the target lesion, this distal 2 to 3 mm of unsampled "dead space" must be kept in mind.

Intraosseous lesions generally require needles specifically designed for bone penetration and the needle sets include both introducing needle and stylet as well as a small gauge hollow trephine-type biopsy needle. The biopsy needle is designed to pass through and extend beyond the introducer needle for lesion sampling. Some bone needle biopsy sets include reusable drills to aid in cortical access.

Of note, the combined employment of both the bone penetration needle system with the soft tissue core needle biopsy system can be a useful technique for sampling lytic bone lesions, improving the likelihood of capturing diagnostic tissue [see **Fig. 5**].

Fine needle aspiration (FNA) of MSK lesions can be performed using any of the above guidance techniques. By using simple needles with sizes that are 22 gauge and smaller, FNA is cost-effective and minimally invasive. These small gauge needles can be safely redirected several times within a lesion to broaden the sampling area. In addition, intraprocedural preliminary diagnostic feedback on the sampled material can be provided when a cytologist is present.[38,39] However, studies evaluating the diagnostic value of FNA versus core needle biopsy in MSK tumors have demonstrated that core biopsy outperforms FNA.[38,39] In our current practice, we will occasionally use FNA before core biopsy, but rarely use FNA alone.

Specimen Handling

Communication of the relevant history and anticipated diagnosis with the pathology team facilitates the most appropriate processing and testing of the sample and can aid the pathologist in diagnosis. At our institutions, a touch-prep analysis of the initial specimen is performed during the procedure which can help confirm diagnostic adequacy real-time and potentially decrease the number of samples needed. Most soft tissue and bone specimens will then be placed in 10% neutral buffered formalin and transported to the pathology department. The pathology team then reviews the patient information to determine how to best process the specimen. Bone specimens will usually require "de-calcification" with ethylenediaminetetraacetic acid (EDTA). However, the touch prep analysis may identify unexpected cytology that spurs the use of different preservation media. For example, in cases of suspected lymphoma, a portion of the specimen is placed in Roswell Park Memorial Institute (RPMI) solution rather than formalin to allow for cytometric flow analysis. Lymphoma biopsy samples initially placed in formalin cannot undergo cytometric flow analysis. Of note, in cases of suspected infection, a portion of the tissue or aspirate is placed into normal saline for culture and a portion is placed in formalin for pathology review. If gout is a consideration, a portion of the sample should be placed in alcohol as formalin can dissolve the uric-acid crystals.[4]

Radiology-Pathology Correlation

The radiologist's involvement in the biopsy process is not complete until after the review of the pathologic diagnosis, which ideally should be reviewed with a multidisciplinary team. This review helps determine whether or not the pathologic diagnosis is concordant with the imaging findings and provides the ability to discuss and give recommendations on the most appropriate next steps in the patient's care based on whether there is concordance or discordance. At our institutions, a weekly radiology-pathology conference is held and attended by the MSK radiology division and pathologists with a special interest in sarcoma. When possible, participation of additional clinical team members from orthopedic oncology, medical oncology, and radiation therapy is helpful. A study of radiology-pathology weekly conferences showed a statistically significant decrease in time to action for discordant results.[40] Another important subjective advantage is the multidisciplinary educational environment provided to the involved

---

> **Box 1**
> **Keys for successful biopsy**
>
> 1. Understand the indication
> 2. Review all relevant imaging
> 3. Select the most aggressive looking component
> 4. Carefully consider needle path
> 5. Become familiar with patient allergies/insensitivities
> 6. Select the most appropriate guidance and biopsy needle system
> 7. Ensure the use of proper preservation media based on the suspected diagnosis
> 8. Correlate pathologic diagnosis with radiology findings

faculty, fellows, residents, and other care team members regarding imaging findings, biopsy approaches, and treatment options. (**Box 1**)

TREATMENT

There are several percutaneous thermal ablation treatment options that can be offered by the radiologist. Most ablation therapies rely on the ability of a device to change the temperature of the tissue to cause irreversible cell damage and can be used to treat many malignant and benign bone or soft tissue tumors. Historically, thermal ablation was considered an alternative treatment option in circumstances whereby surgery, chemotherapy, and radiation therapy had been exhausted or the risks of the other therapies outweighed the benefits. Today, thermal ablation has emerged as a viable treatment of oncology patients, either solely or in combination with other therapies. The 2 indications for thermal ablation with the strongest evidence are (1) local tumor control and (2) pain palliation.

Local tumor control: Ablation can be performed with curative intent with oligometastatic disease (<5 metastases). Many case series have demonstrated the efficacy of thermal ablation in local tumor control. In a retrospective study of 40 patients who underwent cryoablation of 52 tumors, local tumor control was achieved in 45 of 52 tumors (87%) with a median follow-up of 21 months.[41] In another retrospective study by Vaswani and colleagues of 64 metastatic sarcomas treated with cryoablation or radiofrequency ablation (RFA) showed local tumor control in 70% of patients at 1 year, which included 100% control for those with oligometastatic disease.[42]

Pain palliation: Thermal ablation can achieve early and long-lasting pain response. In the same study by Vaswani and colleagues of 64 metastatic sarcomas, the median pain scores decreased from 8/10 preablation to 3/10 at 1-month postablation.[42] A multicenter trial of 61 patients with painful skeletal metastases showed the mean scores dropped from 7.1/10 to 1.4/10 at a longer interval of 24-weeks postprocedure.[43] This pain response translates to significant improvements in the quality of life, decreased opioid use, and maintenance of functional status.[44] Single-institution studies have also shown that the use of RFA and cryoablation in combination with radiation therapy can achieve better pain response compared with either ablation or radiation therapy alone.[45,46]

Treatment of benign bone and soft tissue tumors with thermal ablation is also commonly practiced. Osteoid osteoma was the first bone tumor to be treated with thermal ablation. Given its high level of success, RFA has now become the standard of care for osteoid osteoma treatment given the decreased morbidity and lower cost than surgery[47,48][Fig. 10]. Treatment of osteoid osteomas with other methods of thermal ablation (cryoablation, laser ablation, and high-intensity focused ultrasound (HIFU)) has also been performed.[49–51] For benign soft tissue diseases, thermal ablation of desmoid tumors has shown promise. A single-institution case series of 26 extraabdominal desmoid tumors treated with cryoablation identified only 1 tumor that progressed after a mean follow-up of 16.2 months.[52] A myriad of other benign but painful soft tissue and bone tumors can be successfully treated with ablation, including giant cell tumors of bone, vertebral hemangiomas, chondroblastomas, benign nerve sheath tumors, and nodular fasciitis [Fig. 11].[53,54]

Radiofrequency Ablation

RFA is the most studied method of thermal ablation given its early adoption. An insulated probe with an electrode at the tip is placed into the desired tissue target. An alternating current transmits from the electrode into the adjacent tissue. The ionized molecules in the adjacent tissue attempt to align with the alternating current, creating friction and heat. The electrode itself is not a heat source. At temperatures greater than 60°C, irreversible coagulative necrosis occurs. Older RFA technology was monopolar, meaning a grounding pad had to be placed on the patient. Modern RFA technology uses bipolar probes so no grounding pad is needed. Ablation zones are predicted depending on time and energy, although actual treated volume can differ between tissue types. Multiple RFA probes can be used simultaneously to increase treatment volume [Fig. 12]. Temperature sensors are usually present at or near the probe tip such that tissue temperatures can be monitored during the procedure to ensure adequate heating. Certain RFA probes can articulate to reach difficult locations (ie, posterior vertebral body) and others include a cooled tip to decrease charring and preserve energy transmission. The use of RFA in the spine is attractive because it minimizes the transmission of heat into the spinal canal when the posterior wall is intact.[55,56] One main disadvantage of RFA is the inability to visualize the treatment volume real-time on fluoroscopy or CT imaging.[56,57]

Cryoablation

Cryoablation has become popular for the treatment of bone and soft tissue tumors due to its efficacy and ability to visualize the treatment volume real-time. Most cryo-probes have insulated shafts

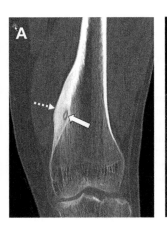
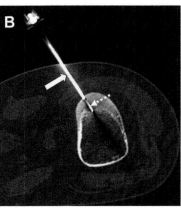

Fig. 10. 20-year-old man with a 2-month history of distal left thigh pain responsive to ibuprofen. CT scan of the left femur (A) shows periosteal reaction along the medial cortex of the distal left femoral shaft (dotted arrow) containing a lucent lesion with central nidus (arrow), consistent with an osteoid osteoma. Intraprocedural CT image of the left distal femur (B) during radiofrequency ablation of the osteoid osteoma shows a coaxial bone access needle (arrow) used to place the tip of the RFA probe (dotted arrow) in the nidus. The patient's left thigh pain completed resolved 1 week following the procedure.

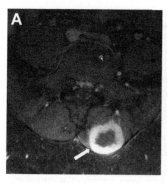
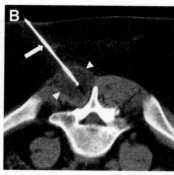

Fig. 11. 35-year-old woman with multiple sclerosis and severe 10/10 lower back pain. Axial postcontrast T1-weighted MR image of the lower lumbar spine (*A*) shows a peripherally enhancing mass (*arrow*) in the left paraspinal musculature. Image-guided biopsy (not shown) was performed with a pathologic diagnosis of nodular fasciitis. The patient was not a good surgical candidate and cryoablation was performed. Intraprocedural axial prone CT image (*B*) obtained during the cryoablation shows the cryoprobe (*arrow*) tip in the left paraspinal mass and ice-ball margins (*arrowheads*) covering the mass. The pain completely resolved 2 weeks following the procedure.

with an uninsulated tip. Once the uninsulated tip is appropriately centered within the tissue target, argon gas is transmitted to the cryo-probe tip which cools the surrounding tissue via the Joule-Thompson effect. Irreversible cell death occurs at temperatures less than -20°C via cell membrane disruption, dehydration, and vascular thrombosis. As with RFA, multiple probes can be used simultaneously, and there are several different designs available that create ice balls of various sizes and shapes, which can allow for optimal coverage of nonuniformly-shaped lesions. Two cycles of freezing are usually performed, in between which the probe(s) can actively thaw. Active thawing can also be used at the end of the procedure before probe removal. An advantage of cryoablation is the ability to see the ice-ball on CT, US, and MRI allowing the operator to ensure adequate tumor coverage [see **Fig. 11**; **Fig. 13**]. Of note, the edge of the ice-ball represents 0°C ice temperature; therefore, the spherical margin of the ice ball should be extended approximately 5 mm

beyond the margin of the tumor to ensure adequate coverage with −20°C ice. A disadvantage of cryoablaton is the prolonged formation of ice that can take up to an hour or 2 to completely thaw; this can result in extended procedure time if cementoplasty is planned immediately following the ablation.[56–58]

Microwave Ablation

Microwave ablation has become popular in the treatment of liver tumors and shows promise in the treatment of bone and other soft tissue tumors. Similar to RFA, microwave ablation heats adjacent tissue via conduction. Microwave probes use antennae to transmit microwave frequency energy from the tip which oscillates adjacent water molecules and heats the tissue. An advantage of microwave is the quick speed at which they can obtain desired heat temperatures and the ability to treat large volumes. In the treatment of liver tumors, microwave ablation has efficacy at least equivalent

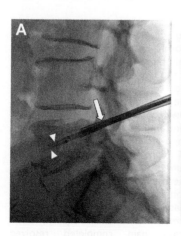
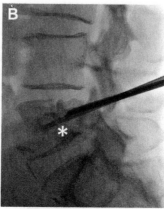

Fig. 12. 50-year-old woman with metastatic renal-cell carcinoma and intractable 10/10 lower back pain. Imaging identified an L5 lesion with pathologic fracture, biopsy proven to represent a metastasis. Intraprocedural lateral fluoroscopic image of the lower lumbar spine (*A*) shows bipedicular access of the L5 vertebral body with coaxial bone access needles (*arrow*) and placement of 2 radiofrequency ablation probes (*arrowheads*) in the vertebral body. Intraprocedural lateral fluoroscopic image of the lower lumbar spine (*B*) shows the existing coaxial needles were used to instill cement into the L5 vertebral body (*asterisk*).

with RFA although can treat larger tumors volumes with less procedural time.[59] As microwave ablation is used more in bone and soft tissues, we expect more insight into its efficacy compared with other modalities.[60–63]

Other Options

HIFU is unique in that it is entirely noninvasive and requires no skin penetration. A transducer is used to apply US energy to desired target and sonications heat the tissue to cytotoxic temperatures.[63,64] HIFU has shown equivalent results to RFA for the treatment of osteoid osteomas in children.[51] Other infrequently used methods of thermal ablation include laser ablation and irreversible electroporation.

Complications of Ablation

Thermal ablation complications are primarily related to the undesired heating or cooling of adjacent vital structures. In circumstances of a closely approximating nerve, displacement is the primary goal to separate the nerve from the ablation zone. This can often be achieved with perineural infiltration of liquid or gas to mechanically displace the nerve while simultaneously insulating the nerve with poorly conductive material (ie, gas with heating or freezing, hypertonic solutions with freezing)

[see **Fig. 13**; **Fig. 14**]. Intraprocedural nerve monitoring via motor and/or sensory evoked potentials is a technique well-established in neurosurgery that can be used during thermal ablation if near an important nerve.[65,66] Additionally, thermocouple probes can be placed near nerves to monitor temperature real-time. In cases of spine RFA, the procedure can be performed with moderate or conscious sedation such that the patient may alert the operator if they develop neuropathic pain during ablation.[56,67]

Skin necrosis is another potential complication that requires proactive preventive measures. Particularly with cryoablation, freezing too close or through the skin can cause irreversible damage. Similar to nerve protection, the primary objective is to displace the skin surface away from the ablation zone with the subcutaneous infiltration of liquid or gas. There are many options to warm the skin during the procedure; gauze soaked in warm saline or sterile procedural gloves filled with warm saline are frequently used at our institutions.

Bone tumors can decrease the integrity of bone and can increase the risk of pathologic fracture. This is particularly true with lytic lesions in weight-bearing bones (lower extremity, portions of the pelvis, and vertebral bodies).[68] Thermal ablation can also negatively impact bone architecture. As bone tumor thermal ablation often requires coaxial

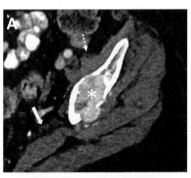
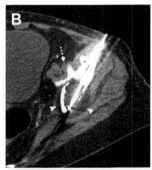
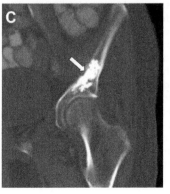
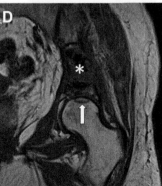

Fig. 13. 65-year-old woman with metastatic renal-cell carcinoma and progressive left hip pain. Axial postcontrast CT image of the pelvis (*A*) shows an enhancing lytic lesion in the supraacetabular region of the left ilium (*asterisk*) with extraosseous tumor extension posteriorly, consistent with a bone metastasis; the sciatic nerve (*arrow*) and femoral nerve (*dotted arrow*) are in proximity to the tumor. Intraprocedural axial CT image (*B*) during cryoablation of the left iliac metastasis shows the ice ball covering the tumor (*arrowheads*); iodinated contrast was infiltrated underneath the iliacus muscle to displace the femoral nerve (*dotted arrow*) and the sciatic nerve was monitored with evoked potentials. Coronal CT image (*C*) shows cement (*arrow*) filling the ablated iliac bone metastasis. Coronal T1-weighted MR image of the left hip at follow-up (*D*) shows the ablation zone (*asterisk*) extending into the femoral head (*arrow*), a known complication of the procedure when lesions are in close proximity to the hip joint.

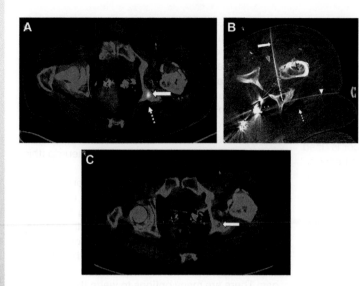

Fig. 14. 80-year-old man with a prostate adenocarcinoma diagnosed 25 years prior and managed with prostatectomy and radiation therapy. Surveillance Choline C-11 PET/CT axial image in the pelvis (A) shows a single focus of increased radiotracer activity in the posterior left-acetabulum (arrow) consistent with oligometastatic disease to the bone, which is in close proximity to the left sciatic nerve (dotted arrow). Intraprocedural CT image (B) during cryoablation of the posterior left acetabular metastasis shows the cryoprobe (arrow) with tip in the lesion; a spinal needle tip (arrowhead) was positioned at the posterior aspect of the posterior acetabulum to displace the sciatic nerve (dotted arrow) with carbon dioxide gas. The sciatic nerve was also monitored with evoked potentials and no sciatic deficit occurred postprocedure. Follow-up Choline C-11 PET/CT axial image in the pelvis (C) shows the focus of increased radiotracer activity in the posterior left-acetabulum (arrow) has resolved 3 months following cryoablation.

bone access, this creates an opportunity to support the bone with cement immediately following the ablation (see cementoplasty section).

Other complications include bowel injury, spinal cord injury, and joint damage[69] [see **Fig. 13**]. Occasionally thermal ablation complications cannot be avoided and may be acceptable given the potential benefits.

Cementoplasty

Cementoplasty is a safe and effective treatment with rare complications whereby poly-methylmethacrylate cement is injected into bone or bone cavities. Cementoplasty is performed to treat fractures or is used prophylactically to prevent fractures in weakened bone. Cementoplasty

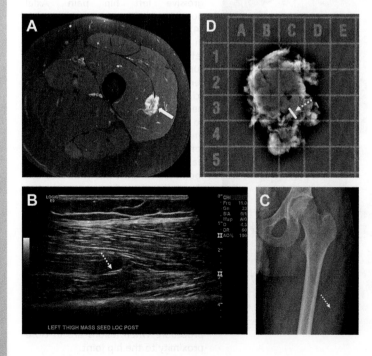

Fig. 15. 30-year-old man with Stage IIA Hodgkin's Lymphoma and a new area of hypermetabolic activity in the left thigh on a surveillance FDG-PET/CT study. Axial postcontrast T1-weighted MR image of the left thigh (A) shows an enhancing lesion (arrow) in the extensor compartment musculature centered in the vastus intermedius and vastus lateralis fascia. This was subsequently diagnosed as nodular fasciitis following biopsy. Given the lesion was not palpable and excision was desired, radioactive seed localization was performed with US guidance (B) showing the seed deployed within the lesion (dotted arrow). Postlocalization radiograph of the left thigh (C) shows the seed (dotted arrow) in the expected location of the lesion. Specimen radiograph (D) following surgical excision shows the specimen contains the radioactive seed (dotted arrow) which then can be disposed of appropriately.

is most often performed in the vertebral bodies whereby it is termed "vertebroplasty." Cementoplasty treatment alone can provide pain relief similar to ablation therapy, which is believed to be secondary to microfracture stabilization of the involved bone.[70] Cementoplasty can also be performed following thermal ablation or radiation therapy in an effort to prevent fractures [see **Figs. 12** and **13**]. The most common complications occur from nontarget cement instillation or "leaks." These can occur through defects in cortical bone or through venous channels. When identified real-time, the proceduralist usually redirects the instillation cannula elsewhere, while the "leaked" cement hardens to prevent progression. Cement leaks into or adjacent to critical structures are the most significant. Cement with mass effect on an adjacent nerve can cause neuropathic pain. This complication can be successfully treated with medication or perineural steroid injection, although surgical intervention may rarely be necessary. In our experience, cement leaks are most often inconsequential.

Tumor Localization

Radiologists can also play a role in localizing tumors before surgical resection or radiation. Hookwire localization and radioactive seed placement are often performed for soft tissue tumors that are difficult to identify clinically before surgical resection[71] [**Fig. 15**]. Fiducial markers can also be placed in soft tissue or bone to guide radiation therapy. Fiducial markers can also be placed in the spine preprocedure to allow guidance to the appropriate vertebral level using fluoroscopy in the surgery,[72] which can help prevent wrong-level spine procedures.

Hardware Fixation

Performing percutaneous techniques to biopsy and intervene on bone requires a similar skillset needed to place hardware with imaging guidance. Using Seldinger technique, screws can be placed with fluoroscopic and CT guidance by drilling an access needle across the target site and exchanging for a cannulated screw over a K-wire. Hardware fixation is advantageous over cementoplasty in bone subject to rotational or torsional forces.[73,74] Hardware fixation as performed by radiologists is growing in North America, although is not performed at most institutions at this time.

SUMMARY

The MSK radiologist functions in the multidisciplinary team not only as diagnostician but also as interventionalist. With minimally invasive image-guided techniques, radiologists are able to diagnose and treat many malignant and benign bone or soft tissue tumors. Knowledge and incorporation of biopsy and ablation best practices aids in optimizing patient care and outcomes.

CLINICS CARE POINTS

- The shortest route to biopsy a bone lesion is not neccesarily considered the safest.
- Weekly Radiology-Pathology Correlation conferences can shorten time to action for discordant results.
- Cryoablation ice-ball volumes are visible with intraprocedural CT.
- Intraprocedural nerve monitoring with sensory and/or motor evoked potentials can alert the interventionalist to thermal nerve injury.

DISCLOSURE

The authors have nothing to disclose.

REFERENCES

1. Le HBQ, Lee ST, Munk PL. Image-guided musculoskeletal biopsies. Semin Intervent Radiol 2010;27(2): 191–8.
2. Filippiadis DK, Charalampopoulos G, Mazioti A, et al. Bone and soft-tissue biopsies: what you need to know. Semin Intervent Radiol 2018;35(4):215–20.
3. Meek RD, Mills MK, Hanrahan CF, et al. Pearls and pitfalls for soft-tissue and bone biopsies: a cross-institutional review. Radiographics 2020;40(1): 226–90.
4. Tomasian A, Hillen TJ, Jennings JW. Bone biopsies: what radiologists need to know. Am J Roentgenol 2020;215(2):523–33.
5. Veltri A, Bargellini I, Giorgi L, et al. CIRSE guidelines on percutaneous needle biopsy (PNB). Cardiovasc Intervent Radiol 2017;40(10):1501–13.
6. Hillen TJ, Baker JC, Jennings JW, et al. Image-guided biopsy and treatment of musculoskeletal tumors. Semin Musculoskelet Radiol 2013;17(2): 189–202.
7. Patel IJ, Rahim S, Davidson JC, et al. Society of Interventional Radiology Consensus Guidelines for the periprocedural management of thrombotic and

bleeding risk in patients undergoing percutaneous image-guided interventions-part II: recommendations: endorsed by the Canadian Association for Interventional Radiology and the Cardiovascular and Interventional Radiology Society of Europe. J Vasc Interv Radiol 2019;30(8):1168–84.

8. Wu JS, Goldsmith JD, Horwich PJ, et al. Bone and soft-tissue lesions: what factors affect diagnostic yield of image-guided core-needle biopsy? Radiology 2008;248(3):962–70.

9. Wallace AN, McWilliams SR, Wallace A, et al. Drill-assisted biopsy of the axial and appendicular skeleton: safety, technical success, and diagnostic efficacy. J Vasc Interv Radiol 2016;27(10):1618–22.

10. Yang SY, Oh E, Kwon JW, et al. Percutaneous image-guided spinal lesion biopsies: factors affecting higher diagnostic yield. Am J Roentgenol 2018;211(5):1068–74.

11. Wiesner EL, Hillen TJ, Long J, et al. Percutaneous CT-guided biopsies of the cervical spine: technique, histopathologic and microbiologic yield, and safety at a single academic institution. AJNR Am J Neuroradiol 2018;39(5):981–5.

12. Tomasian A, Hillen TJ, Jennings JW. Percutaneous CT-guided skull biopsy: feasibility, safety, and diagnostic yield. AJNR Am J Neuroradiol 2019;40(2):309–12.

13. Hillen TJ, Baker JC, Long JR, et al. Percutaneous CT-guided core needle biopsies of head and neck masses: technique, histopathologic yield, and safety at a single institution. AJNR Am J Neuroradiol 2020;41(11):2117–22.

14. Long JR, Stensby JD, Wiesner EL, et al. Efficacy and safety of bone marrow aspiration and biopsy using fluoroscopic guidance and a drill-powered needle: clinical experience from 775 cases. Eur Radiol 2020;30(11):5964–70.

15. Shif Y, Kung JW, McMahon CJ, et al. Safety of omitting routine bleeding tests prior to image-guided musculoskeletal core needle biopsy. Skeletal Radiol 2018;47(2):215–21.

16. Mehta SD, Weber K, Fleisher L, et al. Assessing the need for preprocedural laboratory tests and stopping non-steroidal anti-inflammatory drugs/aspirin in patients undergoing percutaneous bone and soft tissue biopsies. Cardiovasc Intervent Radiol 2019;42(11):1588–96.

17. Tuttle R, Kane JM III. Biopsy techniques for soft tissue and bowel sarcomas. J Surg Oncol 2015;111(5):504–12.

18. Liu P, Valadez SD, Chivers FS, et al. Anatomically based guidelines for core needle biopsy of bone tumors: implications for limb-sparing surgery. Radiographics 2007;27(1):189–205.

19. Espinosa LA, Jamadar DA, Jacobson JA, et al. CT-guided biopsy of bone: a radiologist's perspective. Am J Roentgenol 2008;190(5):W283–9.

20. Mankin HJ, Mankin CJ, Simon MA. The hazards of the biopsy, revisted. Members of the musculoskeletal tumor society. J Bone Joint Surg Am 1996;78(5):656–63.

21. Mohana R, Fausham WI, Zulmi W, et al. The incidence of malignant infiltration in the biopsy tract of osteosarcoma. Malaysian Orthopaed J 2007;1(2):7–10.

22. Oliveira MP, Lima PM, de Mello RJ. Tumor contamination in the biopsy path of primary malignant bone tumors. Rev Bras Orthop 2015;47(5):631–7.

23. Barrientos-Ruiz IB, Ortiz-Cruz EJ, Serrano-Montilla J, et al. Are biopsy tracts a concern for seeding and local recurrence in sarcomas? Clin Orthop Relat Res 2017;475(2):511–8.

24. Siddiqi MA, Kim H, Jede F, et al. Association of core needle biopsy tract resection with local recurrence in extremity soft tissue sarcoma. Skeletal Radiol 2017;46(4):507–12.

25. Seeger LL. Revisiting tract seeding and compartmental anatomy for percutaneous image-guided musculoskeletal biopsies. Skeletal Radiol 2019;48(4):499–501.

26. UyBico SJ, Motamedi K, Omura MC, et al. Relevance of compartmental amnatomic guidelines for biopsy of musculoskeletal tumors: retrospective review of 363 biopsies over a 6-year period. J Vasc Interv Radiol 2012;23(4):511–8.

27. Berger-Richardson D, Swallow CJ. Needle tract seeding after percutaneous biopsy of sarcoma: risk/benefit considerations. Cancer 2017;123(4):560–7.

28. Saghieh S, Masrouha KZ, Musallam KM, et al. The risk of local recurrence along the core-needle biopsy tract in patients with bone sarcomas. Iowa Orthop J 2010;30:80–3.

29. ACR practice parameter on informed consent for image-guided procedures. Available at: https://www.acr.org/-/media/ACR/Files/Practice-Parameters/informedconsent-imagguided.pdf?la=en. American College of Radiology. Accessed April 29, 2021.

30. Hillen TJ, Talbert RJ, Friedman MV, et al. Biopsy of CT-occult bone lesions using anatomic landmarks for CT guidance. Am J Roentgenol 2017;209(1):214–21.

31. Sarti M, Brehmer WP, Gay SB. Low-dose techniques in CT-guided interventions. Radiographics 2012;32(4):1109–19.

32. Kimura T, Naka N, Minato Y, et al. Oblique approach of computed tomography guided needle biopsy using multiplanar reconstruction image by multidetector-row CT in lung cancer. Eur J Radiol 2004;52(2):206–11.

33. Saba L, Saba F, Fellini F. CT-guided biopsy of subdiaphragmatic small renal nodule with the coaxial technique using MRO images. Acta Biomed 2019;90(4):426–31.

34. Carrino JA, Khurana B, Ready JE, et al. Magnetic resonance imaging-guided percutaneous biopsy of musculoskeletal lesions. J Bone Joing Surg Am 2007;89(10):2179–87.

35. Wu HH, Chang C, Chang H, et al. Magnetic resonance imaging guided biopsy of musculoskeletal lesions. J Chin Med Assoc 2012;75(4):160–6.

36. Smith K, Carrino JA. MRI-guided interventions of the musculoskeletal system. J Magn Reason Imaging 2008;27(2):339–46.

37. Liu J, Jiao D, Ren J, et al. Percutaneous bone biopsy using a flat-panel cone beam computed tomography virtual navigation system. Saudi Med J 2018;39(5):519–23.

38. Yang YJ, Damron TA. Comparison of needle core biopsy and fine-needle aspiration for diagnostic accuracy in musculoskeletal lesions. Arch Pathol Lab Med 2004;128(7):759–64.

39. Kaur I, Handa U, Kundu R, et al. Role of fine-needle aspiration cytology and core needle biopsy in diagnosing musculoskeletal neoplasms. J Cytol 2016;33(1):7–12.

40. Banks JS, Garner HW, Chow AZ, et al. Radiology-pathology correlation for bone and soft tissue tumors or tumor-like masses: single institutional experience after implementation of a weekly conference. Skeletal Radiol 2021;50(4):731–8.

41. McMenomy BP, Kurup AN, Johnson GB, et al. Percutaneous cryoablation of musculoskeletal oligometastatic disease for complete remission. J Vasc Interv Radiol 2013;24(2):207–13.

42. Vaswani D, Wallace AN, Eiswirth PS, et al. Radiographic Local Tumor Control and Pain Palliation of Sarcoma Metastases within the Musculoskeletal System with Percutaneous Thermal Ablation. Cardiovasc Intervent Radiol 2018;41(8):1223–32.

43. Callstrom MR, Dupuy DE, Solomon SB, et al. Percutaneous image-guided cryoablation of painful metastases involving bone: multicenter trial. Cancer 2013;119(5):1033–41.

44. Jennings JW, Prologo JD, Garnon J, et al. Cryoablation for Palliation of Painful Bone Metastases: The MOTION Multicenter Study. Radiol Imaging Cancer 2021;3(2):e200101.

45. Di Staso M, Zugaro L, Gravina GL, et al. A feasibility study of percutaneous Radiofrequency Ablation followed by Radiotherapy in the management of painful osteolytic bone metastases. Eur Radiol 2011;21(9):2004–10.

46. Di Staso M, Gravina GL, Zugaro L, et al. Treatment of Solitary Painful Osseous Metastases with Radiotherapy, Cryoablation or Combined Therapy: Propensity Matching Analysis in 175 Patients. PLoS One 2015;10(6):e0129021.

47. Rosenthal D, Callstrom MR. Critical review and state of the art in interventional oncology: benign and metastatic disease involving bone. Radiology 2012;262(3):765–80.

48. Wallace AN, Tomasian A, Chang RO, et al. Treatment of Osteoid Osteomas Using a Navigational Bipolar Radiofrequency Ablation System. Cardiovasc Intervent Radiol 2016;39(5):768–72 [published correction appears in Cardiovasc Intervent Radiol. 2017 Dec 5;:].

49. Rinzler ES, Shivaram GM, Shaw DW, et al. Microwave ablation of osteoid osteoma: initial experience and efficacy. Pediatr Radiol 2019;49(4):566–70.

50. Tomasian A, Cazzato RL, Auloge P, et al. Osteoid osteoma in older adults: clinical success rate of percutaneous image-guided thermal ablation. Clin Radiol 2020;75(9):713.e11-6.

51. Sharma KV, Yarmolenko PS, Celik H, et al. Comparison of noninvasive high-intensity focused ultrasound with radiofrequency ablation of osteoid osteoma. J Pediatr 2017;190:222–8.e1.

52. Schmitz JJ, Schmit GD, Atwell TD, et al. Percutaneous cryoablation of extraabdominal desmoid tumors: a 10-year experience. AJR Am J Roentgenol 2016;207(1):190–5.

53. Koch G, Cazzato RL, Gilkison A, et al. Percutaneous treatments of benign bone tumors. Semin Intervent Radiol 2018;35(4):324–32.

54. Martell B, Jesse MK, Lowry P. CT-Guided Cryoablation of a Peripheral Nerve Sheath Tumor. J Vasc Interv Radiol 2016;27(1):148–50.

55. Dupuy DE, Hong R, Oliver B, et al. Radiofrequency ablation of spinal tumors: temperature distribution in the spinal canal. AJR Am J Roentgenol 2000;175(5):1263–6.

56. Tomasian A, Jennings JW. Hot and Cold Spine Tumor Ablations. Neuroimaging Clin N Am 2019;29(4):529–38.

57. Rybak LD. Fire and ice: thermal ablation of musculoskeletal tumors. Radiol Clin North Am 2009;47(3):455–69.

58. Wallace AN, McWilliams SR, Connolly SE, et al. Percutaneous image-guided cryoablation of musculoskeletal metastases: pain palliation and local tumor control. J Vasc Interv Radiol 2016;27(12):1788–96.

59. Izzo F, Granata V, Grassi R, et al. Radiofrequency ablation and microwave ablation in liver tumors: an update. Oncologist 2019;24(10):e990–1005.

60. Pusceddu C, Sotgia B, Fele RM, et al. Combined microwave ablation and cementoplasty in patients with painful bone metastases at high risk of fracture. Cardiovasc Intervent Radiol 2016;39(1):74–80.

61. Kastler A, Alnassan H, Aubry S, et al. Microwave thermal ablation of spinal metastatic bone tumors. J Vasc Interv Radiol 2014;25(9):1470–5.

62. Khan MA, Deib G, Deldar B, et al. Efficacy and Safety of Percutaneous Microwave Ablation and Cementoplasty in the Treatment of Painful Spinal Metastases and Myeloma. AJNR Am J Neuroradiol 2018;39(7):1376–83.

63. Tomasian A, Jennings JW. Percutaneous minimally invasive thermal ablation for management of osseous metastases: recent advances. Int J Hyperthermia 2019;36(2):3–12.

64. Napoli A, Anzidei M, Marincola BC, et al. Primary pain palliation and local tumor control in bone metastases treated with magnetic resonance-guided focused ultrasound. Invest Radiol 2013;48(6): 351–8.

65. Yoon JT, Nesbitt J, Raynor BL, et al. Utility of Motor and Somatosensory Evoked Potentials for Neural Thermoprotection in Ablations of Musculoskeletal Tumors. J Vasc Interv Radiol 2020;31(6):903–11.

66. Kurup AN, Morris JM, Boon AJ, et al. Motor evoked potential monitoring during cryoablation of musculoskeletal tumors. J Vasc Interv Radiol 2014;25(11): 1657–64.

67. Kurup AN, Morris JM, Schmit GD, et al. Neuroanatomic considerations in percutaneous tumor ablation. Radiographics 2013;33(4):1195–215.

68. Garnon J, Jennings JW, Meylheuc L, et al. Biomechanics of the Osseous Pelvis and Its Implication for Consolidative Treatments in Interventional Oncology. Cardiovasc Intervent Radiol 2020; 43(11):1589–99.

69. Friedman MV, Hillen TJ, Wessell DE, et al. Hip chondrolysis and femoral head osteonecrosis: a complication of periacetabular cryoablation. J Vasc Interv Radiol 2014;25(10):1580–8.

70. Anselmetti GC, Manca A, Ortega C, et al. Treatment of extraspinal painful bone metastases with percutaneous cementoplasty: a prospective study of 50 patients. Cardiovasc Intervent Radiol 2008;31(6):1165–73.

71. Garner HW, Bestic JM, Peterson JJ, et al. Preoperative radioactive seed localization of nonpalpable soft tissue masses: an established localization technique with a new application. Skeletal Radiol 2017;46(2): 209–16.

72. Madaelil TP, Long JR, Wallace AN, et al. Preoperative fiducial marker placement in the thoracic spine: a technical report. Spine (Phila Pa 1976) 2017; 42(10):E624–8.

73. Kurup AN, Callstrom MR. Expanding role of percutaneous ablative and consolidative treatments for musculoskeletal tumours. Clin Radiol 2017;72(8): 645–56.

74. Yevich S, Tselikas L, Kelekis A, et al. Percutaneous management of metastatic osseous disease. Chin Clin Oncol 2019;8(6):62.

Bones and Soft-Tissue Tumors
Considerations for Postsurgical Imaging Follow-up

Zohaib Y. Ahmad, MD[a], Shivani Ahlawat, MD[b], Adam S. Levin, MD[c],
Laura M. Fayad, MD[b],*

KEYWORDS

• Sarcoma • MR imaging • Post-treatment

KEY POINTS

• Imaging follow-up after resection of bone and soft-tissue tumors is vital to assess for post-treatment complications, especially local recurrence of tumor.
• With MR imaging, benign postoperative inflammation can often be distinguished from the local recurrent tumor, especially with the addition of functional sequences.
• Understanding the availability of anatomic and functional MR imaging sequences and how to interpret the findings is critical to finding recurrent tumors within the surgical bed.

INTRODUCTION

The imaging evaluation of patients after treatment for sarcoma is vital to assessing for tumor recurrence. Sarcomas represent a wide group of tumors, varying in both type and grade, and treatment can vary in terms of resection extent and the need for neoadjuvant therapy. As a result, there is a broad range in the rates of recurrence of sarcomas. In the literature, rates have been reported as low as 5%[1] to as high as 50%.[2] The rate of local recurrence is greatest in tumors with size greater than 10 cm, a deep location, high histologic grade, and positive surgical margins.[3] Although recurrence occurs most often within the first 2 years after surgery,[4] more delayed recurrence 5 to 10 years after therapy is possible, particularly in lower grade neoplasms.

Interval MR imaging has proven to be an effective way to assess for recurrent tumor in the surgical bed. MR imaging uses several sequences that when analyzed together can help distinguish local recurrence from typical expected postoperative inflammation and postoperative complications. If MR imaging is contraindicated for any reason, computed tomography (CT) scan with intravenous contrast can be substituted to assess for local recurrence at the treatment site. This can be augmented with whole-body positron emission tomography (PET)–CT, providing anatomic detail with CT and functional tumor metabolic information with the PET portion.

To optimize early detection and treatment of recurrence, there are several factors to consider when prescribing, protocoling, and interpreting postoperative follow-up imaging. We will review how these considerations impact detection of recurrence as well as current general guidelines.

CONSIDERATION #1: TIMING OF SURVEILLANCE

The timing of MR imaging should be determined by a multidisciplinary team that ideally includes medical oncologists, orthopedic oncologists,

[a] Department of Radiology, Columbia University Irving Medical Center, 630 West 168th Street MC 28, New York, NY 10032, USA; [b] The Russell H. Morgan Department of Radiology and Radiological Science, Johns Hopkins University, 601 North Caroline Street, JHOC 3014, Baltimore, MD 21287, USA; [c] Department of Orthopaedic Surgery, Johns Hopkins University, 601 North Caroline Street, JHOC 5255, Baltimore, MD 21287, USA
* Corresponding author.
E-mail address: lfayad1@jhmi.edu

Radiol Clin N Am 60 (2022) 327–338
https://doi.org/10.1016/j.rcl.2021.11.010
0033-8389/22/© 2021 Elsevier Inc. All rights reserved.

radiation oncologists, pathologists, and radiologists.[4] Earlier and more frequent MR imaging examinations are often prescribed for high-risk sarcomas because approximately 80% of high-risk patients will recur in the first 2 to 3 years after treatment. Although controversial, lifelong imaging surveillance has been advocated.[5] For example, in extremity bone tumor patients at high risk, the recommended MR imaging follow-up schedule is:

- every 3 months for the first 2 years
- every 4 months for the next 2 years
- every 6 months for the fifth year
- and then annually after that.[5]

Of note, late relapse after 5 years has been reported in 6.3% of patients with sarcomas.[6] For example, some histologies such as synovial sarcoma are more prone to recurrence after 5 years.[7] Therefore, more aggressive 5- to 10-year surveillance is appropriate, often depending on individual risk. Post-treatment imaging algorithms may also differ depending on whether the tumor was located in the trunk or in an extremity. Importantly, interval imaging would be obtained sooner if the patient begins to experience symptoms outside of the routine imaging surveillance schedule.[5]

CONSIDERATION #2: WHAT TYPE OF THERAPY WAS USED?

An understanding of the types of treatment is crucial to understanding the imaging patterns afterward. The primary treatment methods used for musculoskeletal sarcoma include surgical resection, radiation therapy, and chemotherapy.

Surgical resection techniques include marginal excision, wide excision, or limb amputation. Limb amputation carries a 3-fold increased risk in mortality,[8] therefore wide excision with limb preservation is the preferred surgical method. Of note, wide resection can lead to large soft-tissue defects because of the need to obtain clear margins, which may necessitate the use of pedicled or free flaps for soft-tissue reconstruction.[9] Regardless, when combined with radiation therapy, wide surgical resection has been found to have similar oncologic results as limb amputation.[10] Survival is improved when there is a multidisciplinary approach to management and appropriate imaging surveillance is used.[10]

Depending on the tumor size, histology, and location, radiation therapy may be appropriate for decreasing local recurrence risk. Radiation may be delivered preoperatively or postoperatively. If preoperative radiation therapy is delivered, there occasionally may be a need for a postoperative radiation boost after preoperative

treatment. Although preoperative radiation is associated with a lower dose, a smaller radiation field, and reduced risk of long-term local effects compared with postoperative radiation, there is a higher rate of perioperative wound complications with preoperative radiation.[11]

Chemotherapy has had a significant positive impact on long-term survival in osteosarcoma and Ewing sarcoma when compared with surgery alone[12,13] and is now routinely used in the neoadjuvant as well as the adjuvant settings for both bone tumor types.[14]

In soft-tissue sarcoma, chemotherapy is most often reserved for the management of metastatic disease.[15] However, chemotherapy is used neoadjuvantly and adjuvantly in certain histologic subtypes of soft-tissue sarcoma that are considered chemosensitive, such as synovial sarcoma and myxoid/round cell liposarcoma.[16]

CONSIDERATION #3: HOW CAN MR IMAGING BEST HELP ME NAVIGATE THE TREATMENT BED
Assessment for Local Recurrence

Owing to its high soft-tissue resolution, and in particular its high contrast resolution, MR imaging is the mainstay technique for local postoperative tumor imaging. The ability of MR imaging to provide both anatomic and functional information aids in the differentiation of recurrent tumor from postoperative complications as well as other expected postoperative findings. Table 1 highlights the appearance of recurrence on different sequences.

Noncontrast anatomic sequences
The basis of anatomic evaluation involves T1-weighted and fluid-sensitive sequences, including a fat-saturated T2-weighted sequence or short-tau inversion recovery (STIR) sequence. On T1-weighted images, when the recurrent tumor is in the subcutaneous tissues, it is clearly depicted against a background of subcutaneous fat, and when in muscle, the tumor can be identified by its distortion of the normal striated skeletal muscle morphology. In the case of metastases or recurrence within bone, the T1-weighted sequence optimally delineates the tumor against the background of surrounding normal marrow fat.[17]

Assessment of the treatment area on fluid-sensitive sequences is challenging. T2 hyperintensity is common within the surgical bed because of post-treatment inflammation and granulation tissue (Fig. 1) and can persist for years after surgery. Unfortunately, the recurrent tumor also frequently exhibits T2 hyperintensity. Therefore, it has been

Table 1
Magnetic resonance imaging sequences and findings for local recurrent tumor

MR Imaging Sequence	Finding of Local Recurrent Tumor
Non–contrast-enhanced anatomic	
T1	Architectural distortion
Fluid Sensitive (T2/PD fat-saturated)	Extensive edema
Non–contrast-enhanced functional	
Chemical Shift (in- and out-of-phase)	Bone marrow replacement
Diffusion-weighted/ADC map	Restricted diffusion (low ADC values)
Contrast-enhanced anatomic	
T1 fat-saturated	Nodular or mass-like enhancement
Contrast-enhanced functional	
Dynamic contrast-enhanced	Early arterial enhancement

suggested that only in the absence of fluid signal in the surgical bed can the reader be confident that the recurrent tumor is not present.[17,18]

Noncontrast functional sequences

Proton chemical shift imaging, composed of paired in-phase (IP) and opposed-phase (OP) sequences, can provide valuable information regarding whether a signal abnormality represents a marrow-replacing lesion or non–marrow-replacing mimic, such as hematopoietic marrow reconversion related to treatment.[17] Chemical shift imaging can be interpreted nonquantitatively (visual assessment of signal drop in bone on OP relative to IP) or quantitatively. Compared with the quantitative analysis, the nonquantitative analysis relies solely on subjective visual assessment of signal drop in bone on OP relative to IP. More optimally, the quantitative analysis objectively measures signal intensity (SI) on IP and OP and calculates signal drop between the 2 sequences. SI drops of less than 15% on 3T and less than 20% on 1.5T are reliable thresholds for identifying a marrow-replacing lesion.[19] Chemical shift

imaging is a valuable complement to standard T1-weighted imaging when evaluating bone marrow signal abnormalities.

Quantitative diffusion-weighted imaging (DWI) sequences and apparent diffusion coefficient (ADC) mapping evaluate the Brownian motion of water at the cellular level. Motion is relatively unimpeded extracellularly in a normal cellular environment, but in a tumoral environment with high cellularity, the motion of water is limited or restricted. ADC mapping and measures of restricted water motion are obtained by quantitively measuring the diffusivity of a lesion based on the DWI. The lower the ADC value, the higher the cellularity of a lesion, hence malignant recurrences have low ADC values (**Figs. 2** and **3**).[18] In contrast, scar/granulation tissue in a surgical bed is not highly cellular and will not have a low ADC value. Although there is some debate about whether ADC values can truly measure the differences between benign or malignant disease,[20] ADC measurements have been found to differentiate between recurrent sarcoma and the benign entities of hematoma and postoperative scar.[17]

Contrast-enhanced anatomic sequence

An intravenous gadolinium-enhanced static sequence obtained in the delayed phase can be used to detect nodular or mass-like enhancement that would not be readily apparent on the noncontrast anatomic sequences (T1-weighted and fluid-sensitive sequences; **Fig. 4**).[17] Using high-resolution 3D volumetric sequences with subtraction imaging can further show the presence of an enhancing nodular recurrence with high accuracy.[21] Although there is often ill-defined enhancement in the treatment area from postsurgical and postradiation inflammation and fibrosis, the inflammation and fibrosis may also take the form of nodular and/or mass-like enhancement, with focal-rounded borders.[17] More confident differentiation can be achieved with functional MR imaging sequences or in some cases may require biopsy or close interval follow-up.

Contrast-enhanced functional sequence

Dynamic contrast-enhanced (DCE) MR imaging, a method that can be used to distinguish benign from malignant lesions pretreatment, has also been shown to increase the specificity of detection of recurrent disease when used in conjunction with the other functional sequence, DWI with ADC mapping.[18] DCE MR imaging can be acquired as a fast gradient echo sequence obtained over a certain volume of tissue and repeated after injection of gadolinium-based contrast.[22] Each repetition is obtained after 5 to 10 seconds based on

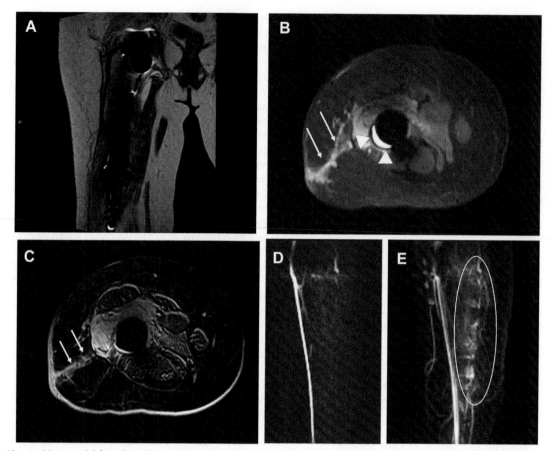

Fig. 1. 28-year-old female with osteosarcoma after distal femoral reconstruction. This follow-up shows no evidence of local tumor recurrence. Coronal PD Warp sequence (A) is without architectural distortion. Axial STIR Warp (B) and postcontrast fat-saturated T1 SEMAC (C) show ill-defined edema and enhancement (arrows) without mass-like enhancement. A pseudocapsular collection surrounding the femoral reconstruction (arrowheads) is commonly seen postoperatively. Dynamic contrast-enhanced maximum intensity projections are shown in the early arterial (D) and late arterial (E) phases. No early arterial enhancement is noted with the enhancement in the surgical bed (circle) progressively enhancing, appearing in the late arterial phase.

the volume of tissue and may be carried out for approximately 3 to 7 minutes. Patterns of enhancement can then be analyzed based on early and late arterial enhancement with malignant lesions more often showing early arterial enhancement as demonstrated in **Figs. 2** and **3**.[17] In one study, although 48% of patients had a mass-like region of enhancement on the static contrast-enhanced sequence, the addition of DCE MR imaging raised the specificity for recurrent tumor detection from 52% to 97%.[18]

Special consideration: MR imaging surveillance in the presence of metal

Primary bone sarcomas often require surgical reconstruction with metal prostheses or other hardware. The presence of metal within the MR imaging field of view frequently causes significant

susceptibility artifacts that can obscure areas of disease recurrence. However, applying metal artifact reduction to T1-weighted precontrast and postcontrast sequences with subtraction imaging increases sensitivity for detection of nodular areas of recurrence. Furthermore, when a DCE sequence is added to the surveillance protocol, the specificity for detection of recurrence around a prosthesis is also increased (see **Fig. 3**).[23]

Assessment for Other Post-treatment Complications

Complications other than recurrence that can occur in the treatment bed are listed in **Table 2**. Local inflammation and fibrosis is a regular occurrence within the area of treatment.[3,18] As noted previously, these inflammatory changes often manifest as an ill-defined enhancement but can

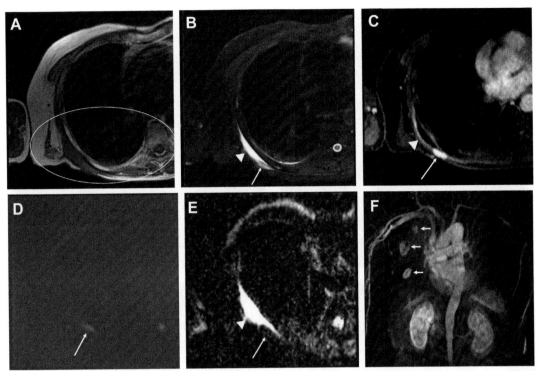

Fig. 2. 73-year-old male with myxofibrosarcoma of the right posterior chest wall after resection. Axial T1 (*A*) shows low signal in the surgical bed with extension to the skin (*circle*). Axial STIR (*B*), postcontrast fat-saturated T1 (*C*), diffusion-weighted (*D*), and ADC map (*E*) show an enhancing nodule (*long arrow*) within the surgical bed with restricted diffusion. On dynamic contrast-enhanced maximum intensity projection (*F*), multiple arterial enhancing nodules (*short arrows*) were discovered. Upon resection, these were confirmed as a local recurrent tumor. A postoperative seroma (*arrowhead*) is also noted in the surgical bed.

also manifest with a nodular morphology similar to recurrence.[18] DCE technique is a valuable tool for accurately distinguishing post-treatment change from recurrence.

In a meta-analysis of extremity soft-tissue sarcomas, there is an overall wound complication rate of 30.2%, with factors such as smoking, diabetes, tumor size, and radiation therapy associated with adverse outcomes.[10] Regarding radiotherapy specifically, preoperative radiation carries a greater risk for wound complications than postoperative radiation.[11] Wound dehiscence will manifest on MR imaging as a skin and subcutaneous soft-tissue defect of variable size along the surgical incision line with associated surrounding reactive edema and enhancement. There may be superimposed infection, which can lead to the formation of peripherally enhancing sinus tracts or abscesses as well as underlying osteomyelitis (Fig. 5). In the setting of a soft-tissue reconstruction flap, there may be a distortion of the flap as well as abnormal ill-defined signal (Fig. 6). Postoperative surgical site infections are seen in approximately 12.2% of patients with malignant tumors.[24]

Factors influencing infection rates include length of surgery, tumor size, amount of blood loss, and the use of preoperative radiation or chemotherapy.

An abscess is usually distinguishable from other postoperative fluid collections based on its morphology, with a thick enhancing wall and heterogeneous nonenhancing internal contents.[15] Of note, unlike the uniformly high ADC values of seromas or hematomas, the ADC values of an abscess may vary. For example, abscesses containing macromolecules typically have low ADC values. Alternatively, abscesses that have completely liquefied will demonstrate higher ADC values because of the increased ability of water to diffuse.[25] As both recurrence and abscess can demonstrate low ADC values, it is important to not over-rely on ADC and correlate the information provided on all the imaging sequences.

Seromas are a common postoperative complication, occurring in approximately 9% to 36% of cases, even in the setting of postoperative drain placement.[26] The exact pathogenesis of seroma formation is unknown, but the 2 leading theories are postoperative lymphatic leakage or fascial

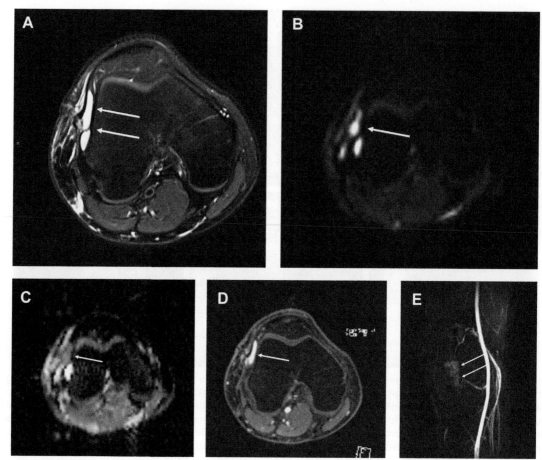

Fig. 3. 18-year-old male with synovial sarcoma status after resection. Axial fat-saturated T2 (*A*), diffusion-weighted images (*B*), ADC map (*C*), and postcontrast fat-saturated T1 (*D*) show a T2-hyperintense, enhancing nodule (*arrow*) with restricted diffusion within the surgical bed. Sagittal dynamic contrast-enhanced maximum intensity projection (*E*) shows the early arterial enhancement of the nodule (*arrow*). This was confirmed as a residual tumor.

shearing with subsequent fluid accumulation. On MR imaging, seromas are usually T2 hyperintense with a rim of hypointensity due to hemosiderin deposition (Fig. 7). However, the appearance of T1-weighted and T2-weighted sequences can be heterogeneous because of the presence of blood products. On static postcontrast imaging, seromas demonstrate peripheral enhancement but lack the internal enhancement and/or early arterial enhancement characteristic of a recurrent tumor. Similarly, hematomas will also demonstrate rim enhancement, with varying signal characteristics on precontrast anatomic imaging. In the absence of contrast administration, DWI with ADC mapping may help with defining a postoperative collection; ADC values will typically be significantly higher in both seromas and hematomas compared with tumor recurrence.[18]

Radiation-related changes in bone

Radiation-induced changes can depend on many factors, including the type of radiation, the location of the radiation field, the dose, and the type of tissue irradiated.[27] Radiation can lead to edema, inflammation, and even compromise of tissue due to cell death. The subsequent body response can create changes over time with radiological signs appearing over a year after the therapy. Such changes include radiation osteitis, where there is cell death of the osteoblasts leading to osteopenia and osteonecrosis.[28] In the acute phase, there will be inflammation of the osseous and nonosseous tissues, depicted as increased T2-weighted/fluid signal (see Fig. 6) and concomitant T1-hypointense signal approaching skeletal muscle. In this setting, chemical shift sequences can serve as a useful adjunct tool to distinguish radiation-related changes from recurrent

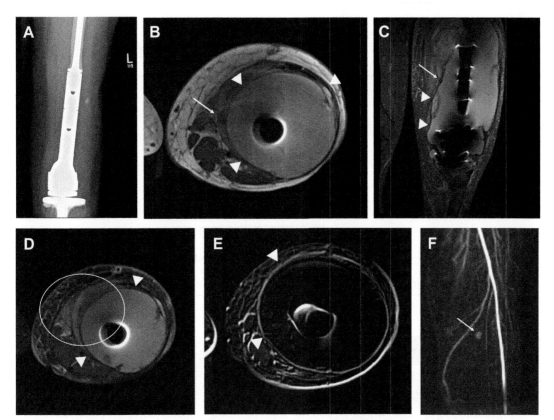

Fig. 4. 17-year-old male with osteosarcoma of the left femur after distal femoral reconstruction. Coronal radiograph (A) shows the femoral hardware. Axial T1 (B) and coronal STIR (C) show a nodule (arrow) in the surgical bed with the axial STIR (D) demonstrating the extensive surrounding edema (circle). Large pseudocapsular fluid collection (arrowheads) surrounding the hardware is noted. Axial postcontrast subtracted T1 (E) confirms the collection as nonenhancing (arrowheads). Dynamic contrast-enhanced maximum intensity projection (F) demonstrates the enhancing nodule (arrow), although the nodule exhibited late arterial enhancement. This nodule was confirmed to be a local recurrent tumor upon subsequent limb amputation.

Table 2
Postoperative complications after resection of tumor with associated findings on Magnetic Resonance Imaging

Postoperative Complications	MR Imaging Appearance	
	Anatomic Sequences	Functional Sequences
Bland fluid collections		
Hematoma	T2 and T1 heterogeneous, peripherally enhancing collection	No early arterial enhancement
Seroma	T2 hyperintense, peripherally enhancing, thin-walled collection	No early arterial enhancement
Lymphocele	T2 hyperintense, peripherally enhancing, thin-walled collection	No early arterial enhancement
Infections		
Cellulitis/Myositis	Ill-defined T2 hyperintensity and enhancement in the subcutaneous and deep muscular tissues	
Abscess	Thick enhancing walls with T2 heterogeneity	Restricted diffusion

(continued on next page)

Table 2
(continued)

Postoperative Complications	MR Imaging Appearance	
	Anatomic Sequences	Functional Sequences
Delayed wound healing and dehiscence	Cutaneous and subcutaneous discontinuity with ill-defined T2 hyperintensity and enhancement	
Deep vein thrombosis	Distended vein with increased intraluminal	
Radiation related	Ill-defined T2 hyperintensity and enhancement within soft tissues and osseous structures. Delayed fatty replacement within osseous structures.	Drop-in signal in chemical shift imaging
Hardware complications	T2 hyperintense rim around prosthesis, periprosthetic fracture	

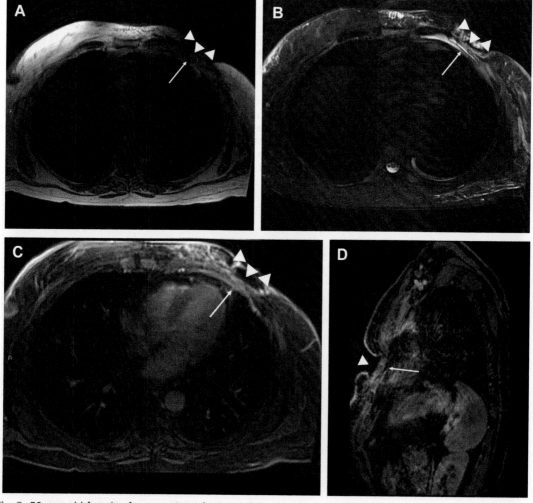

Fig. 5. 56-year-old female after resection of tumor of the left chest wall. Axial T1 (*A*), STIR (*B*), and axial (*C*) and sagittal (*D*) postcontrast fat-saturated T1 demonstrate skin defect (*arrowheads*) that has not been able to heal with subsequent dehiscence. Underlying this skin defect is the left fourth rib that shows edema and enhancement (*long arrow*), raising the suspicion for osteomyelitis.

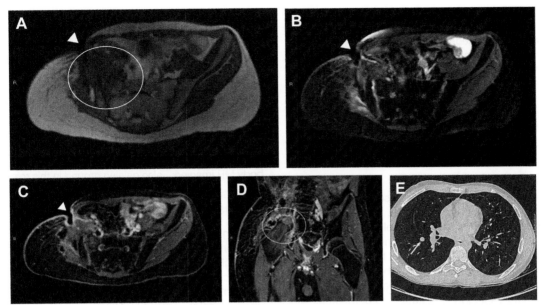

Fig. 6. 14-year-old male with a history of Ewing Sarcoma after radical resection of the pelvis, chemotherapy, and radiation. Axial T1 (*A*), fat-saturated T2 (*B*), and postcontrast fat-saturated T1 (*C*) show delayed wound healing at the muscular flap with wound defect (*arrowhead*). Deeper into the wound, there is extensive architectural distortion (circle) with enhancement from treatment. Coronal postcontrast fat-saturated T1 (*D*) demonstrates post-treatment enhancing synovitis of the right hip with remodeling of the right femoral head (circle). Axial CT (*E*) image of the lung shows metastatic recurrence in the right lower lobe (*arrow*).

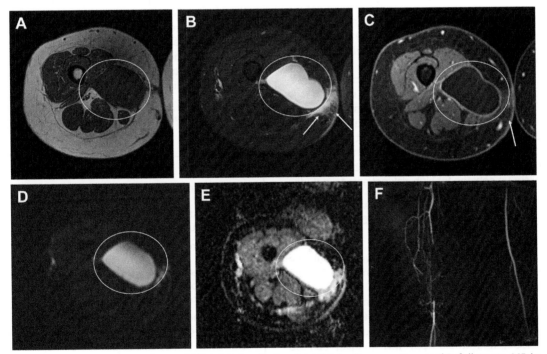

Fig. 7. 32-year-old female with myxoid liposarcoma in the right thigh after resection. In this follow-up, MR imaging, axial T1 (*A*), fat-saturated T2 (*B*), and postcontrast fat-saturated T1 (*C*) show a T2 hyperintense ovoid lesion without enhancement (circle) within the surgical bed compatible with a seroma. Diffusion-weighted imaging (*D*) and ADC map (*E*) confirm there is no restricted diffusion. Coronal dynamic contrast-enhanced maximum intensity projection in the early arterial phase (*F*) shows no nodular or mass-like early arterial enhancing lesion. Within the surgical bed of the medial thigh subcutaneous tissues, ill-defined enhancement (*arrow*) is noted compatible with expected postoperative changes.

neoplasm. After 2 to 6 weeks, fatty transformation will occur within the bone marrow. After 6 months, radiation-induced weakening of the bone can lead to complications such as avascular necrosis and insufficiency fractures. At approximately 9 months after radiotherapy, gelatinous transformation can occur, which will manifest as patchy SI of the bone marrow.[29] Radiation can also affect the joint with development of synovitis, deterioration of the cartilage, and fibrosis of the periarticular ligaments, tendons, and capsule.[29]

Hardware failure

Reconstruction after tumor resection can include the placement of autografts, allografts, and/or hardware.[30] The typical complications related to hardware placement are beyond the scope of this article. However, it is important to note that evaluation of a reconstruction should be made on multiple modalities. Radiographs are helpful for assessing hardware integrity and graft incorporation as well as evaluating for possible osteolysis or fracture. If there is concern for a hardware complication radiographically, CT or MR imaging could be obtained to provide greater clarity.[29,31]

Assessment for Metastatic Disease

Certain histologic subtypes have a predilection for metastatic disease. These include leiomyosarcoma, rhabdomyosarcoma, synovial sarcoma, and epithelioid sarcoma.[32]

Lung metastasis is the most frequent type of metastatic disease and is best evaluated using CT (see **Fig. 6**E).[33] Given that a lung metastasis can be treated with surgical excision and radiofrequency ablation, CT is an effective and cost-efficient tool for assessing metastatic development. The American College of Radiology describes one CT follow-up schema for high-risk patients to include:

- every 3 to 4 months for the first 2 to 3 years
- every 6 months for years 3 to 5
- annually after 5 years.[5]

For low-risk patients, CT follow-up should be obtained every 6 months for the first 3 to 5 years and then annually.[5]

Nonpulmonary distant metastases are less common, ranging from 14% to 20%. Although imaging modalities such as technetium bone scan, PET/CT, and whole-body MR imaging can be used to assess for distant metastasis, they are not often advocated in the asymptomatic patient.

The metastatic potential of specific sarcomas should be noted. Myxoid liposarcoma has been shown to metastasize to extrapulmonary locations, most commonly to the spine and paraspinal soft tissues. A study by Fuglo and colleagues demonstrated that myxoid liposarcoma recurred locally on average 7 years postoperatively and with new metastatic disease 10 years postoperatively.[34] PET/CT has demonstrated low sensitivity for the detection of osseous metastasis of myxoid liposarcoma. Furthermore, Nobel and colleagues found that technetium bone scan had limited use in osseous metastasis without cortical involvement.[35] Therefore, screening MR imaging of the spine has been recommended for follow-up of these patients,[36] with whole-body MR imaging[37] also gaining ground in this role.

SUMMARY

Imaging is a vital tool in the surveillance of patients with bone and soft-tissue sarcoma after treatment. Although there are a variety of post-treatment complications that can occur, tumor recurrence is the most dreaded complication. The ability to discern local recurrence by MR imaging is unparalleled, and awareness of the factors that dictate the most appropriate timing of imaging surveillance is important. In addition, knowledge of the impact of various therapies on the appearance of the postoperative bed and how these appearances can evolve over time is imperative. It is also key to understand the MR imaging methods available that can help differentiate recurrence from other possible post-treatment findings, including functional MR imaging techniques. Lastly, awareness of the metastatic potential for various sarcomas can aid in providing a comprehensive evaluation.

CLINICS CARE POINTS

- Magnetic resonance imaging with functional sequences can help differentiate between postoperative complications and local recurrence of tumor.

- Posttreatment imaging surveillance for recurrent local and metastatic tumor should be determined by a multidisciplinary team and the type of tumor involved, although many surveillance algorithms exist.

- Understanding the types of typical postoperative changes and complications is imperative in not confusing imaging findings for local recurrent tumor.

DISCLOSURE

The authors have nothing to disclose.

REFERENCES

1. James SLJ, Davies AM. Post-operative imaging of soft tissue sarcomas. Cancer Imaging 2008;8(1):8–18.

2. Garner HW, Kransdorf MJ, Bancroft LW, et al. Benign and malignant soft-tissue tumors: Posttreatment MR imaging. Radiographics 2009;29:119–34.

3. Tavare AN, Robinson P, Altoos R, et al. Postoperative imaging of Sarcomas. AJR Am J Roentgenol 2018; 211(3):506–18.

4. Garner HW, Kransdorf MJ. Musculoskeletal sarcoma: Update on imaging of the post-treatment patient. Can Assoc Radiol J 2016;67(1):12–20.

5. Roberts CC, Kransdorf MJ, Beaman FD, et al. Expert Panel on Musculoskeletal Imaging. Follow-up of malignant or aggressive musculoskeletal tumors. ACR Appropriateness Criteria. 2015. 1-15.

6. Kolovich GG, Wooldrige AN, Christy JM, et al. A retrospective statistical analysis of high-grade soft tissue sarcomas. Med Oncol 2012;29(2): 1335–44.

7. Krieg AH, Hefti F, Speth BM, et al. Synovial sarcomas usually metastasize after >5 years: a multicenter retrospective analysis with minimum follow-up of 10 years for survivors. Ann Oncol 2011;22(2): 458–67.

8. Parsons HM, Habermann EB, Tuttle TM, et al. Conditional survival of extremity soft-tissue sarcoma: results beyond the staging system. Cancer 2012; 117(5):1055–60.

9. Slump J, Hofer SOP, Ferguson PC, et al. Flap choice does not affect complication rates or functional outcomoes following extremity soft tissue sarcoma reconstruction. J Plast Reconstr Aesthet Surg 2018;71(7):989–96.

10. Slump J, Bastiaannet E, Halka A, et al. Risk factors for postoperative wound complications after extremity soft tissue sarcoma resection: A systematic review and meta-analyses. J Plast Reconstr Aesthet Surg 2019;72(9):1449–64.

11. O'Sullivan B, Davis AM, Turcotte R, et al. Preoperative versus postoperative radiotheraphy in soft-tissue sarcoma of the limbs: a randomised trial. Lancet 2002;359(9325):2235–41.

12. Dyke JP, Panicek DM, Healey JH, et al. Osteogenic and Ewing sarcoma: Estimation of necrotic fraction during induction chemotherapy with dynamic contrast-enhanced MR imaging. Radiology 2003; 228:271–8.

13. Bierman JS, Chow W, Reed Dr, et al. NCCN guidelines insights: bone cancer, version 2.2017. J Natl Compr Canc Netw 2017;15(2):155–67.

14. Reed DR, Hayashi M, Wagner L, et al. Treatment pathway of bone sarcoma in children, adolescents, and young adults. Cancer 2017;123(12):2206–18.

15. Noebauer-Huhmann IM, Chaudhary SR, Papakonstantinou O, et al. Soft tissue sarcoma follow-up imaging: Strategies to distinguish post-treatment changes from recurrence. Semin Musculoskelet Radiol 2020;24(6):627–44.

16. Pasquali S, Gronchi A. Neoadjuvant chemotherapy in soft tissue sarcomas: latest evidence and clinical implications. Ther Adv Med Oncol 2017;9(6):415–29.

17. Fayad LM, Jacobs MA, Wang X, et al. Musculoskeletal tumors: How to use anatomic, functional, and metabolic MR techniques. Radiology 2012;265(2): 340–56.

18. Del Grande F, Subhawong T, Weber K, et al. Detection of soft-tissue tumor recurrence: Added value of functional MR imaging techniques at 3.0 T. Radiology 2014;271(2):499–511.

19. Kumar NM, Ahlawat S, Fayad LM. Chemical shift imaging with in-phase and opposed-phase sequences at 3 T: what is the optimal threshold, measurement method, and diagnostic accuracy for characterizing marrow signal abnormalities? Skeletal Radiol 2018; 47:1661–71.

20. Einarsdottir H, Karlsson M, Wejde J, et al. Diffusion-weighted MRI of soft tissue tumours. Eur Radiol 2004;14:959–63.

21. Ahlawat S, Morris C, Fayad LM. Three-dimensional volumetric MRI with isotropic resolution: improved speed of acquisition, spatial resolution and assessment of lesion conspicuity in patients with recurrent soft tissue sarcoma. Skeletal Radiol 2016;45:645–52.

22. Sujlana P, Skrok J, Fayad LM. Review of dynamic contrast-enhanced MRI: Technical aspects and applications in the musculoskeletal system. J Magn Reson Imaging 2018;47:875–90.

23. Fayad LM, Levin A, Morris C, et al. Surveillance imaging in patients with tumor prostheses using anatomic and functional metal reduction MRI sequences. Skeletal Radiol 2017;46:1307.

24. Nagano S, Yokouchi M, Setoguchi T, et al. Analysis of surgical site infection after musculoskeltal tumor surgery: Risk assessment using a new scoring system. Sarcoma 2014;2014:645496.

25. Harish S, Chiavaras MM, Kotnis N, et al. MR imaging of skeletal soft tissue infection: utility of diffusion-weighted imaging in detecting abscess formation. Skeletal Radiol 2011;40:285–94.

26. El Abiad JM, Bridgham KM, Toci GR, et al. Postoperative seromas after soft-tissue sarcoma resection: Natural history and progression. Clin Surg 2020;5: 2875.

27. Capps GW, Fulcher AS, Szucs RA, et al. Imaging features of radiation-induced changes in the abdomen. Radiographics 1997;17:1455–73.

28. Bluemke DA, Fishman EK, Scott WW Jr. Skeletal complications of radiation therapy. Radiographics 1994;14:111–21.

29. Bloem JL, Vriens D, Krol ADG, et al. Therapy-related imaging findings in patients with sarcoma. Semin Musculoskelet Radiol 2020;24(6):676–91.

30. Fritz J, Fishman EK, Corl F, et al. Imaging of limb salvage surgery. AJR Am J Roentgenol 2012;198: 647–60.

31. Ahlawat S, McColl M, Morris CD, et al. Pelvic bone tumor resection: post-operative imaging. Skeletal Radiol 2021;50:1303–16.

32. Ezuddin NS, Pretell-Mazzini J, Yechieli RL, et al. Local recurrence of soft-tissue sarcoma: issues in imaging surveillance strategy. Skeletal Radiol 2018;47:1595–606.

33. Miller BJ, Carmody Soni EE, Reith JD, et al. CT scans for pulmonary surveillance may be overused in lower-grade sarcoma. Iowa Orthop J 2012;32: 28–34.

34. Fuglo HM, Maretty-Nielson K, Hovgaard D, et al. Metastatic pattern, local relapse, and survival of patients with myxoid liposarcoma: a retrospective study of 45 patients. Sarcoma 2013;2013:548628.

35. Noble JL, Moskovic E, Fisher C, et al. Imaging of skeletal metastases in myxoid liposarcoma. Sarcoma 2010;2010:262361.

36. Schwab JH, Boland P, Guo T, et al. Skeletal metastases in myxoid liposarcoma: An unusual pattern of distant spread. Ann Surg Oncol 2007;14:1507–14.

37. Visgauss JD, Wilson DA, Perrin DL, et al. Staging and surveillance of myxoid liposarcoma: Follow-up assessment and the metastatic pattern of 169 patients suggests inadequacy of current practice standards. Ann Surg Oncol 2021. https://doi.org/10.1245/s10434-021-10091-1.

Bone and Soft Tissue Tumors
Horizons in Radiomics and Artificial Intelligence

Michael L. Richardson, MD[a],*, Behrang Amini, MD, PhD[b],
Paul E. Kinahan, PhD[c]

KEYWORDS

● Artificial intellligence ● Radiomics ● Soft tissue tumor

KEY POINTS

- AI has the potential to improve the quality of CT, MR and PET/CT images, while simultaneously reducing imaging time, radiation dose and contrast dose.
- AI worklist prioritization systems can improve radiologist workflow and decrease interpretation times.
- The goal of radiomics is achieve "precision medicine", in which radiomic image features, molecular and other biomarkers are used to predict the right diagnosis and the right treatment of the right patient at the right time.
- Accurate segmentation of organs and neoplasms remains the most critical, challenging, and contentious component of radiomics.
- Radiomic information may be helpful in biopsy guidance; tumor classification, grading and prognosis; treatment response; and the prediction of metastasis.

INTRODUCTION

When we first image a bone or soft tissue tumor, we hope that the images will answer a number of important questions:

1. Do we see a tumor?
2. Where is it?
3. How big is it?
4. Is it well-marginated?
5. What important structures does it involve?
6. Is it metabolically active?

With our current imaging tools, we have become fairly good at answering this first group of questions. Answering these questions has led to improved treatment planning, as well as increased patient survival and improved function following limb salvage surgery.[1] However, we are not quite so good at answering a second set of questions:

1. What is it?
2. Is it malignant?

Once treatment has begun, we use imaging to try to answer a final set of important questions:

*This research did not receive any specific grant from funding agencies in the public, commercial, or not-for-profit sectors.
Preprint submitted to Radiologic Clinics of North America June 1, 2021.
a Department of Radiology, University of Washington, 4245 Roosevelt Way NE, Seattle, WA 98105, USA;
b Department of Radiology, The University of Texas MD Anderson Cancer Center, 1400 Pressler Street, Unit 1475, Houston, TX 77030, USA; c Department of Radiology and Bioengineering, University of Washington, Box 357987, Seattle, WA 98105, USA
* Corresponding author.
E-mail address: mrich@uw.edu

1. Is it gone?
2. Is it back?
3. Did it respond to treatment?
4. Did it spread?
5. Are there complications?

Answering this last set of questions can also be problematic. Since radiology imaging is not yet capable of visualizing tumors at the cellular level, we can never be sure that an imaged region does not contain some tiny bit of microscopic tumor. Furthermore, virtually every mode of treatment leaves in its wake some large or small zone of edema.[2,3] These facts, therefore, lead all too often to our standard posttreatment hedge of "Findings are consistent with posttreatment effect, with no definite imaging evidence of recurrent tumor."

The purpose of this article is to review the potential for artificial intelligence (AI) and radiomics to help answer all of the questions posed above—particularly the more difficult ones. We will review recent work in these areas and point out uses on the horizon, that is, aspects that we think will be practical or useful in the near future.

ARTIFICIAL INTELLIGENCE

AI is beginning to have a significant impact on the practice of radiology. AI models can detect and classify musculoskeletal (MSK) tumors on medical images[4] and predict subsequent metastases.[5] There are also many noninterpretive ways in which AI can impact one's radiology practice.[6]

Noninterpretive Uses

Image production and quality control
Tumor imaging often involves multiple imaging modalities, multiple imaging protocols, the use of radiation, hours of scanning time, the administration of a radiotracer or contrast agent, and the creation of hundreds, if not thousands, of medical images. Anything that can reduce imaging time, radiation or contrast dose while maintaining or improving image quality can be considered a big win. Recent developments in the use of AI for image reconstruction for computed tomography (CT), positron-emission tomography (PET), and magnetic resonance (MR) have shown great promise in all of these areas.[7]

Noise reduction Deep learning (DL) techniques have been used to reduce noise and artifacts, to enhance contrast and to improve the conspicuity of disease.[8,9] Some of the first DL techniques used led to over-smoothed images with decreased detail and reduced visibility of anatomic structures.[10–12] However, the use of convolutional neural networks (CNN)[13] and generative-adversarial networks (GAN) has produced in denoised images without losing critical information.[11,14–18]

AI can act directly on a processed image to improve image quality. However, AI can also be used to directly transform the raw sensor data from a scanner into images. Subsequent postprocessing stages can then used to minimize artifacts and noise.[19–22]

Reduction of radiation, contrast dose, and scanning time All radiologists wish they could reduce radiation, contrast dose and scan time while imaging our patients. Any new technique that could cut any one of these in half would be considered big news. Alas, much of our prior experience with tumor imaging suggests to us that we can have 1 or 2 of these wishes granted, but not 3. However, one of the most exciting results from recent AI research suggests that we can, indeed, reduce all 3 of these variables by half or more, while maintaining adequate image quality.

Tumor imaging often involves the use of ionizing radiation. Therefore, the increased utilization of CT and PET imaging has led to significant concerns about patient radiation dose. The easiest way to reduce the radiation dose from CT is by reducing the X-ray tube current. However, this results in fewer X-ray photons per scan and thus noisier images (photon starvation). Multiple algorithmic approaches and iterative reconstruction techniques have been used to ameliorate this problem. However, recent DL techniques have been developed which decrease radiation and contrast doses without the loss of image quality.

One such DL technique teaches an AI model what normal anatomy and abnormal pathology look like at both low and standard radiation doses. The AI model can then create high-quality images directly from low-dose raw sensor data.[10,16] One multi-center study compared the diagnostic quality of low-dose scans versus standard-dose CT scans and found that most of their radiologists deemed the AI-reconstructed low-dose scans to have greater or equal diagnostic quality than the standard-dose images.[23]

Similar techniques can be used to generate high-quality PET images, while significantly reducing patient radiation dosage. One group of investigators was able to decrease the radiation dose to only one-quarter of the original radiation dose by combining the anatomic detail from high-quality, T1-weighted MR images with the metabolic information from low-quality, low-dose PET images.[24] Subsequent studies have used GANs to produce high-quality PET images with only 1% of the standard dose of radiation.[25,26]

Yet another study achieved a 200-fold decrease in the radiotracer dose for ^{18}F-fluorodeoxyglucose (^{18}F-FDG) PET scans in the evaluation of glioblastoma by using deep learning.[27]

DL has also been used to reduce the streak artifacts from low-dose CT scans. After training the AI model on the characteristic artifacts produced from low-dose CT studies using a technique called residual learning, these artifacts could then subtracted from subsequent low-dose CT images to improve image quality.[28]

MR does not use ionizing radiation, but it often involves the use of gadolinium-based contrast agents for MSK tumor imaging.[29] Gadolinium has been shown to accumulate in bone and brain tissue, even in patients with normal renal function.[30] There has therefore been great interest in DL techniques that might reduce the amount of gadolinium required. Such DL techniques have been used to create good quality postcontrast MRI images using only 10% of the standard dose of gadolinium.[31] These images did not have any significant image degradation compared to full contrast dose images and also had lower motion artifacts.

Increasing MR image quality and decreasing scan time DL has been used to improve other aspects of image quality in CT and MR,[32] such as the removal of CT metal artifact,[33] MR banding artifact,[34] and MR motion artifact.[35,36] CNNs have also been used to enhance spatial resolution.[37,38]

MRI imaging involves relatively long acquisition times, which means that one may have to sometimes sacrifice image quality to meet the constraints of limited scanning time. One solution to this issue has been the use of incomplete k-space sampling to shorten MR scan acquisition times. However, DL techniques can train a CNN to learn a mapping between zero-filled and fully sampled MR images.[39] DL and parallel imaging techniques can also been used reduce scan time by reconstructing MR images from clinical multi-coil MR.[40] Diffusion MR imaging, for example, can be accelerated by a factor of 12 when DL is used to optimize q-space data processing.[41]

Improving radiology workflow

Creating study protocols MSK tumor imaging is performed using a wide variety of sometimes complex imaging protocols. Choosing an optimal protocol for each patient is an important task, but is often tedious, time-consuming, and susceptible to human error. Early work suggests that this process might be automated by the use of AI. One large academic center applied rule-based machine learning to order entry information, and substantially decreased the number of studies that needed to be manually protocoled, which in turn improved order turn-around-time.[42] Natural language processing (NLP) algorithms can also be applied to order entry data and used to automated MRI protocol selection[43] and selection of specific MR sequences.[44] Such automation of MR sequence-level protocol information could potentially allow for dynamic sequence selection, instead of a one-size-fits-all approach. DL-based NLP algorithms have been applied to MSK MR protocol selection[45] and general radiology protocol selection[46] with some success.

AI could also be used for protocol development, by experimentally determining the optimal pulse sequence for a particular clinical indication. Optimal sequences are currently chosen by radiologists, following a tedious, side-by-side comparison of multiple pulse sequences. However, a properly trained CNN might provide an acceptable surrogate for human readers when performing such a protocol optimization study.[47] The use of a CNN could not only reduce the tedious aspects of such studies but could also greatly increase the practical number of sequence combinations that could be tested.

Hanging protocols Hanging protocols can have a large impact on a radiologist's workflow. A lean 6 sigma study performed by General Electric Healthcare in 2010 observed that 9% of a radiologist's average task time was spent on modifying the image layout.[48] Efficient hanging protocols could, therefore, reduce the lag time between study selection and the point at which a radiologist could actually start to review the images. Automation of hanging protocols can be challenging, due to inconsistencies in Digital Imaging and Communications in Medicine (DICOM) metadata among institutions, sequence names among vendors, and individual preferences among radiologists. It would, therefore, be a great help to have a system that could dynamically create a hanging protocol based on image content, rather than metadata alone. To this end, there is ongoing work using AI to automatically create hanging protocols based on users' prior manual hanging patterns.[48,49]

Worklist prioritization AI can improve radiologist workflow by means of worklist prioritization. An appropriately trained radiology preprocessor (RP) can assigning higher priorities to cases on the worklist that may contain emergent abnormalities (**Figs. 1–3**). In this paradigm, there is an image interpretation component to the RP's task, but the role of the RP is not to primarily render an interpretation but to alert radiologists to potential critical findings and improve turnaround time for reporting of potentially actionable abnormalities. RP systems can currently triage chest

original worklist

AI	priority	name	MRN	Modality	hospital location	exam type
	STAT	Twain, M	12345	CT	ED	head
	STAT	Poe, EA	23456	CT	ED	abdomen
	STAT	Faulkner, W	34567	CT	Inpatient	C-spine
		Heinlein, R	45678	CT	Outpatient	abdomen
		Asimov, I	56789	CT	Inpatient	C-spine
		Christie, A	67890	MR	Outpatient	C-spine
		Tolstoy, L	78901	CT	Inpatient	abdomen
		Chekhov, A	89012	CT	Outpatient	chest

Fig. 1. An fictitious radiology worklist, sorted by clinician-classified level of urgency.

radiographs,[50] abdominal CT,[51] and head CTs[52] for emergent findings. However, an RP could also be trained to triage for relevant oncologic issues, such as new lesions on follow-up studies (**Fig. 4**), or impending pathologic fractures (**Fig. 5**). An RP system can also be used to assist radiologists in oncologic imaging in the detection of target lesions and estimating tumor burden. One recently described RP improved concordance with target lesions measurements (68 vs. 23%), decreased clinician notification times (median time = 1 hour) and decreased radiologist interpretation times (37%).[53]

Diagnosis of Disease

AI researchers have successfully trained AI models to diagnose MSK disorders. In 1965, Lodwick described a probabilistic approach to the diagnosis of bone tumors, using a näive Bayesian model and radiologist input of patient age and four radiographic features (size, matrix, periosteal reaction and pattern of bone destruction)[54–56] (**Fig. 6**). Within its limited differential range of only 9 different bone tumors, its average accuracy was 80%. In 2017, this work was extended to similar but larger Bayesian model using 18

AI-identified priority studies

AI	priority	name	MRN	Modality	hospital location	exam type
	STAT	Twain, M	12345	CT	ED	head
	STAT	Poe, EA	23456	CT	ED	abdomen
!	STAT	Faulkner, W	34567	CT	Inpatient	C-spine
		Heinlein, R	45678	CT	Outpatient	abdomen
		Asimov, I	56789	CT	Inpatient	C-spine
		Christie, A	67890	MR	Outpatient	C-spine
!		Tolstoy, L	78901	CT	Inpatient	abdomen
!		Chekhov, A	89012	CT	Outpatient	chest

Fig. 2. An AI radiology preprocessor has reviewed the images in these cases and classified two additional cases on the list as being urgent.

worklist re-sorted by AI priority

AI	priority	name	MRN	Modality	hospital location	exam type
❗	STAT	Faulkner, W	34567	CT	Inpatient	C-spine
❗		Tolstoy, L	78901	CT	Inpatient	abdomen
❗		Chekhov, A	89012	CT	Outpatient	chest
	STAT	Twain, M	12345	CT	ED	head
	STAT	Poe, EA	23456	CT	ED	abdomen
		Heinlein, R	45678	CT	Outpatient	abdomen
		Asimov, I	56789	CT	Inpatient	C-spine
		Christie, A	67890	MR	Outpatient	C-spine

Fig. 3. The AI radiology preprocessor has resorted the worklist to account for these additional urgent cases.

demographic and radiographic features and a differential list of 66 possible bone tumors.[4] For the top 10 most common diagnoses, primary accuracy was 62% and differential accuracy was 80%. In the past 5 years, work has shifted away from radiologists entering features into AI models, and toward models for which the image is presented directly to a CNN-based AI model. With nontumor imaging, AI models have been trained to detect femoral neck fractures on radiographs better than orthopedic surgeons,[57] and displaced wrist fractures with a sensitivity of 0.953 and a specificity of 0.993.[58] Other models can diagnose anterior cruciate ligament (ACL) and meniscal lesions with performance similar to that of human radiologists[59,60] and recognize osteonecrosis of the femoral head with a sensitivity noninferior to that of experienced radiologists.[61] Despite these early successes, current AI models are trained to recognize only a tiny fraction of the many lesions a MSK radiologist will see during a day's work, and may miss even egregious examples of findings for which they have not been trained (**Fig. 7**).

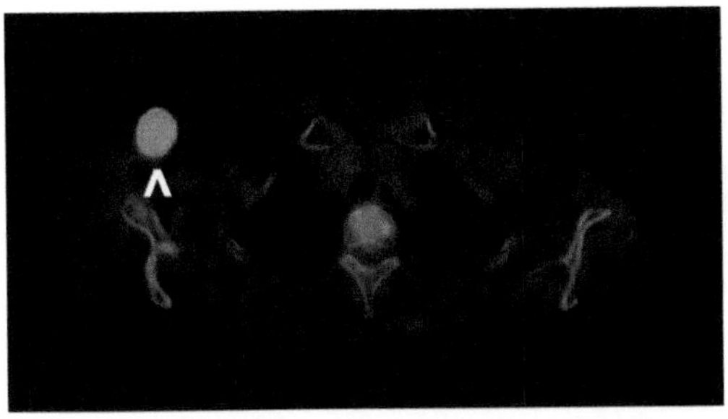

A small dose of perspective

A brief review of past computer-aided detection (CAD) efforts can give us a useful dose of perspective on CAD of the future. In 2000, the U.S. Congress established national Medicare coverage for CAD in breast imaging, based on promising but limited evidence that CAD might lead to better clinical outcomes than routine film mammography.[62] This led to a rapid proliferation of CAD technology into U.S. mammography practices. Unfortunately, this has not resulted in an increase in radiologist performance,[63] and systematic reviews reveal persistent uncertainty as to whether CAD has any clinically important impact on key breast cancer outcomes.[64,65] With a positive predictive value of only 0.1%,[66] it is not surprising that radiologists ignore the vast majority of correct computer detections of breast cancers on a mammogram,[67] possibly due to alert fatigue.[66] It remains to be seen whether MSK CAD systems will fare any better with radiologists. For the moment, the European Society of Radiology has concluded that second or concurrent-reader status is appropriate for CAD, but that CAD should never be used as an independent reader.[68]

RADIOMICS

Radiomics: Promise and Problems

We will start by defining the term "radiomics." The "-omics" portion of radiomics originated in the field of molecular biology, but has recently been applied to other disciplines. Today, when one

Fig. 4. Our fictitious AI radiology preprocessor has pointed out a possible new lesion in this patient with melanoma.

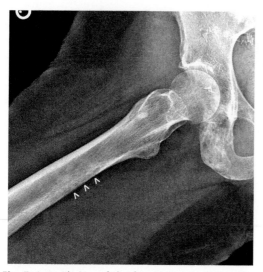

Fig. 5. Lateral view of the femur shows a lesion that results in severe thinning of the posterior cortex, placing the patient at increased risk for impending pathological fracture. Our fictitious AI radiology pre-processor has placed cursors on the image pointing out this worrisome area.

sees the suffix "-omics," it indicates a type of data that can be mined by an automated process. Radiomics, therefore, refers to the extraction of features from medical images which can then be used to support decision-making.[69] This is of special interest in the field of oncology, since gigabytes of digital images are obtained for almost every patient with cancer.

Why should one care about radiomics? We will answer that question with a sartorial metaphor: much of current cancer therapy is "off-the-rack" and "one-size-fits-all." This is unfortunate, as most clinically relevant solid tumors are highly heterogeneous at the phenotypic, physiologic, and genomic levels[70–72] and continue to evolve over time. It is, therefore, understandable if standard treatment protocols result in therapeutic sleeves that are too long, waistlines that are too tight, and garments that are quickly outgrown over time. We should care about radiomics because of its potential to create bespoke diagnoses and treatment plans that fit a patient exactly. This tailored approach is sometimes called "precision medicine," in which molecular and other biomarkers are used to predict the right diagnosis

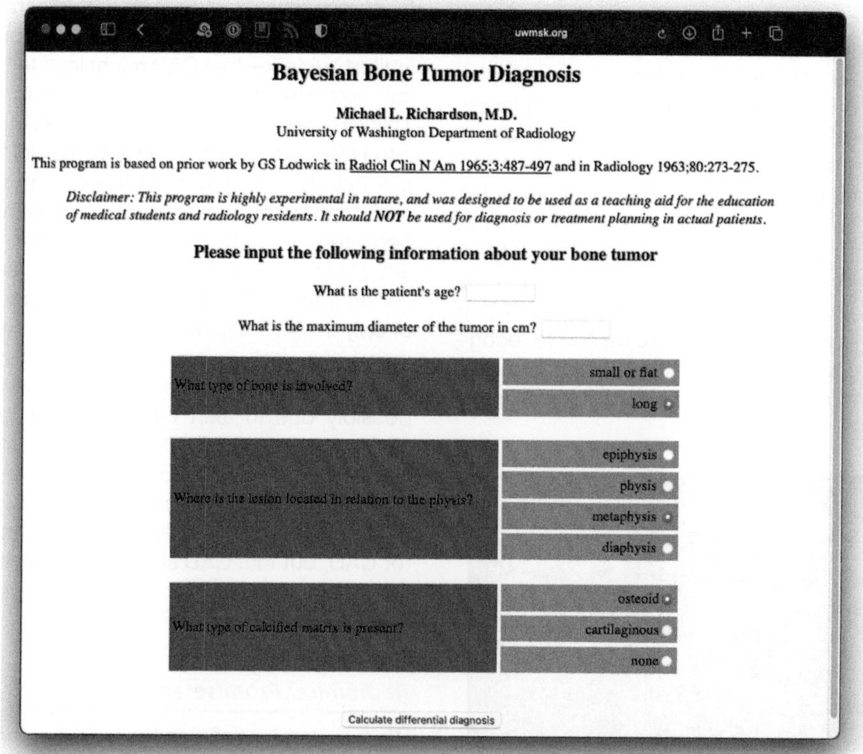

Fig. 6. An online calculator for radiographic diagnosis of bone tumors using a naïve Bayesian model (http://uwmsk.org/bayes/bonetumor.html).

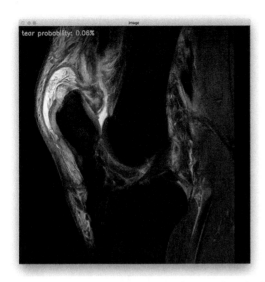

Fig. 7. An AI model trained by one of the authors had absolutely no trouble correctly classifying this patient's ACL as normal. However, it was completely oblivious to the huge tear of the quadriceps tendon.

and the right treatment of the right patient at the right time.[12,69,73–75]

This would be a good time to issue a spoiler alert: radiomics cannot currently deliver this kind of precisely tailored diagnosis or therapy. However, the great progress in genomics, radiomics, molecular imaging and DL over the past 10 years suggests that these capabilities are drawing tantalizingly closer every year.

Radiologists can play a prime role in moving radiomics from the theoretic into the practical realm. Radiologists are critically needed to meet one of the biggest challenges in radiomics research: the current lack of large-scale, high-quality databases of radiomic data. The creation

and curation of such a database can be extremely time-consuming—totaling about 3 hours per patient in one radiomics study.[69] A much more viable solution to this curation problem is for radiologists to capture more and more data prospectively, at the point of care. One step in this direction is the development of the Soft Tissue Tumor Reporting and Data System (ST-RADS) (Table 1).[76] The goal of this initiative is to develop and validate a soft-tissue tumor reporting and data system that will assist in stratifying benign from potentially malignant soft tissue tumors and provide management guidelines, in a manner similar to that of the numerous American College of Radiology Reporting and Data Systems.[77]

Radiologists should not be daunted by the prospect of learning radiomics. Indeed, every radiologist has already committed multiple acts of radiomics during their career. Every time one queries a region of interest (ROI) on a CT scan for its mean Hounsfield value, one has extracted a radiomic data point. Radiologists have long used tissue-specific Hounsfield values from CT to distinguish bone, air, fluid, fat and soft tissue. We have also used long-used these values to estimate bone mineral density, and have more recently extended this concept to the estimation of muscle quantity and quality.[78]

The mean Hounsfield value is one of the several first order statistics of the histogram of an ROI. One can extract other first-order statistics from the histogram, such as the median, maximum, minimum, uniformity or randomness (entropy), skewness (asymmetry), and kurtosis (flatness). One can also derive second order statistics such as Haralick[79] and other textures,[80] which contain information about the spatial distribution of intensity values in the ROI. Higher-order statistical methods involving wavelets, Laplacian transforms, Minkowski functionals, and fractal dimensions can be imposed on the image.[69] To this list, one might also add metabolic information, such as contrast enhancement, apparent diffusion coefficient (ADC) and the standardized uptake value (SUV) of a radiotracer. Finally, a radiologist could add semantic information, such as shape, location, heterogeneity, vascularity, or spiculation of a lesion. These radiomic features can be combined with genomic data and clinical outcome information to offer a seemingly limitless (currently thousands) supply of biomarkers.

One of the great hopes of radiomics is that there are many useful patterns buried in this gigantic trove of radiomic features—patterns that may be imperceptible to a human eye, but visible to a computer. With this hope in mind, a variety of statistical, AI and ML techniques have been invoked.

Table 1
Proposed ST-RADS grades and MRI categories.[76]

ST-RADS Grade	Category
0	Incomplete imaging
I	Negative
II	Definitely benign
III	Probably benign
IV	Indeterminate or suspicious for malignancy
V	Highly suggestive of malignancy
VI	Known biopsy proven malignancy or recurrence

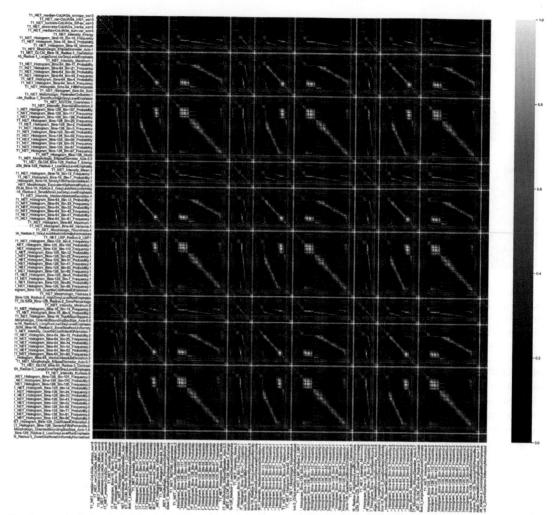

Fig. 8. Correlation matrix of radiomic features of glioblastoma. A total of 2360 MR features were extracted from tumors in 31 patients. Across all tumors, each feature was individually compared with all other features, generating squared correlation coefficients (R^2). Individual features were then clustered and plotted along both axes, with R^2 shown as a heat map, whereby low correlations are black and high correlations are white. Each of the white squares contains a pair of features that are highly correlated with one another and are thus redundant. (*Data from* Clark K, Vendt B, Smith K, Freymann J, Kirby J, Koppel P, et al. The cancer imaging archive (tcia): maintaining and operating a public information repository. J Digit Imaging 2013;26(6):1045–57; Pati S, Verma R, Akbari H, Bilello M, Hill VB, Sako C, et al. Reproducibility analysis of multi-institutional paired expert annotations and radiomic features of the Ivy Glioblastoma Atlas Project (Ivy GAP) dataset. Medical Physics 2020;47(12):6039–52. URL: https://aapm.onlinelibrary.wiley.com/ doi/abs/10.1002/mp.14556; Pati S, Verma R, Akbari H, Bilello M, Hill VB, Sako C, et al. Data from the multi-institutional paired expert segmentations and radiomic features of the ivy gap dataset. 2020. URL: https://wiki.cancerimagingarchive.net/display/DOI/Multi-Institutional+Paired+Expert+Segmentations+ and+Radiomic+Features+of+the+Ivy+GAP+Dataset.)

When one analyzes a large collection of numbers (ie, biomarkers), there is a strong possibility of arriving at spurious correlations by chance alone. For example, the latitude and longitude of the University of Washington Medical Center (47.6490°N, 122.3061°W) occur, respectively, 205 and 23 times within the first 200 million digits of the numerical constant π—purely by chance.[81]

Another aspect of radiomic data is that it is higher-dimensional, that is, the number of radiomic features exceeds the number of observations.[82] This leads to a common statistical problem known as multicollinearity, in which many of the radiomic features are highly correlated (**Fig. 8**). One way to deal with this problem is to collapse clusters of highly-correlated features

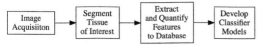

Fig. 9. Steps in the process of radiomics.

down to one representative feature, usually the one with the largest inter-subject variability or highest dynamic range.[69] One can also prioritize features based on their reproducibility.[83–86]

Reproducibility is another major challenge for radiomics. There are wide variations in acquisition and image reconstruction protocols among CT, MR, and PET/CT scanners, and standardization of these protocols across medical imaging centers is typically lacking. When images are analyzed numerically to extract meaningful data, variations in acquisition and image reconstruction parameters can introduce significant changes that are not due to any underlying biological effects. In fact, radiomic features are sensitive to almost all factors involved in the PET/CT workflow, from the generation of the images, to the radiomics implementation choices.[87] Initiatives such as the Quantitative Imaging Biomarkers Alliance have, therefore, begun the work of establishing a consensus on the measurement accuracy of a quantitative imaging biomarker for a specific use, as well as the requirements and procedures needed to achieve an acceptable level of measurement accuracy.[88]

Image Segmentation

Radiomics involves a set of discrete steps (**Fig. 9**). We will focus herein on the second of these steps:

segmentation. The other 3 steps are all worthy topics, but are a bit outside the scope of this review.

Segmentation is the process of partitioning an image into multiple segments, each of which could represent a cell, a tissue, an organ or a disease process. Ac- curate segmentation of muscle boundaries allows one to estimate muscle quantity and quality in patients with suspected sarcopenia.[78,89] Sarcopenia is not only common in patients with cancer [90] but is also an important prognostic factor for complications and surivival.[91] Accurate segmentation of a tumor informs the oncologist of the patient's tumor burden and allows the radio-oncologist to precisely localize the dose of radiation to that tumor and its surrounding tissues.[92–94]

Segmentation remains the most critical, challenging, and contentious component of radiomics. If segmentation is not done properly, it is hard to trust any of the feature data derived from the segmented volumes. Segmentation can be relatively easy in tissues such as bone or fat, with distinctive mean Hounsfield values. However, segmentation is often quite difficult in patients with cancer, because many tumors have indistinct margins. Manual segmentation of tumors continues to demonstrate high interoperator variability.[95–97]

Following imaging acquisition, images are segmented to reduce the image to a set of essential components by manual (**Fig. 10**), automated, or semiautomated methods (**Figs. 11–15**).

Image segmentation and volumetric assessment are commonly used, and are becoming an important component of diagnostic imaging

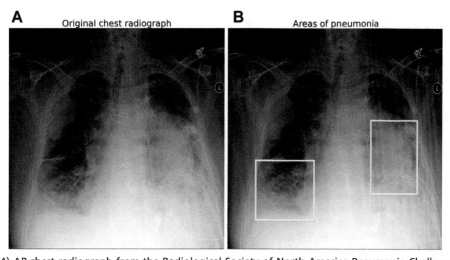

Fig. 10. (A) AP chest radiograph from the Radiological Society of North America Pneumonia Challenge dataset without annotations. [97] (B). The same radiograph with annotations. Yellow bounding boxes outline areas of medium to high probability of pneumonia, as annotated by members of the Society of Thoracic Radiology.

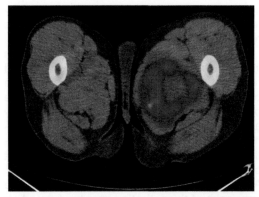

Fig. 11. ¹⁸F-FDG PET/CT scan of a 50 year-old man with a high-grade, pleomorphic liposarcoma of the left adductor magnus muscle. (*Data from* Clark K, Vendt B, Smith K, Freymann J, Kirby J, Koppel P, et al. The cancer imaging archive (tcia): maintaining and operating a public information repository. J Digit Imaging 2013;26(6):1045–57; Vallières M, Freeman CR, Skamene SR, El Naqa I. A radiomics model from joint FDG-PET and MRI texture features for the prediction of lung metastases in soft-tissue sarcomas of the extremities. Phys Med Biol 2015;60(14):5471–96.)

interpretation. These tasks are mostly performed by radiologists or specially-trained technologists on dedicated workstations under a radiologist's supervision. Segmentation can be a tedious and time-consuming task. Fortunately, the

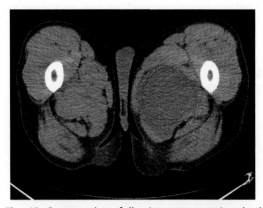

Fig. 12. Same patient following segmentation (*red contour lines*) by an expert radiation oncologist. (*Data from* Clark K, Vendt B, Smith K, Freymann J, Kirby J, Koppel P, et al. The cancer imaging archive (tcia): maintaining and operating a public information repository. J Digit Imaging 2013;26(6):1045–57; Vallières M, Freeman CR, Skamene SR, El Naqa I. A radiomics model from joint FDG-PET and MRI texture features for the prediction of lung metastases in soft-tissue sarcomas of the extremities. Phys Med Biol 2015;60(14):5471– 96.)

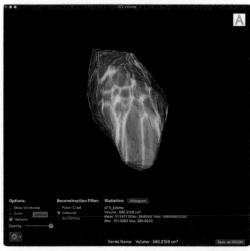

Fig. 13. 3D reconstruction of segmented tumor and tumor volume calculation from the same patient (*Data from* Clark K, Vendt B, Smith K, Freymann J, Kirby J, Koppel P, et al. The cancer imaging archive (tcia): maintaining and operating a public information repository. J Digit Imaging 2013;26(6):1045–57; Vallières M, Freeman CR, Skamene SR, El Naqa I. A radiomics model from joint FDG-PET and MRI texture features for the prediction of lung metastases in soft-tissue sarcomas of the extremities. Phys Med Biol 2015;60(14):5471–96.)

segmentation process itself can be automated to a certain extent through use of DL algorithms.[12] The current consensus is that optimal and reproducible segmentation is achievable with computer-aided edge detection followed by manual curation.[69]

Subsequently, feature extraction is performed to obtain quantitative data to characterize the volumes of interest. The imaging-derived data can be combined with clinical or genomic data to build databases that can be later mined. AI can be applied to these databases in either unsupervised learning approaches (eg, to identify patterns) or supervised learning approaches (in which outcome data or confirmed pathologic diagnoses are used to train a learning model).

AI models have been used to successfully localize and annotate organs such as the kidney, segmental anatomy such as lobes of the liver or lung, and automated detection and labeling of vertebral bodies.[98,99] This is extremely useful when volumetric assessment of a lesion or organ is needed (see **Fig. 13**), particularly for tumor treatment planning and response (see **Figs. 14** and **15**).

Segmentation remains an important component in oncologic clinical trials whereby lesions (target or nontarget) are followed from baseline at various

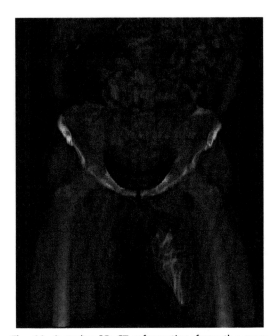

Fig. 14. Anterior 3D CT reformation from the same patient data. The tumor has been superimposed over the original CT data as an example of how this information might be used for treatment planning. (*Data from* Clark K, Vendt B, Smith K, Freymann J, Kirby J, Koppel P, et al. The cancer imaging archive (tcia): maintaining and operating a public information repository. J Digit Imaging 2013;26(6):1045–57; Vallières M, Freeman CR, Skamene SR, El Naqa I. A radiomics model from joint FDG-PET and MRI texture features for the prediction of lung metastases in soft-tissue sarcomas of the extremities. Phys Med Biol 2015;60(14):5471– 96.)

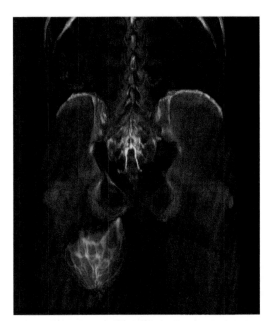

Fig. 15. Posterior 3D CT reformation from the same patient data. The tumor has been superimposed over the original CT data as an example of how this information might be used for treatment planning. (*Data from* Clark K, Vendt B, Smith K, Freymann J, Kirby J, Koppel P, et al. The cancer imaging archive (tcia): maintaining and operating a public information repository. J Digit Imaging 2013;26(6):1045–57; Vallières M, Freeman CR, Skamene SR, El Naqa I. A radiomics model from joint FDG-PET and MRI texture features for the prediction of lung metastases in soft-tissue sarcomas of the extremities. Phys Med Biol 2015;60(14):5471– 96.)

time points to assess treatment response. These studies require precise and consistent evaluation of the lesions across different readers at different time points, and can be best optimized using annotations and in some instances automated/semi-automated segmentation or volumetric assessment. Studies have shown that DL can efficiently monitor changes and perform quantitative analysis before, during, and after treatment and can also help to predict prognostic endpoints.[100–102]

CURRENT APPLICATIONS OF ARTIFICIAL INTELLIGENCE AND RADIOMICS IN MUSCULOSKELETAL TUMORS

There has been considerable enthusiasm about using CNN models for the evaluation of bone and soft tissue tumors. For decades of tumor imaging, the final diagnosis was made by a combination of the radiologic and histologic appearances of a lesion. In the past 10 years, however, there has been a shift away from morphological features alone and toward adding information from immunohistochemical, radiomic and genetic markers.

We will now briefly review recent work in the use of AI models to diagnose, classify and grade MSK tumors, as well as to predict treatment response, metastasis and patient outcome. This review includes several summary tables, which we will preface with a few general caveats. The reader can readily see that many of the studies cited involve a relatively small number of patients, which reduces their reliability. Every biomarker study should be validated against a completely independent data set, preferably from another institution. Very few of the studies cited here have performed such validation. Clinical endpoints used by these studies are quite variable. The most common figure of merit in these tables the area under the receiver operating characteristic curve (AUC). The other figure of merit listed

Table 2
Classification of soft tissue tumors with ultrasound

Author, Year	Tumor	Imaging Modality	n	AUC	Outcome
Wang et al,[111] 2021	multiple soft tissue masses	US	227	0.91	benign vs malignant
Wang et al,[111] 2021	soft tissue subset	US	83	0.86	lipoma vs other
Wang et al,[111] 2021	soft tissue sub-set	US	83	0.68	nerve sheath tumorvs other
Wang et al,[111] 2021	soft tissue sub-set	US	83	0.73	vascular malformation vs other

is the C-index (aka concordance index), which is a generalization the AUC that can take into account censored data. For a perfect test, both of these indices will be 1.0. For a useless test which performs no better than chance, both indices will be 0.5. At some level between 0.5 and 1.0, we begin to consider a test to be "good". While this exact level is somewhat subjective, we suggest that a test should score at least 0.75 to rise above the level of mediocrity.[103]

Biopsy Guidance

Image-guided biopsies are already an important part of an MSK radiologist's practice. Quantitative radiomic features can refine this process by identifying locations within complex tumors that are most likely to contain important diagnostic, prognostic, or predictive information. Prostate segmentation is used by urologists for targeted biopsy in suspected MR findings of high-risk prostate cancer. Studies have shown high accuracy in prostate segmentation using deep learning.[104,105] In another study, patients with metabolically active bone disease, PET/CT-guided biopsies changed the previously planned treatment in 56%.[106] Radiomics information could also be useful following the biopsy, as the estimated error rate of cancer histopathology may be as high as 23%.[107–110] Radiomic information could support or contradict histopathologic findings and possibly suggest the need for a pathology review in non-concordant cases.

Tumor Classification

One recent study trained several CNN models to classify soft tissue masses based on their ultrasound (US) appearance (**Table 2**). One model was able to distinguish between benign and

Table 3
Recent radiomic studies of tumor classification

Author, Year	Tumor	Imaging Modality	n	AUC	Outcome
Hsu et al,[112] 2018	Hodgkin's lymphoma & Ewing sarcoma	18F-FDG PET/CT	38	0.8	normal tissue high-FDG uptake vs tumor uptake
Li et al,[113] 2019	chordoma & chondrosarcoma	MR	210	0.87	chordoma vs chondrosarcoma
Yin et al,[114] 2019	chordoma & giant cell tumor	CT	95	0.79	chordoma vs chondrosarcoma
Dai et al,[115] 2020	osteosarcoma & Ewing sarcoma	MR	210	0.77–0.88	osteosarcoma vs Ewing sarcoma
Hong et al,[116] 2021	Osteoblastic metastases	CT	177	0.96	bone islands vs osteoblastic metastases

Abbreviations: AUC, area under the ROC curve; n, number of subjects; STS, soft tissue sarcoma.

Table 4
Recent radiomic studies of tumor grading

Author, Year	Tumor	Imaging Modality	n	C-Index	Outcome
Corino et al,[118] 2018	STS	MR	19	0.87	Intermediate vs high-grade
Gitto et al,[119] 2019	Chondroid	MR	68	0.78	Low vs high-grade
Zhang et al,[120] 2019	STS	MR	35	0.92	Low vs high-grade
Peeken et al,[121] 2019	STS	MR	225	0.78	Low vs high-grade
Xu et al,[122] 2020	STS	MR	70	0.92	Low vs high-grade
Wang et al,[123] 2020	STS	MR	95	0.96	Low vs high-grade

Table 5
Recent radiomic studies of tumor treatment prognosis

Author, Year	Tumor	Imaging Modality	n	C-Index	Outcome
Wu et al,[124] 2018	Osteosarcoma	CT	150	0.84	5-y survival
Chen et al,[125] 2020	Osteosarcoma	MR	93	0.81	Early relapse (<1 year)
Morvan et al,[126] 2020	Multiple myeloma	^{18}F-FDG PET/CT	66	0.64	Progression-free survival
Crombé et al,[127] 2020	Desmoid tumor	MR	42	0.84	Progression-free survival
Peeken et al,[128] 2021	High-grade soft tissue sarcoma	MR	179	0.64	Overall survival

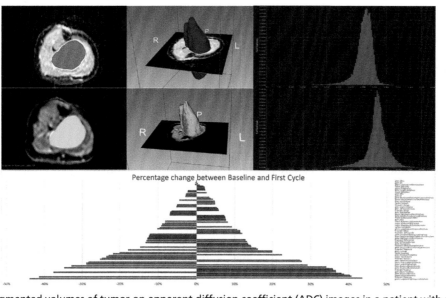

Fig. 16. Segmented volumes of tumor on apparent diffusion coefficient (ADC) images in a patient with a myxoid sarcoma before (magenta) and after (cyan) one cycle of chemotherapy. There was no significant change in size or volume of the lesion, but radiomics features were helpful in assessing response. Specifically, first-order (histogram) analysis showed a clear rightward shift of the histogram following treatment, as well as significant changes in skewness (40%) and kurtosis (25%). Although diffusion-weighted imaging (DWI) is considered by many to be of limited utility in assessment of myxoid tumors (due to the absence of restricted diffusion), radiomic analysis allows for assessment of therapeutic response. Bottom panel shows the changes noted in multiple radiomic features following treatment.

Table 6
Recent radiomic studies of tumor treatment response

Author, Year	Tumor	Imaging Modality	N	AUC	Outcome
Li et al,[131] 2019	Acute leukemia	^{18}F-FDG PET/CT	41	0.89	Bone marrow involvement in suspected relapse
Tagliafico et al,[132] 2019	Soft tissue sarcoma of limbs	MR	11	0.96	Local recurrence
Dufau et al,[133] 2019	Osteosarcoma	MR	69	0.98	Response to neoadjuvant chemotherapy
Peng et al,[134] 2020	Osteosarcoma	CT	191	0.87	Response to neoadjuvant chemotherapy
Crombé et al,[135] 2020	Myxoid/round cell liposarcoma	CT	35	0.64–0.94	Metastatic relapse

Abbreviations: AUC, area under the ROC curve; n, number of subjects.

Table 7
Recent radiomic studies of tumor metastasis

Author, Year	Tumor	Imaging Modality	N	AUC	Outcome
Vallières et al,[136] 2015	Soft tissue sarcoma	MR & ^{18}F-FDG PET/CT	51	0.98	Prediction of lung metastasis
Peng et al,[134] 2019	Soft tissue sarcoma	^{18}F-FDG	51	0.85	Prediction of distant metastasis
Sheen et al,[137] 2019	Osteosarcoma	PET/CT ^{18}F-FDG PET/CT	83	0.80	Prediction of metastasis

Abbreviations: AUC, area under the ROC curve; n, number of subjects.

malignant soft tissue masses with an AUC of 091, matching the performance of 2 expert readers. Another model was trained to differentiate among an 83 mass subset of 3 commonly-observed benign masses (26 lipomas, 30 nerve sheath tumors and 27 vascular malformations). This model fared less well, with an overall accuracy of 71%).

Several recent studies have used radiomic features to classify different tissue and tumor types with acceptable AUC values (Table 3). One model was able to distinguish high-uptake normal tissues (brain, heart, kidneys, and bladder) versus high-uptake in tumors (Hodgkin's lymphoma and Ewing sarcoma).[112] Other radiomic models were trained to distinguish among several different osseous lesions (chordoma, chondrosarcoma, giant cell tumor, Ewing sarcoma, osteosarcoma, bone islands, and osteoblastic metastases).[113–116]

Tumor Grading and Prognosis

Tumor grading is an essential element in the classification of sarcomas. It correlates with the prognosis of the disease and the risk of metastasis. The differentiation between high-grade and low-grade lesions drives therapeutic decision-making. The question remains what and how much role imagers can take in aiding the clinicians and pathologists toward an accurate, noninvasive evaluation of tumor grade and subsequent management.[117] Eleven recent studies with small to medium numbers of patients have used radiomic features to predict tumor grade (**Table 4**), and prognosis (**Table 5**) with varying degrees of success.

Treatment Response and Prediction of Metastasis

Several investigators have found that imaging phenotypes[129] and MR textures[130] correlated with subsequent chemotherapy response (**Fig. 16**. Eight studies with small to medium numbers of patients used radiomic features to predict treatment response (**Table 6**) and the development of metastasis (**Table 7**) with moderate success.

SUMMARY

The ultimate goal of AI and radiomics in medical imaging is to improve patient outcomes. As we have discussed in this review, the application of AI and radiomics can provide detailed characteristics of the radiographic characteristics of underlying tissues. These tools can be used at many locations in the clinical care path to improve diagnosis, treatment planning, and assessment of treatment response. Additional goals include the reduction of time, cost and radiation dose. This tremendous potential for clinical translation has led to a increase in the number of research studies published in this field by over an order of magnitude—a number that will likely continue to rise sharply.

Many studies have reported robust and meaningful findings. However, a growing number also suffer from flawed experimental or analytical designs. Such errors could result not only in invalid discoveries but also may lead others to perpetuate similar flaws in their own work.[138] Although The FDA has granted approval for several AI-based diagnostic software packages to be used in clinical practice, the critical appraisal and independent evaluation of these technologies are still in their infancy.[139] Even within seminal studies in the field, there remains wide variation in design, methodology and reporting that limits the generalizability and applicability of their findings.[140] Regardless of which of these techniques are ultimately adopted, we hope that our review will provoke thought in the wider community of radiologists, and perhaps help lead to even newer and more intriguing applications of AI and radiomics.

CLINICS CARE POINTS

The purpose of this article is to review the potential for artificial intelligence (AI) and radiomics that are out on the horizon, that is, aspects that we think will be practical or useful in the near future.

Although this work seems promising, it is still at the research stage and therefore speculative. Thus, there is not yet sufficient evidence to make evidence-based recommendations for the use of AI or radiomics at the point of care.

REFERENCES

1. Han G, Bi WZ, Xu M, et al. Amputation versus limb-salvage surgery in patients with osteosarcoma: A meta-analysis. World J Surg 2016;40(8):2016–27.
2. Kuno RC, Richardson ML, Zink-Brody GC, et al. Prevalence of muscle injury following intra-arterial chemotherapy. Skeletal Radiol 1996;25(4):345–8.
3. Richardson ML, Zink-Brody GC, Patten RM, et al. MR characterization of post-irradiation soft tissue edema. Skeletal Radiol 1996;25(6):537–43.
4. Do BH, Langlotz C, Beaulieu CF. Bone tumor diagnosis using a näive bayesian model of demographic and radiographic features. J Digit Imaging 2017;30(5):640–7.
5. Deng J, Zeng W, Shi Y, et al. Fusion of FDG-PET image and clinical features for prediction of lung metastasis in soft tissue sarcomas. Comput Math Methods Med 2020;2020:8153295.
6. Richardson ML, Garwood ER, Lee Y, et al. Noninterpretive uses of artificial intelligence in radiology. Acad Radiol 2020. https://doi.org/10.1016/j.acra.2020.01.012.
7. Langlotz CP, Allen B, Erickson BJ, et al. A roadmap for foundational research on artificial intelligence in medical imaging: From the 2018 NIH/RSNA/ACR/The Academy Workshop. Radiology 2019;291(3):781–91.
8. Dargan R. AI-based applications boost image quality. Revolution in AI will benefit image quality and 3D print modeling. 2019. Available at: https://www.rsna.org/news/2019/may/ai-based-applications-boost-image-quality. Accessed December 5, 2021.
9. Higaki T, Nakamura Y, Zhou J, et al. Deep learning reconstruction at CT: Phantom study of the image characteristics. Acad Radiol 2020;27(1):82–7.
10. Chen H, Zhang Y, Kalra MK, et al. Low-dose CT with a residual encoder-decoder convolutional neural network. IEEE Trans Med Imaging 2017;36(12):2524–35.
11.. Dong C, Loy CC, He K, et al. Image super-resolution using deep convolutional networks. IEEE Trans Pattern Anal Machine Intelligence 2016;38(2):295–307.
12. Ronneberger O, Fischer P, Brox T. U-net: Convolutional networks for biomedical image segmentation. abs/1505.04597. CoRR 2015. Available at: http://arxiv.org/abs/1505.04597. arXiv:1505.04597.

13. Jiang D, Dou W, Vosters L, et al. Denoising of 3D magnetic resonance images with multi-channel residual learning of convolutional neural network. Jpn J Radiol 2018;36(9):566–74.

14. Yang Q, Yan P, Zhang Y, et al. Low-dose CT image denoising using a generative adversarial network with Wasserstein distance and perceptual loss. IEEE Trans Med Imaging 2018;37(6):1348–57.

15. Kang E, Chang W, Yoo J, et al. Deep convolutional framelet denoising for low-dose CT via wavelet residual network. IEEE Trans Med Imaging 2018; 37(6):1358–69.

16. Chen H, Zhang Y, Zhang W, et al. Low-dose CT via convolutional neural network. Biomed Opt Express 2017;8(2):679.

17. Ledig C, Theis L, Huszar F, et al. Photo-realistic single image super-resolution using a generative adversarial network. abs/1609.04802. CoRR 2016. Available at: http://arxiv.org/abs/1609.04802. arXiv:1609.04802.

18. Lakhani P, Prater AB, Hutson RK, et al. Machine learning in radiology: applications beyond image interpretation. J Am Coll Radiol 2018;15(2): 350–9.

19. Wang G, Ye JC, Mueller K, et al. Image reconstruction is a new frontier of machine learning. IEEE Trans Med Imaging 2018;37(6):1289–96.

20. Zhu B, Liu JZ, Cauley SF, et al. Image reconstruction by domain-transform manifold learning. Nature 2018;555(7697):487–92.

21. Quan TM, Nguyen-Duc T, Jeong WK. Compressed sensing MRI reconstruction using a generative adversarial network with a cyclic loss. IEEE Trans Med Imaging 2018;37(6):1488–97.

22. Gözcü B, Mahabadi RK, Li YH, et al. Learning-based compressive MRI. IEEE Trans Med Imaging 2018;37(6):1394–406.

23. .. Cross N, DeBerry J, Daniel Ortiz D, et al. Diagnostic quality of machine learning algorithm for optimization of low dose computed tomography data. Leesburg, VA: Society of Imaging Informatics in Medicine; 2017.

24. Xiang L, Qiao Y, Nie D, et al. Deep auto-context convolutional neural networks for standard-dose PET image estimation from low-dose PET/MRI. Neurocomputing 2017;267:406–16.

25. Ouyang J, Chen KT, Gong E, et al. Ultra-low-dose PET reconstruction using generative adversarial network with feature matching and task-specific perceptual loss. Med Phys 2019;46(8):3555–64.

26. Chen KT, Gong E, de Carvalho Macruz FB, et al. Ultra-low-dose 18F-Florbetaben amyloid PET imaging using deep learning with multi-contrast MRI inputs. Radiology 2019;290(3):649–56.

27. Xu J, Gong E, Pauly JM, Zaharchuk G. 200x low-dose PET reconstruction using deep learning. CoRR 2017;abs/1712.04119. Available at: http://

arxiv.org/abs/1712.04119. arXiv:1712.04119. Accessed December 5, 2021.

28. Xie S, Zheng X, Chen Y, et al. Artifact removal using improved GoogLeNet for sparse-view CT reconstruction. Sci Rep 2018;8(1):6700.

29. Amini B, Murphy WA Jr, Haygood TM, et al. Gadolinium-based contrast agents improve detection of recurrent soft-tissue sarcoma at MRI. Radiol Imaging Cancer 2020;2(2):e190046.

30. Ramalho J, Semelka RC, Ramalho M, et al. Gadolinium-based contrast agent accumulation and toxicity: an update. AJNR Am J Neuroradiol 2016; 37(7):1192–8.

31. Gong E, Pauly JM, Wintermark M, et al. Deep learning enables reduced gadolinium dose for contrast-enhanced brain MRI. J Magn Reson Imaging 2018;48(2):330–40.

32. Higaki T, Nakamura Y, Tatsugami F, et al. Improvement of image quality at CT and MRI using deep learning. Jpn J Radiol 2019;37(1):73–80.

33. Zhang Y, Yu H. Convolutional neural network based metal artifact reduc- tion in X-ray computed tomography. IEEE Trans Med Imaging 2018;37(6): 1370–81.

34. Kim KH, Park SH. Artificial neural network for suppression of banding ar- tifacts in balanced steady-state free precession MRI. Magn Reson Imaging 2017;37:139–46.

35. Hauptmann A, Arridge S, Lucka F, et al. Real-time cardiovascular MR with spatio-temporal artifact suppression using deep learning — proof of concept in congenital heart disease. Magn Reson Med 2019;81(2):1143–56.

36. Nguyen XV, Oztek MA, Nelakurti DD, et al. Applying artificial intelligence to mitigate effects of patient motion or other complicating factors on image quality. Top Magn Reson Imaging 2020; 29(4):175–80.

37. Liu C, Wu X, Yu X, et al. Fusing multi-scale information in convolution network for MR image super-resolution reconstruction. Biomed Eng Online 2018;17(1):114.

38. Park J, Hwang D, Kim KY, et al. Computed tomography super-resolution using deep convolutional neural network. Phys Med Biol 2018;63(14): 145011.

39. Wang S, Su Z, Ying L, et al. Accelerating magnetic resonance imaging via deep learning. In: 2016 IEEE 13th International Symposium on Biomedical Imaging (ISBI). IEEE. San Francisco, April 13-16, 2016. p. 514–7.

40. Hammernik K, Klatzer T, Kobler E, et al. Learning a variational network for reconstruction of accelerated MRI data. CoRR 2017;abs/1704.00447. Available at: http://arxiv.org/abs/1704.00447. arXiv: 1704.00447. Accessed December 5, 2021.

41. Golkov V, Dosovitskiy A, Sperl JI, et al. q- space deep learning: twelve-fold shorter and model-free diffusion MRI scans. IEEE Trans Med Imaging 2016;35(5):1344–51.

42. Tajmir SH, Alkasab TK. Toward augmented radiologists: changes in radiology education in the era of machine learning and artificial intelligence. Acad Radiol 2018;25(6):747–50.

43.. Brown AD, Marotta TR. A natural language processing-based model to automate MRI brain protocol selection and prioritization. Acad Radiol 2017;24(2):160–6.

44. Brown AD, Marotta TR. Using machine learning for sequence-level automated MRI protocol selection in neuroradiology. J Am Med Inform Assoc 2017; 25(5):568–71.

45. Trivedi H, Mesterhazy J, Laguna B, et al. Automatic determination of the need for intravenous contrast in musculoskeletal MRI examinations using IBM Watson's natural language processing algorithm. J Digital Imaging 2018;31(2):245–51.

46. Goel A, Shih G, Rasiej M, et al. Deep learning for comprehensive automated radiology protocolling. Leesburg, VA: Society for Imaging Informatics in Medicine; 2018. Available at: https://cdn.ymaws. com/siim.org/resource/resmgr/siim2018/abstracts/ 18ml-productivity-Goel.pdf.

47. Richardson ML. MR protocol optimization with deep learning: a proof of concept. Current problems in diagnostic radiology 2019. https://doi.org/ 10.1067/j.cpradiol.2019.10.004. Available at:.

48. Wang T, Iankoulski A, Mullarky B. Intelligent tools for a productive radiologist workflow: how machine learning enriches hanging protocols. White paper. Boston, MA: GE Healthcare; 2013. Available at: https://silo.tips/queue/intelligent-tools-for-a-produ ctive-radiologist-workflow-how-machine-learning- enr?&queue_id=-1&v=1619921610&u=MjYwMTo 2MDI6OWMwMDoxYjAwOmE1NmU6YWRiNDo0O DZjOjlyMzg%3D"\ \ o".

49. Bergström P. Automated setup of display protocols. Master's thesis. Linköping, Sweden: Linköping University; 2015. Available at: http://www. diva-portal.org/smash/record.jsf?pid=diva2: 810660.

50. Rajpurkar P, Irvin J, Ball RL, et al. Deep learning for chest radiograph diagnosis: a retrospective comparison of the CheXNeXt algorithm to practicing radiologists. PLoS Med 2018;15(11):e1002686.

51. Winkel DJ, Heye T, Weikert TJ, et al. Evaluation of an AI-based detection software for acute findings in abdominal computed tomography scans: Toward an automated work list prioritization of routine CT examinations. Invest Radiol 2019;54(1):55–9.

52. Prevedello LM, Erdal BS, Ryu JL, et al. Automated critical test findings identification and online

53. Do HM, Spear LG, Nikpanah M, et al. Augmented radiologist workflow improves report value and saves time: a potential model for implementation of artificial intelligence. Acad Radiol 2020;27(1): 96–105.

54. Lodwick G, Haun CL, Smith WE, et al. Computer diagnosis of primary bone tumors: a preliminary report. Radiology 1963;80(2):273–5.

55. Lodwick GS. A probabilistic approach to the diagnosis of bone tumors. Radiol Clin North Am 1965; 3(3):487–97.

56. Richardson ML. Bayesian bone tumor diagnosis. 2005. Available at: https://uwmsk.org/bayes/ bonetumor.html. Accessed December 5, 2021.

57. Urakawa T, Tanaka Y, Goto S, et al. Detecting intertrochanteric hip fractures with orthopedist-level accuracy using a deep convolutional neural network. Skeletal Radiol 2019;48(2):239–44.

58. Thian YL, Li Y, Jagmohan P, et al. Convolutional neural networks for automated fracture detection and localization on wrist radiographs. Radiol Artif Intell 2019;1(1):e180001.

59. Bien N, Rajpurkar P, Ball RL, et al. Deep-learning-assisted diagnosis for knee magnetic resonance imaging: Development and retrospective validation of MRNet. PLoS Med 2018;15(11):e1002699.

60. Liu F, Guan B, Zhou Z, et al. Fully automated diagnosis of anterior cruciate ligament tears on knee MR images by using deep learning. Radiol Artif Intell 2019;1(3):1–10.

61. Chee CG, Kim Y, Kang Y, et al. Performance of a deep learning algorithm in detecting osteonecrosis of the femoral head on digital radiography: A comparison with assessments by radiologists. AJR Am J Roentgenol 2019;213(1):155–62.

62. Fenton JJ, Foote SB, Green P, et al. Diffusion of computer- aided mammography after mandated medicare coverage. Arch Intern Med 2010; 170(11):987–9.

63. Lehman CD, Wellman RD, Buist DSM, et al. Diagnostic accuracy of digital screening mammography with and without computer-aided detection. JAMA Intern Med 2015;175(11):1828–37.

64. Noble M, Bruening W, Uhl S, et al. Computer-aided detection mammography for breast cancer screening: systematic review and meta-analysis. Arch Gynecol Obstet 2009;279(6):881–90.

65. Taylor P, Potts HWW. Computer aids and human second reading as in- terventions in screening mammography: two systematic reviews to compare effects on cancer detection and recall rate. Eur J Cancer 2008;44(6):798–807.

66. Nishikawa RM, Bae KT. Importance of better human-computer interac- tion in the era of deep learning: Mammography computer-aided

diagnosis as a use case. J Am Coll Radiol 2018; 15(1 Pt A):49–52.

67. Nishikawa RM, Schmidt RA, Linver MN, et al. Clinically missed cancer: how effectively can radiologists use computer- aided detection? AJR Am J Roentgenol 2012;198(3):708–16.

68. European Society of Radiology (ESR). What the radiologist should know about artificial intelligence — an ESR white paper. Insights Imaging 2019; 10(1):44.

69. Gillies RJ, Kinahan PE, Hricak H. Radiomics: Images are more than pictures, they are data. Radiology 2016;278(2):563–77.

70. Gerlinger M, Rowan AJ, Horswell S, et al. Intratumor heterogeneity and branched evolution revealed by multiregion sequencing. N Engl J Med 2012;366(10):883–92.

71. Sottoriva A, Spiteri I, Piccirillo SGM, et al. Intratumor heterogeneity in human glioblastoma reflects cancer evolutionary dynamics. Proc Natl Acad Sci U S A 2013;110(10):4009–14.

72. Yachida S, Jones S, Bozic I, et al. Distant metastasis occurs late during the genetic evolution of pancreatic cancer. Nature 2010;467(7319):1114–7.

73. Kickingereder P, Bonekamp D, Nowosielski M, et al. Radiogenomics of glioblastoma: Machine learning-based classification of molecular characteristics by using multiparametric and multiregional MR imaging features. Radiology 2016;281(3): 907–18.

74. Kumar D, Shafiee MJ, Chung AG, et al. Discovery radiomics for computed tomography cancer detection. abs/1509.00117. CoRR 2015. Available at: http://arxiv.org/abs/1509.00117. arXiv: 1509.00117.

75. Li Z, Wang Y, Yu J, et al. Deep learning based radiomics (DLR) and its usage in noninvasive IDH1 prediction for low grade glioma. Sci Rep 2017; 7(1):5467.

76.. Ratakonda RB, Chhabra A, Ashikyan O, et al. Soft-tissue tumor reporting and data system (ST-RADS): Multi-institutional and multi-reader validation study. Scientific Session SSO5-04. Oak Brook, IL: Association of University Radiologists; 2021.

77. American College of Radiology. ACR reporting and data systems (RADS). 2021. Available at: https://www.acr.org/Clinical-Resources/Reporting-and-Data-Systems.

78. Boutin RD, Lenchik L. Value-added opportunistic CT: Insights into osteoporosis and sarcopenia. AJR Am J Roentgenol 2020;215(3):582–94.

79. Haralick RM, Shanmugam K, Dinstein IH. Textural features for image classifi- cation. IEEE Trans Syst Man Cybern 1973;(6):610–21.

80. Peeken JC, Wiestler B, Combs SE. Image-guided radiooncology: The po- tential of radiomics in clinical application. Recent Results Cancer Res 2020;216:773–94.

81. Andersen D. The Pi-search page. 2021. Available at: https://www.angio.net/pi/. Accessed December 5, 2021.

82. Peeters CFW, Ubelhor C, Mes SW, et al. Stable prediction with radiomics data. 2019. Available at: https://arxiv.org/abs/1903.11696. arXiv:1903. 11696. Accessed December 5, 2021.

83. Balagurunathan Y, Kumar V, Gu Y, et al. Test- retest reproducibility analysis of lung CT image features. J Digit Imaging 2014;27(6):805–23.

84. Clark K, Vendt B, Smith K, et al. The cancer imaging archive (TCIA): maintaining and operating a public information repository. J Digit Imaging 2013;26(6):1045–57.

85. Pati S, Verma R, Akbari H, et al. Reproducibility analysis of multi-institutional paired expert annotations and radiomic features of the Ivy Glioblastoma Atlas Project (Ivy GAP) dataset. Med Phys 2020; 47(12):6039–52. Available at: https://aapm.onlinelibrary.wiley.com/doi/abs/10.1002/mp.14556.

86. Pati S, Verma R, Akbari H, et al. Multi-institutional paired expert segmentations and radiomic features of the Ivy gap dataset. 2020. Available at: https://wiki.cancerimagingarchive.net/display/DOI/Multi-Institutional+Paired+Expert+Segmentations+and+Radiomic+Features+of+the+Ivy+GAP+Dataset. Accessed December 5, 2021.

87. Lovinfosse P, Visvikis D, Hustinx R, et al. FDG PET radiomics: a review of the methodological aspects. Clin Translational Imaging 2018;6:379–91.

88. Buckler AJ, Bresolin L, Dunnick NR, et al, Group. A collaborative enterprise for multi-stakeholder participation in the advancement of quantitative imaging. Radiology 2011;258(3):906–14.

89. Hemke R, Buckless CG, Tsao A. Deep learning for automated segmentation of pelvic muscles, fat, and bone from CT studies for body composition assessment. Skeletal Radiol 2020;49(3): 387–95.

90. Anjanappa M, Corden M, Green A, et al. Sarcopenia in cancer: risking more than muscle loss. Tech Innov Patient Support Radiat Oncol 2020;16:50–7.

91. Joglekar S, Nau PN, Mezhir JJ. The impact of sarcopenia on survival and complications in surgical oncology: a review of the current literature. J Surg Oncol 2015;112(5):503–9.

92. Bibault JE, Xing L, Giraud P, et al. Radiomics: A primer for the radiation oncologist. Cancer Radiother 2020;24(5):403–10.

93. Giraud N, Popinat G, Regaieg H, et al. Positron-emission tomography-guided radiation therapy: ongoing projects and future hopes. Cancer Radiother 2020;24(5):437–43.

94. Wang M, Zhang Q, Lam S, et al. A review on application of deep learning algorithms in external beam radiotherapy automated treatment planning. Front Oncol 2020;10:580919.

95. Rios Velazquez E, Aerts HJWL, Gu Y, et al. A semiautomatic CT-based ensemble segmentation of lung tumors: comparison with oncologists' delineations and with the surgical specimen. Radiother Oncol 2012;105(2):167–73.

96. van Dam IE, van Sörnsen de Koste JR, Hanna GG, et al. Improving target delineation on 4-dimensional CT scans in stage I NSCLC using a deformable registration tool. Radiother Oncol 2010;96(1):67–72.

97. Radiological Society of North America. RSNA Pneumonia detection challenge 2018. Available at: https://www.rsna.org/education/ai- resources-and-training/ai-image-challenge/RSNA-Pneumonia-Detection-Challenge-2018.

98. Gaonkar B, Hovda D, Martin N, et al. Deep learning in the small sample size setting: cascaded feed forward neural networks for medical image segmentation. In: Tourassi GD, Armato SGIII, editors. Medical imaging 2016: computer-aided diagnosis, vol 9785. Bellingham, WA: International Society for Optics and Photonics; 2016. p. 97852I.

99. Forsberg D, Sjoblom E, Sunshine JL. Detection and labeling of vertebrae in MR images using deep learning with clinical annotations as training data. J Digit Imaging 2017;30(4):406–12.

100. Arbour KC, Anh Tuan L, Rizvi H, et al, ml- RECIST. Machine learning to estimate RECIST in patients with NSCLC treated with PD-(L) 1 blockade. J Clin Oncol 2019;37(15 suppl):9052.

101. Huang C, Clayton EA, Matyunina LV, et al. Machine learning predicts individual cancer patient responses to therapeutic drugs with high accuracy. Scientific Rep 2018;8(1):16444.

102. Xu Y, Hosny A, Zeleznik R, et al. Deep learning predicts lung cancer treatment response from serial medical imaging. Clin Cancer Res 2019;25(11):3266–75.

103. Richardson ML. The zombie plot: A simple graphic method for visualizing the efficacy of a diagnostic test. AJR Am J Roentgenol 2016;207(4):W43–52.

104. Cheng R, Roth HR, Lu L, et al. Active appearance model and deep learning for more accurate prostate segmentation on MRI. Medical imaging 2016: image processing 2016;9784:97842I. Available at. https://www.spiedigitallibrary.org/proceedings/Download?fullDOI=10.1117%2F12.2216286. Accessed December 5, 2021.

105. Klein S, van der Heide UA, Lips IM, et al. Automatic segmentation of the prostate in 3D MR images by atlas matching using localized mutual information. Med Phys 2008;35(4):1407–17.

106. Klaeser B, Wiskirchen J, Wartenberg J, et al. PET/CT-guided biopsies of metabolically active bone lesions: applications and clinical impact. Eur J Nucl Med Mol Imaging 2010;37(11):2027–36.

107. Clauson J, Hsieh YC, Acharya S, et al. Results of the lynn sage second-opinion program for local therapy in patients with breast carcinoma. changes in management and determinants of where care is delivered. Cancer 2002;94(4):889–94.

108. Kronz JD, Westra WH, Epstein JI. Mandatory second opinion surgical pathology at a large referral hospital. Cancer 1999;86(11):2426–35.

109. Nguyen PL, Schultz D, Renshaw AA, et al. The impact of pathology review on treatment recommendations for patients with adenocarcinoma of the prostate. Urol Oncol 2004;22(4):295–9.

110. Staradub VL, Messenger KA, Hao N, et al. Changes in breast cancer therapy because of pathology second opinions. Ann Surg Oncol 2002;9(10):982–7.

111. Wang B, Perronne L, Burke C, et al. Artificial intelligence for classification of soft-tissue masses at us. Radiol Artif Intell 2021;3(1):e200125.

112. Hsu CY, Doubrovin M, Hua CH, et al. Radiomics features differentiate between normal and tumoral high-FDG up- take uptake. Sci Rep 2018;8(1):3913.

113. Li L, Wang K, Ma X, et al. Radiomic analysis of multiparametric magnetic resonance imaging for differentiating skull base chordoma and chondrosarcoma. Eur J Radiol 2019;118:81–7.

114. Yin P, Mao N, Zhao C, et al. Comparison of radiomics machine-learning classifiers and feature selection for differentiation of sacral chordoma and sacral giant cell tumour based on 3D computed tomography features. Eur Radiol 2019;29(4):1841–7.

115. Dai Y, Yin P, Mao N, et al. Differentiation of pelvic osteosarcoma and Ewing sarcoma using radiomic analysis based on T2- weighted images and contrast-enhanced T1-weighted images. Biomed Res Int 2020;2020:9078603.

116. Hong JH, Jung JY, Jo A, et al. Development and validation of a radiomics model for differentiating bone islands and osteoblastic bone metastases at abdominal CT. Radiology 2021;299(3):626–32.

117. Fisher SM, Joodi R, Madhuranthakam AJ, et al. Current utilities of imaging in grading musculoskeletal soft tissue sarcomas. Eur J Radiol 2016;85(7):1336–44.

118. Corino VDA, Montin E, Messina A, et al. Radiomic analysis of soft tissues sarcomas can distinguish intermediate from high-grade lesions. J Magn Reson Imaging 2018;47(3):829–40.

119. Gitto S, Cuocolo R, Albano D, et al. MRI radiomics-based machine-learning classification of bone chondrosarcoma radiomics-based machine-

learning classification of bone chondrosarcoma. Eur J Radiol 2020;128:109043.

120. Zhang Y, Zhu Y, Shi X, et al. Soft tissue sarcomas: Preoperative predictive histopathological grading based on radiomics of MRI. Acad Radiol 2019; 26(9):1262–8.

121. Peeken JC, Spraker MB, Knebel C, et al. Tumor grading of soft tissue sarcomas using MRI-based radiomics. EBioMedicine 2019;48:332–40.

122. Xu W, Hao D, Hou F, et al. Soft tissue sarcoma: Pre-operative MRI-based radiomics and machine learning may be accurate predictors of histopatho-logic grade. AJR Am J Roentgenol 2020;215(4): 963–9.

123. Wang H, Chen H, Duan S, et al. Radiomics and ma-chine learning with multiparametric preoperative MRI may accurately predict the histopathological grades of soft tissue sarcomas. J Magn Reson Im-aging 2020;51(3):791–7.

124. Wu Y, Xu L, Yang P, et al. Survival prediction in high-grade osteosarcoma using radiomics of diag-nostic computed tomography. EBioMedicine 2018; 34:27–34.

125. Chen H, Liu J, Cheng Z, et al. Development and external validation of an MRI-based radiomics nomogram for pretreatment prediction for early relapse in osteosarcoma: A retrospective multi-center study. Eur J Radiol 2020;129:109066.

126. Morvan L, Carlier T, Jamet B, et al. Leveraging RSF and PET images for prognosis of multiple myeloma at diagnosis. Int J Comput Assist Radiol Surg 2020; 15(1):129–39.

127. Crombé A, Kind M, Ray-Coquard I, et al. Progres-sive desmoid tumor: Radiomics compared with conventional response criteria for predicting pro-gression during systemic therapy-a multicenter study by the French sarcoma group. AJR Am J Roentgenol 2020;215(6):1539–48.

128. Peeken JC, Neumann J, Asadpour R, et al. Prog-nostic assessment in high-grade soft-tissue sar-coma patients: a comparison of semantic image analysis and radiomics. Cancers (Basel) 2021; 13(8).

129. Kuo MD, Gollub J, Sirlin CB, et al. Radiogenomic analysis to identify imaging phenotypes associated with drug response gene expression programs in hepatocellular carcinoma. J Vasc Interv Radiol 2007;18(7):821–31.

130. Teruel JR, Heldahl MG, Goa PE, et al. Dynamic contrast-enhanced MRI texture analysis for pre-treatment prediction of clinical and pathological response to neoadjuvant chemotherapy in patients with locally advanced breast cancer. NMR Biomed 2014;27(8):887–96.

131. Li H, Xu C, Xin B, et al. 18F-FDG PET/CT radiomic analysis with machine learning for identifying bone marrow involvement in the patients with suspected relapsed acute leukemia. Theranostics 2019;9(16): 4730–9.

132. Tagliafico AS, Bignotti B, Rossi F, et al. Local recur-rence of soft tissue sarcoma: a radiomic analysis. Radiol Oncol 2019;53(3):300–6.

133. Dufau J, Bouhamama A, Leporq B, et al. [predic-tion of chemotherapy response in primary osteo-sarcoma using the machine learning technique on radiomic data]. Bull Cancer 2019;106(11): 983–99.

134. Peng Y, Bi L, Guo Y, et al. Deep multi-modality collaborative learning for distant metastases pred-ication in PET-CT soft-tissue sarcoma studies. Annu Int Conf IEEE Eng Med Biol Soc 2019;2019: 3658–88.

135. Crombé A, Le Loarer F, Sitbon M, et al. Can radio-mics improve the prediction of metastatic relapse of myxoid/round cell liposarcomas? Eur Radiol 2020;30(5):2413–24.

136. Vallières M, Freeman CR, Skamene SR, et al. A ra-diomics model from joint FDG-PET and MRI texture features for the prediction of lung metastases in soft-tissue sarcomas of the extremities. Phys Med Biol 2015;60(14):5471–96.

137. Sheen H, Kim W, Byun BH, et al. Metas- tasis risk prediction model in osteosarcoma using metabolic imaging pheno-types: A multivariable radiomics model. PLoS One 2019;14(11):e0225242.

138. Aerts HJWL. Data science in radiology: a path for-ward. Clin Cancer Res 2018;24(3):532–4.

139. Beam AL, Kohane IS. Big data and machine learning in health care. JAMA 2018;319(13): 1317–8.

140. Aggarwal R, Sounderajah V, Martin G, et al. Diag-nostic accuracy of deep learning in medical imag-ing: a systematic review and meta-analysis. NPJ Digit Med 2021;4(1):65.

Moving?

Make sure your subscription moves with you!

To notify us of your new address, find your **Clinics Account Number** (located on your mailing label above your name), and contact customer service at:

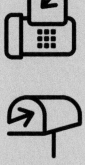

Email: journalscustomerservice-usa@elsevier.com

800-654-2452 (subscribers in the U.S. & Canada)
314-447-8871 (subscribers outside of the U.S. & Canada)

Fax number: 314-447-8029

Elsevier Health Sciences Division
Subscription Customer Service
3251 Riverport Lane
Maryland Heights, MO 63043

*To ensure uninterrupted delivery of your subscription, please notify us at least 4 weeks in advance of move.

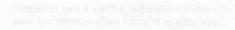